Controversies in Analytical Psychology

T0187719

Analytical psychology is a broad church, and influences areas such as literature, cultural studies and religion. However, in common with (Freudian) psychoanalysis, there are many different schools of thought and practice which have resulted in divisions within the field. *Controversies in Analytical Psychology* picks up on these and explores many of the most hotly contested issues in and around analytical psychology.

A group of leading international, mainly Jungian authors have contributed papers from contrasting perspectives on a series of key controversies. Some of these concern clinical issues such as what helps patients get better, or how closely analysts should work with transference. Other contributions focus on the relationship between analytical psychology and other disciplines, including evolutionary theory, linguistics, politics and religion. A critical eye is cast over Jungian theories and practices, and a number of questions are raised:

- Are they homophobic?
- Do they denigrate women?
- Do they confuse absolute with narrative truth?
- Is the frequency of sessions chosen for political rather than clinical reasons?

Controversies in Analytical Psychology encourages critical thinking on a variety of issues, helping to foster dialogue and investigation in a climate of mutual respect and understanding. It will be invaluable for Jungian analysts, psychoanalysts and psychotherapists in training and practice.

Robert Withers is a Jungian analyst in private practice and is a member of the Society of Analytical Psychology. He is also Senior Lecturer at the University of Westminster.

Controversies in
Analytical Psychology

Edited by Robert Withers

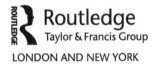

Routledge
Taylor & Francis Group

LONDON AND NEW YORK

Published 2003 by Routledge
27 Church Road, Hove, East Sussex, BN3 2FA

Simultaneously published in the USA and Canada
by Routledge
711 Third Avenue, New York, NY 10017

Routledge is an imprint of the Taylor & Francis Group, an informa business

© 2003 Selection and editorial matter, Robert Withers; individual
chapters, the contributors.

Typeset in Times by Keystroke, Jacaranda Lodge, Wolverhampton
Paperback cover design by Lisa Dynan

All rights reserved. No part of this book may be reprinted
or reproduced or utilized in any form or by any electronic,
mechanical, or other means, now known or hereafter
invented, including photocopying and recording, or in any
information storage or retrieval system, without permission in
writing from the publishers.

British Library Cataloguing in Publication Data
A catalogue record for this book is available from the British Library

Library of Congress Cataloging in Publication Data
Controversies in analytical psychology/[edited by] Robert Withers.
        p. cm.
    Includes bibliographical references and index.
    ISBN 0–415–23304–6 (hbk) — ISBN 0–415–23305–4 (pbk)
    1. Psychoanalysis. 2. Jungian psychology.
    3. Psychoanalytic counseling. I. Withers, Robert, 1952–
BF173 .C569 2002
150.19′5—dc21   2002066749

ISBN 13: 978-0-415-23305-7 (pbk)

For Polly, Craig, Imogen and Leo

Contents

Biographical details of contributors

Robert Caper is an Assistant Clinical Professor of Medicine (Psychiatry) at the UCLA School of Medicine. He is the author of over 30 publications on psychoanalysis and the psychotherapy of adults, adolescents and children, and two books: *Immaterial Facts: Freud's Discovery of Psychic Reality and Klein's Development of His Work* (Routledge), and *A Mind of One's Own* (The New International Library of Psychoanalysis).

Richard Carvalho is a psychiatrist by origin. He studied concurrently at the Tavistock Clinic and at the Society of Analytical Psychology, following which he held the post of Consultant Psychotherapist at St Mary's Hospital in London for several years. He is currently in private analytic practice.

Warren Colman is a Professional Member of the Society of Analytical Psychology. He was a Senior Marital Psychotherapist at the (mainly Kleinian) Tavistock Marital Studies Institute until 1997, since when he has been in full-time private practice in St Albans, UK. He is a teacher and supervisor for psychotherapy trainings in England, Poland and Russia, and is an Assistant Editor of the *Journal of Analytical Psychology*. He has published numerous articles, mainly on couples, gender/sexuality and the Self.

JoAnn Culbert-Koehn is a Jungian analyst in private practice with adults and children in Beverly Hills, California. She is a former director of training at the C. G. Jung Institute of Los Angeles and former Co-Director of the Hilde Kirsch Children's Center. She has published and lectured in the United States and Europe on issues of separation and birth trauma and has taught in an innovative programme in Santa Fe, New Mexico, integrating Jung, Klein and Bion.

Julian David trained in Zurich. He was a founder member and one-time Convenor of IGAP. He was also the founding analyst of SAAJA, the Cape Town Jungian group, starting in the period of apartheid in 1988, and going on through the changes up to, in some small degree, the present. He has links now with the C. G. Jung Study Centre of Southern California, and is currently applying to the IAAP for permission to bring classical Jungian psychology back to Los Angeles. He practises principally in South Devon.

Chess Denman, MBBS, MRCPsych., is consultant psychiatrist in psychotherapy at Addenbrookes Hospital and clinical lecturer at Cambridge University. She is a member of the Society of Analytical Psychology and a founder-member of the Association of Cognitive Analytic Therapists.

Moira Duckworth is a professional member, training analyst and supervisor for the Association of Jungian Analysts (AJA). She is also an honorary member and professional member of the Foundation for Psychotherapy and Counselling (FPC), and a teacher and supervisor for several counselling and psychotherapy trainings. With Martin Stone, she has done research into qualitative and quantitative outcomes of therapy related to frequency of work.

Christopher Hauke is a Jungian analyst, trained at the Society of Analytical Psychology, and Lecturer in Psychoanalytic Studies at the University of London, Goldsmiths College. He teaches and supervises for several psychotherapy trainings and lectures widely. He has recently completed a book on the relationship between the ideas of C. G. Jung and corresponding strands in postmodern thought called *Jung and the Postmodern: The Interpretation of Realities*, published by Routledge in February 2000. His collection of Jungian writings on movies – *Post-Jungian Takes on the Moving Image* – edited in conjunction with Ian Alister was published by Brunner-Routledge in June, 2001.

Robert Hinshelwood is a psychoanalyst trained at the British Psycho-analytical Society. He has published and written on many aspects of Kleinian theory. He was previously Clinical Director of the Cassel Hospital, and is currently Professor in the Centre for Psychoanalytic Studies, University of Essex.

Verena Kast is Professor of Psychology at the University of Zurich and training analyst and lecturer at the C. G. Jung Institute of Zurich. From 1995 to 1998 she was president of IAAP. She lectures throughout the world and is the author of numerous books on psychological issues, among others: *The Dynamics of Symbols: Fundamentals of Jungian Psychology, Imagination as Space of Freedom, Growth through Emotions: Interpretation of Fairy Tales* (all Fromm International, New York), and *Father–Daughter, Mother–Son: Freeing Ourselves from the Complexes that Bind Us* (Element, Dorset).

Paul Kugler, Ph.D., is a Jungian analyst in private practice in East Aurora, New York. He is a Past-President of the Inter-Regional Society of Jungian Analysts and has served as a member of the Executive Committee of the International Association of Analytical Psychologists. His is the author of numerous publications, including Supervision: Jungian Perspectives on Clinical Supervision (Diamon Verlag, 1995), 'Psychic Images: A Bridge between Object and Subject' in *The Cambridge Companion to Jung*, edited by Polly Young-Eisendrath and Terence Dawson (Cambridge University Press, 1997) and 'Childhood Seduction: Material and Immaterial Facts', in *The Alchemy of Seduction*, edited by Stanton Marlan (Chiron Press, 1997).

Roderick Main, Ph.D., is Lecturer in Psychoanalytic Studies at the University of Essex. He is the editor of *Jung on Synchronicity and the Paranormal* (Routledge, 1997) and the author of articles on Jungian psychology, religion, divination and synchronicity.

Barry Proner is a Training and Supervising Analyst of the Society of Analytical Psychology. He trained originally in the United States as a psychiatrist and a child psychiatrist, and then in the UK in both child and adult analysis. He is interested in early emotional life and the links between post-Kleinian psycho-analysis, notably the work of W. R. Bion, and analytical psychology. He writes and lectures extensively.

Andrew Samuels is Professor of Analytical Psychology at the University of Essex and a training analyst with the Society of Analytical Psychology. His most recent book was *Politics on the Couch: Citizenship and the Internal Life* (London: Profile Books. New York: Other Press, 2001).

Joy Schaverien, Ph.D., is a member of the Society of Analytical Psychology in London. She is Professor Associate at the University of Sheffield, Visiting Fellow of Goldsmiths College, University of London, and a professional member of the West Midlands Institute of Psychotherapy. In private practice as a Jungian analyst in Leicestershire, she lectures widely in Britain and abroad on gender issues and the links between art and psychoanalysis. She is the author of *The Revealing Image: Analytical Art Psychotherapy in Theory and Practice* (1991) and *Desire and the Female Therapist: Engendered Gazes in Psychotherapy and Art Therapy* (1995), and co-editor of Art, *Psychotherapy and Psychosis* (1997).

Ann Shearer is a senior analyst and past Convenor of the Independent Group of Analytical Psychologists, with a private practice in London. Before training with IGAP, she worked as a journalist and international consultant in aspects of social welfare. Her most recent books are *Athene: Image and Energy* (1996) and *When a Princess Dies* (1998), co-edited with Jane Haynes.

Anthony Stevens has practised as a psychiatrist and Jungian analyst for the last thirty years. He is a graduate of Oxford University and in addition to his DM has two degrees in psychology. He is the author of 12 books. His latest, *Archetype Revisited: an Updated Natural History of the Self*, was published by Routledge in March, 2002.

Martin Stone is a Jungian analyst in private practice in London. He is a supervisor and training analyst for the Association of Jungian Analysts (AJA), and researches with Moira Duckworth into qualitative and quantitative outcomes of therapy in relation to the frequency of therapy sessions.

Elizabeth Urban is a professional member of the Society of Analytical Psychology and a member of the Association of Child Psychotherapists. She works with adults, adolescents and children and has a particular interest in early infancy and psychic development, about which she has written a number of papers.

Edward Whitmont originally trained as a homeopath before going on to become a Jungian analyst. He taught and published widely in both fields and pioneered various aspects of their integration. He died in September 1998.

Melanie Withers is a lecturer in psychodynamic counselling, psychoanalytic psychotherapy, counselling psychology and clinical supervision at the University of Sussex. She is Clinical Director and co-founder of the Rock Clinic Association, Brighton, where she has a large private practice.

Robert Withers is a member of the Society of Analytical Psychology in private practice. He is also senior lecturer at the University of Westminster where he lectures, researches and publishes on the interface between psychoanalysis and complementary medicine, in which he originally trained.

Acknowledgements

I would like to thank the *International Journal of Psycho-analysis* for permission to republish Robert Caper's article, Blackwell Publishers for permission to republish the Edward Whitmont article, and Routledge for permission to republish the articles by Elizabeth Urban and Andrew Samuels. I would also like to thank those authors or their heirs for allowing me to use their papers in this book. Full publication details can be found at the end of each of the articles in question.

I am indebted to Professor Andrew Samuels, not only for the initial insight that led to this book, but also for his assistance in its compilation. Thanks are also due to Warren Colman, Marcus West, Mary Addenbrooke, Fiona Ross, Jean Thomson, and Hazel Robinson, my colleagues in the publications committee at the SAP, for their invaluable editorial and emotional support. Thanks too to the Brighton analytic discussion group, especially my colleagues Eogain Gallagher and Jenny Leeburn, to Christopher Hauke, Mary-Jayne Rust, and Robert Snell, to The Auckland Family Consultation and Psychotherapy Centre who allowed me to practise an early version of one of my papers on them, to my patients and my former analyst's relatives for their kind permission to use related clinical material, to the many contributors without whom the book could not have happened, and, last but not least, to my family for their long-suffering forbearance while I have laboured over this manuscript.

February 2002   **Robert Withers**

Introduction

Robert Withers

The field of analytical psychology and psychoanalysis has been bedevilled with more than its fair share of controversies, splits and schisms. These range from the original Freud/Jung split, whose ghost can still be discerned haunting the current volume, through to the present-day proliferation of analytic trainings, organizations and ideologies – most of them jealously staking their own claim to truth. The bitterness of some of the resultant disputes would stand unique among the sciences, were it not for the fact that we are unable to agree that analysis is a science, or, if it is, what kind. That controversy too stalks this book.

It is of course deeply ironic that in a therapeutic discipline that styles itself a talking cure, we are generally so bad at talking (and listening) to one another. But perhaps this has something to do with our chosen subject matter, which most, though by no means all, of us would agree is the unconscious. We are by definition unable to verify the truth of claims about our own unconscious, while claims made about the contents of someone else's can be disputed on the grounds that they are not open to falsification and therefore rest on some arbitrary presumption of authority. Perhaps it should not be wondered at then, if we sometimes respond to these doubts by adopting compensatory positions of 'certainty' with which we identify and to which we defensively cling. Clearly we will all have to sacrifice the sense of security that comes from such clinging if we are to enter into a genuine dialogue with one another. Despite this loss, the potential benefits of such dialogue are great – both in terms of the potential for creative interchange thus fostered and the strength that can emerge from collaborative exploration and mutual understanding. It is to the furtherance of that process of dialogue that this book is dedicated.

The book was originally inspired by a short series of lectures given by Andrew Samuels in 1983 in which it became clear that many of the complexities of the analytic field as a whole could be effectively grasped by contrasting simple assumptions underlying the theories and practices of the various analytic schools. The book then continues in this spirit of celebrating controversy as an effective way of promoting understanding. It consists of a series of papers, written from contrasting perspectives, that attempt to explore some of the major issues facing analytical psychologists today. Many of these issues concern psychoanalytically orientated therapists as well. And although analytical psychologists have written most of the papers, some are written from a specifically psychoanalytic perspective, where this best illuminates the subject matter. Each chapter has a short introduction, which outlines the arguments underlying the specific controversy under discussion. Some authors have taken up the invitation to respond to their paired paper, while others have chosen not to. What though are the fault lines that lie beneath the book as a whole?

One recurrent theme already touched on concerns analytical psychology's relationship to psychoanalysis. The book opens with the discussion of some case material from a Fordhamian perspective. Michael Fordham of course, was instrumental in establishing the 'Developmental School' (Samuels, 1985 *Jung and the Post-Jungians*. London: Routledge & Kegan Paul) of analytical psychology, which attempts to bring some of Jung's insights into line with developments in psychoanalysis. Reactions to Fordham's innovations within the Jungian world have varied from relief and admiration on the one hand to suspicion and downright hostility on the other. But if Fordham attempted a rapprochement between analytical psychology and psychoanalysis, further effects of the original rift can be discerned underlying our differences of approach to the transference, to religion, to early trauma and to the place of interpretation within the analytic relationship. These issues are discussed in Controversies Three, 'Transference, countertransference and beyond', Six, 'Approaching religion', Two, 'The status of developmental theory', and Eleven, 'The role of interpreting and relating in analytic therapy', respectively.

Another 'fault line' already mentioned concerns our relationship to science. One place this is seen particularly clearly is in Controversy Eight, 'The contemporary status of archetypal theory', where Anthony Stevens argues strongly that we should ground our theories in the hard sciences of genetics and ethology. Paul Kugler on the other hand makes a contrasting claim for the importance of incorporating the findings of the soft sciences of linguistics and sociology into our theories. The same theme is developed in Controversy Five, 'Analysis and implicit homophobia', where the epistemological basis of our appeal to the 'centrality of the conjunctio' is considered in relation to analytic attitudes about homosexuality. Controversies Two, 'The status of developmental theory', and Nine, 'Reflections on the anima and culture', reiterate aspects of the same argument in relation to memory and the feminine respectively.

Splits, boundaries and controversies are closely linked concepts. So it will not be a surprise to learn that boundaries are another recurrent theme in this book. One school's sound clinical practice can constitute acting out from another's perspective. It all depends on where our boundaries are drawn. Boundary issues thus not only underlie the discussion of clinical material throughout the book, they also importantly determine many differences of opinion on theory. This can be seen especially clearly in Controversies One, 'Prospects for the Jung/Klein synthesis', Four, 'The political in analysis', and Seven, 'The body, analysis and homeopathy', where analytical psychology's relationship to Kleinian theory, to politics and to complementary medicine is discussed. It also features in Controversy Three, 'Transference, countertransference and beyond', in relation to the transference; while in Controversy Ten, 'Frequency of sessions and the analytic frame', boundary issues that determine the practice and definition of analysis itself are considered.

If the book generates thought and discussion on this wide variety of topics, it will have amply served its purpose.

Prospects for the Jung/Klein synthesis

Introduction

A tension exists within the world of Jungian analysis between the wish to preserve the distinctive features that constitute our Jungian identity, and the wish to relate to the broader field of psychoanalysis. This tension especially contributes to conflicting attitudes towards the theoretical and clinical formulations of Michael Fordham, who attempted to integrate Jungian thinking with some of the findings of Kleinian and post-Kleinian psychoanalysis.

In this chapter Elizabeth Urban, herself an adherent of Fordham's 'developmental school' of analytical psychology, presents a piece of clinical material with the intention of clarifying certain aspects of Fordham's work. She is concerned in particular to illustrate how his model can be applied to practice. At the same time she hopes to draw attention to conceptual differences and similarities between his theories and those of Melanie Klein.

The chapter elicits two distinctive responses. On the one hand (or wing) is the classically trained Jungian analyst, Julian David. David points out that Jung thought of himself as a phenomenologist and treated analytic theory with suspicion, despite his fascination with the world of the archetypes and the collective unconscious. David reiterates Jung's suspicion of theory when he questions the weight that Kleinian theories of early infancy are asked to carry in both Fordham's model and Urban's work with her patient, Ruthie. He wonders, for instance, whether Urban's theoretical preoccupation with infantile issues and with the transference could have blinded her to evidence of sexual material in Ruthie's analysis. Urban later picks up on this issue in her own response to the commentaries.

The other response to Urban's chapter comes from the Kleinian analyst Robert Hinshelwood. He too remarks on the apparent absence of sexual material in Ruthie's analysis, but is far more willing than David to engage in a discussion of theoretical issues. In fact he makes a particular effort to clarify some of the differences and similarities between the Kleinian and Fordhamian theoretical positions, as he understands them. He argues for instance that terms like 'the self' and 'the depressive position' have become subject to a kind of conceptual drift within the different schools of analysis. As a result of this, the same word can end up referring to different things as it is required to perform different functions within the two theoretical systems.

This could give rise to the pessimistic conclusion that analysts of different orientations are likely to end up thinking they are talking to one another, when in fact they are not. And this probably does sometimes happen. But a careful reading of all four contributions to this chapter could equally yield the opposite conclusion. It is possible for instance to conclude that Hinshelwood and Urban use the term 'depressive position' to describe the same phenomenon from an inter- and intra-psychic perspective respectively – rather than to describe completely different phenomena. Likewise it is possible to make clear links between Klein's concept of self, as ego plus internal objects, and Jung's concept of self, as ego plus archetypes. On a practical level too it is possible to identify many areas of consensus between the contributors, despite their contrasting attitudes to theory.

(a) With healing in her wings: integration and repair in a self-destructive adolescent

Elizabeth Urban

INTRODUCTION

One of the most important of Jung's concepts is that of the self. Although he used the term in a number of different ways, the one that predominates is Jung's definition of the self as the totality of the personality: mind and body, conscious and unconscious, ego and archetypes (Jung, 1971). As a phenomenon, the self is characterized by totality and wholeness, and is the source of meaning. Functionally it is an organizer and integrator, bringing together and structuring the inner world. Because the self is the totality of the personality, it contains or, rather, transcends opposites.

For Jung, meaning and the pressure to become whole are the motivating drives behind development. From his work with adults in mid-life, he conceived development as a process, termed 'individuation', in which the individual becomes more deeply and truly himself. Individuation is ongoing; one individuates but is never individuated. Technically, it is a process by which the ego, the centre of perception, time and again confronts conflicting and opposite forces, say between good and evil, or being dependent and being separate. The consequence of the conflict between opposites is – and here is Jung's optimism (Fordham, 1985a) – a new resolution, symbol or insight arising in the ego. Individuation thus involves the ego and a pair of opposites, and this triangulation is a cornerstone in Jungian understanding of development (Jung, 1955–6, 1959; Fordham, 1985b).

FORDHAM'S MODEL

Drawing upon Jung's concept of the self, Fordham postulated a *primary* integrate before birth, which he termed the primary self. Taking Jung's concept of the self as a psychic integrator and organizer, he added his own original concept, that the primary self divides up, or deintegrates, in order to relate to the environment. The self then assimilates the experience by reintegrating it (Fordham, 1976, 1994).

Freud used the protozoa amoeba as an analogy for the ego (Laplanche and Pontalis, 1973), and it can also be used as a model for the deintegrating and reintegrating primary self. The pseudopod of the amoeba reaches out into the environment and takes in food (deintegration). What is taken in is then assimilated into the nucleated endoplasm (reintegration). The pseudopod does not become detached from the rest of the amoeba, but remains part of it; just as deintegrates remain part of the primary self. If the deintegrate (experience) becomes cut off from the self, then splitting occurs. In other words, according to Fordham, splitting refers to experiences that have pathologically become detached from the self (Fordham, 1987, 1993).

Fordham cites a typical example of deintegration and reintegration in infancy. An infant wakes up from sleep, a state of integration, and relates to the breast during a feed. Following the feed, the baby sleeps again, assimilating, or reintegrating, the milk and the experience (Fordham, 1987). A fuller description, which takes into account the interactive dimension of Fordham's model, would be as follows. The infant wakes from a state of integration, having an archetypal predisposition towards that which fills his need (cf. Bion's preconception (Bion, 1962)). He gives signals, such as crying, to his mother. The mother takes these signals into herself, does something with them, and then responds to her baby, such as putting him to the breast. The baby feeds, and takes in not only the milk but something of the mother's way of feeding and responding. In assimilating the milk and the experience, the baby adds something of his own, such as meaning, the way the mother added something of her own, such as alpha function, when she took in the baby's signals. What is done within the baby is the result of actions of the self. I shall return to this.

The organizing functions of the self differ from those of the ego. It is the self that accounts for the overall, archetypally shaped unfolding of the personality, and for the organization of the infant's personality. However, infants also exhibit rapidly fluctuating states, which Fordham understands as evidence of the fragile and unstable infant ego. There are bits of ego at birth, because early experiences (deintegrates) include bits of perception or awareness. Only in the course of development, that is, as the self deintegrates and reintegrates, do they coalesce into a stable ego.

The unfolding of the personality proceeds in surges, which can be understood as periods of massive deintegration. The findings of experimental researchers indicate that surges within the first year occur at birth, at about two months, to a lesser degree at three to five months, and again at ten to twelve months (Stern, 1985; Trevarthen, 1980; Trevarthen and Marwick, 1986).

I should now like to focus on three corollaries of Fordham's postulate of a deintegrating and reintegrating primary self, which pertain to whole and part objects and the depressive position. I shall attempt to expand upon each by drawing upon infant studies.

FIRST COROLLARY: WHOLE OBJECTS PRECEDE PART OBJECTS

For Fordham, the primary self begins before birth. Unlike Freud's primary narcissism with its libidinous and destructive energies, the energy of the primary self is neutral. Interaction between archetypally (biologically) determined expectations and the intra-uterine environment produces the first objects, which Fordham terms 'self objects' (Fordham, 1994). These are pre-image and pre-symbol, and, as I understand them, are what Alvarez is describing when she refers to the pre-objects of autistic children (Alvarez, 1992).

Self objects are imbued with the self, that is, with feelings of wholeness, at-oneness, altogetherness, together-with-me-ness. At the beginning of life, these qualities pervade experiences, thus creating states of fusion via the processes of projective and introjective identification, early processes that initially are probably very close to one another. Foetal swallowing provides a picture of how the experience of being at one with that which one *is* inside (projective identification) can be very close to that of being at one with that which one *has* inside (introjecitive identification). According to Milakovic, the foetus 'at will' swallows amniotic fluid in order to regulate the imbalance of fluids in its body (Milakovic, 1967). It is easy to imagine that, because what provides relief is of minimum texture and the same temperature as the foetus, what envelops and what is taken in is experienced by the foetus as being part of itself.

After birth, early feeds (deintegrations) are typified by the infant's total absorption in the experience, eyes closed, body still, and mouth sucking rhythmically, as if the breast were the whole of his universe and he was giving himself entirely to it. Visual, aural and tactile aspects of the mother become incorporated into the wholeness characterizing early self objects. From the observer's point of view, the baby is relating to parts of the mother, but from the infant's point of view, the part *is* the whole (Fordham, 1987; Astor, 1989).

Earlier, I stated that, when the infant assimilates an experience (reintegration), he adds something to it. An example is amodal perception and cross-modal fluency. Because the newborn can fluently translate amodal experiences from one sense into another, Stern concludes that the 'seen' breast is experienced by the infant to be the same as the 'sucked' breast (Stern, 1985). In Fordham's model, the global, whole nature of the infant's perceptions is an expression of actions of the self that make them so. According to the infant's experience, self objects are whole objects. However, even in infancy, self objects come and go, and so do experiences of wholeness and fusion (Fordham, 1985b).

SECOND COROLLARY: PART OBJECTS ARE A RESULT OF DEINTEGRATION AND REINTEGRATION

Self objects arise out of and represent the satisfied needs of the foetus and, later, the infant, and quickly develop into good objects. Early on, other concurrent sense data, for example, commotion from an older sibling, do not become integrated (Stern, 1985; Brazelton, 1991), or are experienced as not-self: if not-self objects are felt to be frustrating or unpleasant, they initially are rejected, attacked or evacuated (Fordham, 1976), and can later become bad objects. The intensification of and differentiation between 'good' and 'bad', which can be observed in young infants, is a result of early actions of the self, creating parts out of the whole.

At about six weeks to two months, dramatic changes occur in the infant, indicating a new surge of deintegration. Trevarthen details the considerable changes that occur in the area of communication. He describes in fascinating detail the intricate, alternating behaviours of infant and mother that develop into protoconversations. Later, at three to five months and given a secure relationship with a present mother, the infant turns away from face-to-face conversations in order to engage with an object animated by the mother (Trevarthen, 1980; Trevarthen and Marwick, 1986). Psychoanalytic baby observations show how babies this age explore objects on their own through mouthing and handling. Taken all together, these observations show how animate and inanimate become firmly differentiated.

Stern describes the gradual differentiation between self and other. He details how the infant sifts invariant from variant features of experience and organizes them into clusters of experiences associated with self and experiences associated with another, resulting in the infant's sense of core self and sense of core other: 'Somehow, the different invariants of self-experience are integrated. . . . Similarly, [the different invariants of different experiences of the mother] all get disentangled and sorted. "Islands of consistency" somehow form and coalesce' (Stern, 1985: 98).

In Fordham's model, the sorting of invariant from variant features and the organization of them into discrete clusters are actions of the integrating and organizing functions of the primary self. Fordham would consider Stern's description of the coalescence of 'islands of consistency' into a sense of self to be a description of ego formation. For Fordham, having a sense, a perception or an awareness – no matter how primitive – is a function of the ego (Fordham, 1994).

The self not only shapes the ego, it also adds something to the clustering of perceptions. This means that there is a fundamental difference between Fordham's and Stern's concepts of the ego. This can be seen in their different views about self-representations, which arise in the ego. Stern's representations of interactions that have been generalised (RIGS) are mental prototypes of lived experience, that is, memories of actual experiences. For Fordham, the ego is born out of the self and despite the gradual boundary that is built up between them, the self remains partially represented in the ego. Hence self representations contain aspects of the self, and are more than memories of actual experiences (Fordham, 1985b).

In summary, through deintegration and reintegration, the original wholeness of self objects divides up into parts, such as good and bad, inside and outside, animate and inanimate, and self and other.

THIRD COROLLARY: INDIVIDUATION BEGINS WITH THE DEPRESSIVE POSITION

At about ten to twelve months there is another surge of new developments, or deintegrations. In the period Trevarthen terms 'secondary intersubjectivity', play between mother and infant becomes a shared activity. The baby begins to cooperate with the mother, anticipating her intentions and learning from her the purposes of certain objects, for instance, what to do with a comb. When the meaning of an object can be shared, the object becomes a potential symbol (Trevarthen, 1980; Trevarthen and Marwick, 1986). According to Stern, this is the period of establishing a sense of subjective self. As the infant discovers that inner experiences are shareable, he begins to relate to his mother's mind and acquires 'a "theory" of separate minds' (Stern, 1985: 124). Thus, Trevarthen and Stern demonstrate the enormous potential for cognitive development that comes out of the bringing together of self/other, animate/inanimate, and inside (the mind)/outside (behaviour).

Psychoanalytic baby observations during this period are usually concerned with the infant's final weaning from the breast. An example is from the observation of Edward, at twelve months, one week. I am grateful to the observer in the BAP training who allowed me to use the following extracts from her notes.

Edward was completely weaned from the breast only a few weeks before. At the beginning of the observation, the observer watched him being given lunch from a bowl. When the bowl was emptied and taken away, Edward suddenly let out an intense wail, 'mouth open wide and crying bitterly so that he was just exhaling in bursts. He was inconsolable'.

His mother offered him the bowl and then juice, which he refused. Then she tried to hold him. Each effort on her part to comfort or distract seemed to escalate his screams. Eventually the mother took him into the lounge and cleared a space for him on the floor, while she sat close by. 'For fifteen or twenty minutes, he rolled on the floor and screamed, [writhing] back and forth.' Throughout this time the mother remained close and attentive.

> Slowly the intensity of the screaming eased but did not stop, and Edward seemed able to tolerate his mother's soothing. The screams had changed into something more regular and rhythmic, but [eventually] they stopped altogether and at last he lay still and quiet. . . . He stared at the ceiling, exhausted. . . . His mother bent over him after a while and he smiled slowly in response. Within minutes he was smiling and seemed quite happy.

The seminar group found this observation quite upsetting, and considered that Edward's loss of the bowl might be an expression of his loss of the breast. Nothing external in the observation accounted for the unreachable depth and intensity of his response; he was responding to something internal. In thwarting his mother's efforts to console or distract, he seemed to be 'true' to his experience of his loss and to show a depth of character. Eventually and of its own accord, the intensity subsided, disappeared, and a good relationship with the mother was restored. When his mother went into the kitchen, he played happily with the observer, something he had never done before and which seemed to mark an increased awareness of reality and affection. These are hallmarks of the depressive position.

The classical Kleinian idea of the depressive position is that the infant comes to experience that the good, satisfying breast is the same as the one he recognizes as bad and frustrating and which he attacks. Consequently he comes to feel that he has destroyed that which he loves most (Segal, 1979). Fordham describes the sequence that follows:

> He pines and becomes absorbed in himself so that he is inaccessible to his mother. After a variable and distressing period of time, he gradually recovers; now he has reconstructed the breast internally. In short, he has accomplished a rather wonderful act of reparation. After this sequence, the baby's sense of reality takes a step forward and his mental life is enriched. The transformation is called the *depressive position* and, in my view, constitutes the first step in individuation. (Fordham, 1989: 68)

When Fordham states that the depressive position marks the beginning of individuation, he understands that the opposites of good and bad and love and hate are brought together in such a way that a new symbol (an internal breast) is formed, thereby enriching inner life and, equally, leading to an increased sense of reality.

These three corollaries, taken in the order presented here, demonstrate the development of the internal world. The original wholeness of self objects divides up into parts, and then the parts come into relationship with one another.

CLINICAL MATERIAL

The girl I shall call Ruthie was 13 when she was referred because of her excessive and irrational terror of pigeons. Ruthie could not walk from home to the nearby tube nor from school to the bus stop without being frightened that she might encounter a pigeon.

A psychoanalytic understanding of a phobia would usually include sexuality. Although treatment included the gradual understanding of emotional, cognitive and sexual aspects of what the pigeons represented to Ruthie, in what follows I shall focus on the aspects of the phobia that related to certain states of confusion. These states were not only the subject of much of Ruthie's treatment but also referred to her self-destructiveness and what stood in the way of her development. I should like to use Ruthie's treatment to describe how Fordham's model of development helped me to help Ruthie to integrate the experiences represented by the pigeons and how, therefore, splitting became deintegration.

When Ruthie and I first met, she reported in detail how abhorrent and repulsive she found pigeons. I asked her to draw a picture of one and she made an attempt but stopped short of completing the picture because it aroused such strong fear and revulsion. Closing her eyes and shaking her head, she shuddered and flapped her hands while expelling repeated 'oohs' of disgust. We established that what was unthinkable for her was that a pigeon would fly up on big flapping wings and rush into her face.

Once-weekly treatment started, and Ruthie eventually filled me in on some of the details of her external life. She started to become frightened of pigeons after her family moved to London from a smaller community, when she was about ten. Unhappy and friendless, she remained the 'new girl' in school until secondary transfer.

Most of the sessions during the first months were detailed, repetitious accounts of her day-to-day encounters with pigeons, which left me feeling sleepy, cut off and useless. For her part, Ruthie found me cold and unfriendly. When I tried to offer an interpretation, she frequently would ask me to repeat or to say more. When I tried to do so, I often discovered that I was unable to restate my thoughts coherently; my sentencing broke up into nonsense.

Eventually I suggested that she was frightened of getting into a flap. Having had some experience of her mother's anxiety and volatility, I felt I could picture what Ruthie might feel like when her mother was upset. I wondered if, when her mother got in a flap, Ruthie became frightened that the flap in her mother's mind would get into her mind. This line of thinking seemed to mean something to Ruthie. She became increasingly aware of her worry that my muddle or lack of understanding might become her mixed-upness and confusion. She told me dreams, and then worried about the parts she could not remember for sure. What if I got the wrong idea about the dream and based my interpretation on a misconception? She feared that she would then have this wrong understanding in her mind, and believe in it. This implied that Ruthie felt that knowledge and understanding needed to be linked to the truth.

After about five months, Ruthie left for an extended holiday abroad, and, when she returned, her mother stopped the treatment because there had been no change in the pigeon phobia. The mother arranged for Ruthie to see a behaviour therapist, and over a year passed before this broke down. The mother contacted me again, thus beginning a second period of treatment that, in retrospect, roughly corresponded to the school year prior to her taking her GCSEs.

Ruthie returned to treatment livelier and more motivated, and with a positive transference to me. Mostly she spoke to me of her fear of failing her exams, and from week to week she faced one assignment or exam after another, fraught with an anxiety bordering on panic. She spent more and more time over her studies and turned down invitations to be with friends over the weekend in order to do home-work. She became exhausted from these efforts, which seemed her only protection against the dread of failure.

As her exams approached, any changes in my room were noted and treated with deep suspicion. For instance, during a break my consulting room was redecorated, and I moved a vase containing a willow branch from a position opposite to one alongside where Ruthie sat. She became frightened of this, frequently looking across her shoulder as she spoke. I made a number of interpretations, including that the spreading branches were felt by her to be the spreading wings of a flapping pigeon. Just saying this seemed to vivify and intensify her fears. The terror on the streets was now in my room.

This period of treatment came to an end when she passed her GCSEs with virtually all As. The confirmation of the competence of her own thinking seemed to parallel her developing confidence in mine.

A-level developments

Soon after starting her A-levels, Ruthie's accounts of her anxiety about schoolwork began to include fights she had with her mother. The rows tended to arise when her younger sister got attention from their mother that Ruthie felt was her due. The fights usually occurred at bedtime, when Ruthie demanded that her mother see her to sleep. Arguments also arose from Ruthie's demand for a vegetarian diet, different from what the rest of the family ate.

Some of the fights became violent, with Ruthie furiously decanting non-vegetarian food from the fridge, throwing things and, occasionally, hitting her mother. The emotional violence could keep the family awake until the early hours of the morning. Just what occurred was difficult to ascertain because Ruthie got confused and forgot what happened. Gradually a pattern could be described. As the anger and hate escalated, Ruthie would tip into feeling out of control, and screaming, hitting, crying, swearing and vomiting. Rage became violence, which became chaos.

I did not appreciate the extent of Ruthie's destructiveness at home until the parents contacted me, asking to meet. Ruthie had anticipated this, saying she hoped I would see them because they were upset and needed my help to understand what was happening. After I heard the parents' accounts, I explained that Ruthie's pigeon phobia represented a condensation of intense emotions that were now beginning to break up and be experienced as feelings in relation to the family. We discussed how Ruthie needed boundaries in order to help her manage the violence of her feelings and to limit psychological, personal and material damage that she might inflict. By the end of the interview I was impressed with the parents' ability to work together to draw limits that, by the mother's admission, had not before been established.

When Ruthie and I next met, she was in a flap. Her parents had told her of the boundaries they were going to set, and she was overwhelmingly persecuted by the awareness that her parents were not under her control. At one point, she spluttered out through her tears, '*I can't stand being ordinary!*' Tearful, frightened and outraged, she was reluctant to go home after her session. In order to restore her omnipotence, she threatened to cut herself. That night she carried out the threat, the first of several instances of self-inflicted wounding.

There was a long period of intense and turbulent emotion, as limits became set and tested both at home and in her sessions. But there was evidence of change. Her relationship with her father improved, she spent more time with her friends, and she used her therapy to avoid fights with her mother. From time to time she indicated that her fear of pigeons was subsiding. These changes happened alongside evidence of her increased dependency on her treatment and the thinking she associated with it. For example, there was a crisis during the summer break between her first and second years of A-level study. She had been given homework to complete over the summer, but she got into such a state over it that the family holiday abroad had to be cut short.

There was a very real question about whether she would be able to continue with her A-level work and her sessions were increased to twice weekly. Her return to A-level studies was accompanied by heightened anxiety about failing because of the incomplete homework. She studied increasingly late into the night, which left her so tired after school that she had to sleep and then wake up in the late evening to begin her work. As this pattern became set, rows about her mother putting her to bed became replaced by arguments about whether the mother would wake Ruthie up in time for school in the morning. I pointed out how days and nights, holidays and term times were all mixed up.

When studying for her GCSEs, Ruthie had been compelled to check and recheck that she had gathered up all her papers when leaving class. She was deeply anxious that her papers would get all mixed up, and spent considerable time sorting them. With A-levels, her 'obsessionality', as she herself called it, increased. If she threw away a wasted sheet of paper, she would spend long periods frightened that she was throwing away good work needed for class. Sorting out dirty laundry could take hours, because she repeatedly had to check that the pockets were empty.

I had taken a number of approaches to this material, but it became clearer that these yet-to-be-understood phenomena had to do with mixed-upness and confusion. My comments along this line seemed to produce relevant, guiding dreams. In one of the first, her mother was wearing Ruthie's swimsuit while diving into what I interpreted was their fused and confusing pool of emotional life. In another dream about the same time, Ruthie was in a house associated with mine talking on the telephone to me, who was in the house of one of her best friends. I interpreted that the Ruthie in me was talking to the me in Ruthie. Not surprisingly, the confusion the dream was describing spilled into our discussion, so that we both had to struggle to disentangle the muddle.

Following these dreams, new images arose expressing internal development. In one dream, two birds flew into her room, which was at the top of the house. They settled, one above her desk and one above her bed. Ruthie left and went into the room of her younger sister, whom Ruthie had described as a 'go-with-the-flow' kind of person. This was not long before a holiday break, and I understood it to be an expression of her worry about getting into a flap without her two sessions. What was important was that she had another state of mind to which to go. That was to the room of the easygoing, that is, unflappable sister.

In another dream, I was visiting her in her room. She was pointing out that there were two piles: one of a messy stack of schoolwork and the other of dirty laundry. When she told me the dream, she said she had sorted this laundry over the weekend. What seemed significant was that she could take my thinking into her mind – her room at the top of the house – without the previous worry about being contaminated. Also, there was a sorting out of internal objects, between schoolwork done during the week and household chores done during the weekend. Because I was concerned about Ruthie's confusion, I focused on evidence of underdeveloped differentiation – *the separate piles* – rather than on what was in need of processing – *the messy homework* and the *unwashed laundry*.

Still another dream pictured her father showing her mother a series of lottery cards that looked like bingo cards. The mother commented that there were so many cards and so many numbers that it was confusing and one could not tell them apart. I interpreted that 'lottery' referred to 'lots and lots', and that the dream was about having lots and lots of feelings about her parents and their relationship. In her father's hands they were, upon discernment, distinct and separate items. Although for her mother these were overwhelming and confusing, there seemed to be a new thought – a Bingo! – namely, that there is a difference between a single mass of confusion and a plurality of distinct thoughts and feelings.

These dreams occurred alongside her increasing interest in my mind, which she found calm and settled. Her curiosity was evoked: how do I remember what she says? Do I keep notes on her? Are they in the filing cabinet across the room? Is that a dictionary on top of the table? Gradually we established that she perceived my mind as containing things that were organized. The filing cabinet was my mind with ordered contents, and the dictionary was my mind where everything has a meaning, all in order. Although these were rather sterile pictures of a mind, they were a development from the threatening chaos of misperception, wrong understanding and a mind in a flap.

After the Christmas break there were other views of my mind and thinking, which arose out of an emerging negative transference. Although the apparent trigger for the change in the transference was moving one of her session times, there were other factors. Deepening supportive friendships and other advantages of being 'ordinary' had begun to compensate for the loss of omnipotence over her parents. Also, as Ruthie began to see beyond her A-level exams, there was a dawning awareness that going to university meant that she would leave home and, of course, her therapy.

About this time there were two sessions in which her negative transference was evident. Each was followed by other events, and it was noticeable that those following the second session resulted in a state of confusion while those following the first did not. I should therefore like to compare these two sessions and their subsequent events.

In the first, Ruthie had been squeezing one of her fingers with a string, while talking in a teasing and manic way about clever people who knew things she wished she did. I interpreted that she wanted to squeeze information out of me that would explain why I was changing the session time. She agreed, and the jokey teasing and wheedling escalated, until eventually, in answer to her direct question, I said I did not intend to tell her why. The giggly mania abruptly became rage. She attacked me with the criticism that I was just like her mother; I was inconsistent, sometimes I answered questions and sometimes I did not, and session times changed. She exclaimed, 'I never know what to expect from you!'

A week later, she briefly referred to what had happened in our session, but was preoccupied with something that had happened at school the same day as the giggliness-turned-rage session. She had got into a similar teasing with a teacher, with whom, as with me, she had become friendly only after a difficult period. Although that school day ended in a spirit of high jinks, the atmosphere of the next day (the day after the session) was very different. She thought the teacher had become distant and disapproving, and that their good relationship was damaged. Yet he also seemed still to be interested. Several times at school she burst uncontrollably into tears, and yearned to talk to him to get the problem sorted out. Later at home she again experienced waves of intense pain and unstoppable crying. When I suggested that she was worried and hurt that she had damaged our relationship, she denied this, protesting that she was still angry at me.

Not long after, she again became angry at me, for what I thought was the changed session. Her anger in this session was expressed as criticism that I would not make up sessions she intended to miss over the summer because she planned to have two summer holidays after her A-levels. She told me that I was stupid not to make up important sessions, and, in the same breath, that I was too intelligent to do so without a good reason. She demanded to know what it was, and when I did not offer one acceptable to her, she again attacked me for being inconsistent and irrational, like her mother.

Following that session, she was scheduled for some minor surgery with a doctor she admired. She had broken her toe at Christmas, and this required a brief hospitalization. When she later told me about this, she was full of praise for the doctor and the hospital staff. She anticipated a similar good experience from the follow-up surgery, but at the last minute the day of the operation was changed. She had planned to stay in overnight, but this too was changed, in part because the experience had become so 'horrible'. Before going to hospital she had cleared up her room in a brief twenty minutes. When she came home, she returned to her old obsession of checking and rechecking what needed sorting out in her room. Worried, she wanted to know why this was.

I compared the two sessions I have described here. In the first, a clearly perceived bad, injurious me was experienced in contrast to a good but injured (by her) teacher. In the second, a similar bad me was experienced in contrast to what might have been a clearly perceived skillful and good doctor, but his goodness had become mixed up with badness because he had unpredictably changed the time. That was just what I had done to make me bad. The good and the bad had become all mixed up and she was compelled to try and sort them out. This interpretation had a noticeably calming effect upon Ruthie.

As the end of school approached, and as her exams were eventually taken and passed, Ruthie's material increasingly focused on leaving her family and her friends to go to university, and drawing her therapy to a close.

DISCUSSION

I have described the treatment of an adolescent girl, who was eventually able to integrate a split-off part of herself. What was split off held not only unwanted aggressive parts of herself, but also projective and introjective identification with unprocessed 'bits' of an anxious maternal mind. Ruthie's fears about psychic contamination had therefore to be dealt with first. Ruthie then faced her anxieties about her own destructive phantasies, which were split off from both her loving relationships and a primitive form of guilt. I should add that I view her Herculean efforts to get good marks to be a way of warding off this primitive superego.

I have just suggested that Ruthie had split off 'bad' parts of herself from 'good' parts, but in another sense 'bad' and 'good' had not developed into distinctly differentiated qualities. It was as if the distinction between bad and good rested on a precariously held foundation. This foundation was an infantile state of fusion with a mother-in-a-flap, a state of projective and introjective identification analogous to the foetus swallowing some if its amniotic environment. When tested against the weight of change – of moving to London and of puberty – the foundation became split off and the pigeon phobia developed. Although her self-inflicted wounding could have become dangerous if not dealt with, I consider that it was of secondary importance compared to the destructiveness of splitting and states of primitive projective and introjective identification. Self-wounding was a conscious effort to punish her parents, while splitting and confusion were unconscious phenomena that interfered with Ruthie's mental processes and development, and impoverished her internal world and her external relationships.

With treatment and consequent deintegration and reintegration, confusion developed into differentiated qualities of experience. When parts became distinguishable, they could then come into relation to one another, as I think they did when Ruthie's 'bad' therapist came into relation with her 'good' teacher. The pain, pining and remorse she felt in relation to him, and for which what actually happened did not fully account, are reminiscent of little Edward. I viewed my therapeutic role to be similar to that of Edward's mother: to allow space, to monitor the degree of persecution, and to process the fluctuating states of mind, even if the process was sometimes unspoken.

I should now like to turn to the theme of my paper, Jungian concepts relevant to integration and repair. First, although Ruthie was well defended against the part that had become split off, I also think that she was just as drawn to the pigeons as she was repelled by them. In being drawn to them, I think that she was seeking wholeness. According to Jung, wholeness is a characteristic of the self, and the pressure to become whole is the motivation behind individuation. It is out of my understanding that the self seeks to integrate that I have titled this paper 'With healing in her wings'.[1]

---

1 'But unto you that fear my name shall the Sun of righteousness arise with healing in his wings; and ye shall go forth, and grow up as calves in the stall' (Malachi iv, 2).

Second, what was integrated was a self-representation of what I consider to be something like a self object, and thus referred to primitive aspects of Ruthie's experience. The image of the pigeons was characterized by wholeness, because they were *totally* bad. Ruthie was preoccupied by pigeons for a long time, and spoke to me of little else, which indicates how much *meaning* they had for her. The image also included reference to states of projective and introjective identification with a mother who was in a flap, and thus referred to *states of fusion*. As with self objects, the representation contained enormous *potential*, which gradually began to unfold.

What early on was experienced as chaos and confusion was acted upon by the self and organized into discernible objects and experiences that then developed and complexified. My understanding and handling of the dreams of differentiation were informed by my understanding of how the self, in the Jungian sense, operates to differentiate and organize. I suppose that one could say that these were unconscious operations, but for a Jungian it is more meaningful to refer to the self.

This brings me to the concept of repair. Within a Jungian framework, 'repair' is seen as making whole. Ruthie's personality was 'repaired' when the split-off part became a deintegrate and experienced by Ruthie as a part of herself. In other words, to use a model I described earlier, the pseudopod got reattached to the amoeba. This is also what is meant by integration in a developed personality, like Ruthie's, in contrast to a small infant, for whom integration would refer to states of at-oneness.

As what the pigeons represented became a deintegration, Ruthie became more open to deintegrative and reintegrative processes. In this the ego is just as important as the self. As Fordham writes, 'the ego contributes and ensures that the dynamic sequences in the self [deintegration and reintegration] do not prove unproductive and circular, but are changed by ego activity, which in turn increases its strength' (Fordham, 1994: 73). Hence, the treatment could be seen to have facilitated actions of the self that restored the dynamic processes of deintegration and reintegration, thereby enriching Ruthie's ego, her personality and her life.

I should like to make a distinction between 'repair' and 'reparation'. I understand 'reparation' to arise creatively out of guilt, born out of the conflict of opposites in the depressive position. With Ruthie, when feelings of persecution occurred alongside deep remorse and apparent pining in the 'bad' therapist/'good' teacher episode, her internal organization seemed close to that of the depressive position. It is difficult to say whether reparation was involved. Fordham points out that in infancy the depressive position does not occur 'in a clear-cut form' (Fordham, 1995: 72), and it is likely that the same applies to adolescence.

Finally, having distinguished deintegration from splitting, I should like briefly to comment upon 'disintegration'. Fordham holds that, in a fundamental sense, the self is indestructible, and points to the persistence of the individual's uniqueness and continuity, which are expressions of the self. 'Disintegration' refers to the ego. It was Ruthie's ego, not her self, that from time to time disintegrated in the face of overwhelming fear, rage, persecution and confusion.

NOTES

This chapter was originally presented at the Association of Child Psychotherapists' Conference, London, March 1995. It was subsequently published in *The Journal of Child Psychotherapy*, Vol. 22, no. 1, 1996: pp. 64–81.

REFERENCES

Alvarez, A. (1992) *Live Company*. London: Routledge.

Astor, J. (1989) 'The breast as part of the whole: theoretical considerations concerning whole and part objects'. *Journal of Analytical Psychology*, Vol. 34, no. 2, 117–128.

Bion, W. (1962) *Learning from Experience*. London: Heinemann.

Brazelton, B. (1991) *The Earliest Relationship*. London: Karnac.

Fordham, M. (1976) *The Self and Autism*. London: Heinemann Medical.

Fordham, M. (1985a) 'Abandonment in infancy'. *Chiron*, Vol. 2, no. 1, 1–21.

Fordham, M. (1985b) *Explorations into the Self*. London: Academic Press.

Fordham, M. (1987) 'Action of the self', in P. Young-Eisendrath and J.A. Hall (Eds), *The Book of the Self*. New York: New York University Press.

Fordham, M. (1989) 'The infant's reach'. *Psychological Perspectives*, Vol. 21, 58–76.

Fordham, M. (1993) 'Notes for the formation of a model of infant development'. *Journal of Analytical Psychology*, Vol. 38, no. 1, 5–12.

Fordham, M. (1994) *Children as Individuals*. London: Free Association Books. Revised and amplified edition of the 1969 edition, London: Hodder & Stoughton.

Fordham, M. (1995) In R. Hobdell (Ed.), *Freud, Jung, and Klein: the Fenceless Field*. London: Routledge.

Jung, C. G. (1955–6) *Mysterium Coniunctionis. Collected Works*, Vol. 14. London: Routledge & Kegan Paul.

Jung, C. G. (1959) 'A study in the process of individuation', *Collected Works*, Vol. 9 ii. London: Routledge & Kegan Paul.

Jung, C. G. (1971) 'Definitions', *Collected Works*, Vol. 6. London: Routledge & Kegan Paul.

Laplanche, J. and Pontalis, J.-B. (1973) *The Language of Psycho-Analysis*. London: Hogarth.

Milakovic, I. (1967) 'The hypothesis of a deglutitive (prenatal) stage in libidinal development'. *International Journal of Psycho-Analysis*, Vol. 48, 76–82.

Segal, H. (1979) *Klein*. Glasgow: Collins.

Stern, D. (1985) *The Interpersonal World of the Infant*. New York: Basic Books.

Trevarthen, C. (1980) 'The foundations of intersubjectivity: development of interpersonal and cooperative understanding in infants', in D. Olson (Ed.), *The Social Foundations of Language and Thought*. New York: Norton.

Trevarthen, C. and Marwick, H. (1986) 'Signs of motivation for speech in infants, and the nature of a mother's support for development of language', in B. Lindblom and R. Zetterstrom (Eds), *Precursors of Early Speech*. Basingstoke: Macmillan.

(b) Classical Jungian comment

Julian David

It is difficult to compare a classical Jungian theory with a developmental one since Jung to the end had no clinical theory. This may be why those Jungians who wanted one have had to get it from other sources. But absence of a clinical theory is itself a considerable theory, so that is a very great step to take. Jung was strictly a phenomenologist, to that extent a postmodern before postmodernism – though only to that extent, for postmodernism with an archetypal theory is very different to postmodernism without it. Moreover he was disappointed (by 1936) that it was not taking on in the psychological community.

> Nevertheless it cannot be maintained that the phenomenological viewpoint has made much headway. Theory still plays far too great a role, instead of being included in phenomenology, as it should. Even Freud, whose empirical attitude is beyond doubt, coupled his theory as a *sine qua non* with his method, as if psychic phenomena had to be viewed in a certain way in order to mean something. (Jung, *Collected Works*, Vol. 9i, p. 112)

Phenomena are, in Jung's view, intrinsically new and unique (nature never makes exactly the same thing twice) but archetypal in their structure. That, therefore (the empirical study, and *experience*, of archetypal structures), was where a psychotherapist's training should occur. That is what he would *mean* by depth psychology. So beyond such injunctions as: 'A genuine participation going right beyond professional routine is absolutely imperative . . .'(Jung, *Collected Works*, Vol. 16, p. 400) he had no clinical theory.

But more than that, can even his vast study of psychic phenomena be called a theory? This makes a real problem between Jung and the modern (and modernist) world. There is no way that alchemy, for example, is a theory. It is a piling of metaphor upon metaphor, each as provisional as the many grips that a man must have on Proteus, in which can perhaps be held, as in a net, the elusive quality of the psyche – which if held as a sea lion turns into a serpent; and if held as a serpent turns into a tree or a leopard or a stream of water. Any honest thinker is familiar with Proteus. Theories, like metaphors, take one as far as they can go and then must be abandoned and another one taken, or they become an obstacle to understanding. This is so with nature and so with the psyche.

Therefore I have no quarrel with the theoretical preamble to this study, much of which is a phenomenological study of the first year of life and as such deeply interesting. But when it comes to applying it to the situation of a thirteen-year-old I do have a quarrel. I would need present phenomena, and plenty of them, dreams, symptoms, fantasies as well as irrational terrors such as the pigeon phobia. All these things *say themselves*; and from collating them it is generally possible to get an intuitive picture of what needs to be done in a particular therapy. So one cannot do that without material; and though I do not imagine the developmental school to believe that theory makes the therapist, one might almost, from this case study, get that impression.

Therapists need to develop a sharp eye for the many stages of development. That cannot be controversial. They include death, and also puberty. Different archetypes arise at different stages, different driving images. There is in this case no stated recognition that though she only came into therapy at thirteen the phobia had started at ten! There is an absence of dreams in the account of this period, so only this single phenomenon from which to judge the quality of the forces then moving in the psyche. There are always dream-memories if one looks for them. I would need them, and if I did not have at least one I would struggle, as Elizabeth Urban says she struggled. The father, also, is not less than a phenomenon. There is no mention of him either, until much later we learn that the relationship has 'improved', which is at last a clear statement that it was not good before. Yet the first passionate dynamic of mother and child *must* be complicated by the emergence of the opposite archetype, the father, which *must* become active very soon after the first year, if not within it – and be present increasingly at puberty. The psychic, or feeling quality of the father is simply different to that of the mother, and a child is well able to pick it up. It is a hand-hold outside her and could well be considered the beginning of all differentiation – this great *other* in the family.

The same issue (the different *quality* of the male) arises later when Ms Urban confuses the transference to a male teacher with the transference to her. It seems to me (with respect – genuine respect, as I shall explain later) the price exacted by an over-powerful theory. The *assimilation* of a life-story to the dynamics of the first year seems to me to be of the same order as the assimilation of psyche itself to 'mother'. This is the most serious criticism I have to make of this case. For if the original purpose of this chapter was to use clinical material to illustrate a theory then it is an abuse of the material – precisely that imposition of theory upon phenomena which *must* be avoided if we are to interpret those phenomena.

I say 'with respect' not as a mere formula of words, for the case as a whole seems to have worked. How much the theory matters, whether right or wrong, is exactly the question. We are often in the dark and yet manage to remain still there with the patient – and the therapy works. Goethe remarks somewhere that people of good will are not impeded by apparent errors in theory, and it may well be like that between client and therapist. The little research that we have on the effectiveness of psychotherapy seems to be in line with that done by David Orlinsky and colleagues at Chicago (Orlinsky, 1986), which is (to quote from Anthony Stevens's overview of this work) that over the whole field, from frequent analysis on the couch to once-a-week counselling, the factor of crucial importance is the quality of the therapeutic bond.

> It is essential that this alliance should be experienced as positive and supportive and that it should be based on a 'collaborative sharing of responsibility', as both participants focus on the patient's feeling, experiences and difficulties. It is also important that the therapist should be conceived as skilful as well as sympathetic and that the patient should be open, non-defensive and actively committed to the therapeutic process. (Stevens, 1998: 172)

But since most of us believe that insight is also a factor, even if left in the psychic field where the consciousness of the therapist is still active, we must have a go at the phobia. Let us start with Elizabeth Urban's excellent description.

> When Ruthie and I first met she reported in detail how abhorrent and repulsive she found pigeons. I asked her to draw a picture of one and she made an attempt but stopped short of completing the picture because it aroused such fear and revulsion. Closing her eyes and shaking her head, she shuddered and flapped her hands while expelling repeated 'oohs' of disgust. We established that what was unthinkable for her was that a pigeon should flap up on big flapping wings and rush into her face.

In some quarters the repeated 'oohs' of disgust and the image of the flapping wings forcing itself into the face, would be taken as conclusive proof of sexual abuse. Much of what goes on in such quarters is, admittedly, tomfoolery – rising from the need, within Freud's model of the psyche, to assume that everything in the unconscious was once conscious and then repressed. Nevertheless, the sexual aspect must be present, though not necessarily in such a crass and concrete fashion. Recently a girl of ten (not in therapy) dreamt that a big bird came down from the sky and mated with her. That is the sort of image that is moving at puberty. There is a ferment in the psyche, a spiritual dimension shouldering its way in – an instinctual upwelling in which instinct and spirit form, in Jung's words, 'an impenetrable mass – a veritable magma sprung from the depths of primeval chaos' (Jung, *Collected Works*, Vol. 16: 363). The big bird in the sky is not a million miles from the angel that comes to Mary, the swan to Leda. Like them it bears the charge of symbolic incest, for the swan is a disguise for Zeus, and the angel is a messenger from the great Father and bears his seed. Pigeons are not so big, but they are in this girl's mind. They spend much of their day sitting together cooing, or chasing each other noisily through trees. Traditionally they belong to the goddess of love and it is easy to see why. Ruthie must have wondered, sometimes, what they were doing. Elizabeth Urban claims that 'a significant part of the phobia was an infantile state of projective and introjective identification with the mother'. This is true in that the strength and security of the mother-relationship mediates the great mystery of the opposite sex. Her attitude to it is picked up by her daughter, for their psyches are still porous to each other (and I believe should be). But the problems are different now.

So I do not see the pigeon phobia as 'mother in a flap'. It probably includes that but it is far too powerful to be just that. What we must conclude is that the part-formed ego is fighting with huge energies in the unconscious, just recently emerged – and that it is under threat from them. When Elizabeth Urban tells the parents, some time later, that the phobia represents 'a condensation of intense emotions', I would say, yes, that is well put. The move from a small town to London would certainly have increased the uncertainty of the ego, for it was a loss of the familiar walls and corners, and the familiar friends, which give support in crisis. The most disturbed children are often those of policemen or diplomats who have had to move too often. Some girls adjust to puberty with very little problem. Others have very great problems. All possibilities should be considered, particularly that the decisive factor may be in the parents – as they *are* at the moment. Is there a place laid for sex at the family table? Does it officially exist? Or is it the Thirteenth Fairy? I would need pointers to their states of mind, and would get hints, at least, in the dreams – because of that porousness that I have mentioned of the child's psyche to what is moving not only in the mother's psyche but in the walls of the house. I should want to know, at a conscious level, if she *feels* her father is *there*, that he is emotionally present? For if he is *there*, in an ordinary, banal, discreet, affectionate and un-invasive way, then the image of the opposite sex is much less alarming when it rises in the fantasies of a girl-child. And many fathers in our culture are so frightened of incest that they give their daughters *nothing*. Some incest fantasies arise, as we know well, from his *neglect* rather than his over-intrusiveness. The burden of work, too, often in our culture makes it impossible for a father to be a father; but his human presence is important at this stage. I would want to know about that, and also how effective the mother feels to Ruthie, as an aid in facing the great transition. A daughter's puberty is a test of both parents' relation to the issue of instinct, sexuality, and the unconscious. And if there were any chance of getting some of this through to the parents I would have a go.

In a primal culture Ruthie would be making a retreat right back into the world of the ancestors. An example occurs to me from a missionary account of the puberty rites for girls of the Tacuna tribe:

> As soon as a girl detects signs of her first period, she takes off all her ornaments, hangs them in an obvious place on the posts of her hut and goes off to hide in a nearby bush. When her mother arrives she sees the ornaments, realises what has happened and sets off to look for her daughter. The latter replies to her mother's call by striking two pieces of dry wood together. The mother then loses no time in erecting a partition around the girl's bed and takes her there after nightfall. From that moment the girl remains in seclusion for two or three months without being seen or heard by anyone except her mother and her paternal aunts. (Lévi-Strauss, 1973)

The tribe is matrilineal, that is the huts pass through the female line. This is the world of the mother and all the mothers back to the beginning, the world of instinct and the world also of ghosts and spirits – exactly that 'magma' of which Jung speaks, in which it is impossible to distinguish spirit from instinct. In our culture a girl only has her mother as access to all that; and if the way through her is blocked by a state perhaps accurately described as 'mother in a flap', she needs a relationship with some other woman. As a male therapist I would look round for such a one. Ruthie got it in Elizabeth Urban, and I believe that that is why the therapy succeeded.

Let me draw a picture of how I think it *may* have worked. In the first five months little progress is made in understanding or reducing the phobia; but a relationship *is* made – strong enough to survive an extended holiday and an excursion into behaviour therapy of more than a year's duration – and then bring her back with a positive transference so that the real work can begin. That is remarkable. In this five months a connection was made, which did not occur in a much longer period with another therapist. It is now the year before GCSEs. Ruthie is intelligent, and Elizabeth Urban's quality as an intelligent, perhaps quite academic person who is also a woman, fits her to be a guide into this aspect of adulthood. Week after week she helps her face the panics which occur with her assignments and exams. The ego gains in confidence and as it does so the chaos in the unconscious becomes less alarming. The second stage of the treatment ends with her passing her exams with virtually all As – a classic initiation process completed.

But there is much more to do. Soon Ruthie begins to make life at home impossible for everyone, fighting with her mother and furiously throwing food out of the fridge. A meeting between both parents and therapist occurs, and a further stage of progress begins. The relationship to her father improves, maybe simply because he begins to believe that he might matter to her and she to him; while Ruthie uses her relationship with her therapist 'to avoid fights with her mother'. Boundaries on her behaviour are set, principally now by her father. They anger her to the extent of enraged self-wounding, but in the end they make her feel more secure. She now has something to push against. It is a relationship.

In the accounts of the later stages of the work there is far greater access to the unconscious material than earlier. As well as Ruthie's improved contact with her father there is a steady strengthening, it seems to me, of her *unconscious identification* both with her female analyst and her mother. It is normal, I believe, for the improvement in the relation to one sex to go hand in hand with the improvement in the relation to the other. This unconscious identification can be followed in the dreams. They are generally interpreted negatively by the therapist, but I do not believe that 'unconscious' is in itself negative. A living dynamic between conscious and unconscious is the object of 'classical' Jungian work – because it conceives that to be nature's own object in the human creature. In one dream Ruthie's mother is wearing Ruthie's swimsuit while diving into a pool. In another, Ruthie is in Elizabeth Urban's house, speaking to her on the telephone, since she is installed in the house of one of Ruthie's best friends (presumably female). In a third dream her therapist is visiting her in her own bedroom. They are all classical signs of the transference as Jung conceived it, where boundaries blur and a shared identity develops – deeply nourishing and just the regression that Ruthie needs to make. What is happening, it seems to me, is that her therapist is *doing her best* for her – something like that commitment *beyond professional routine* which Jung believed is the active ingredient in any cure. One imagines that her mother is doing her best too, perhaps now in a less rationalist way. She *picks it all up* in the unconscious; she is nourished by it, and at a deeper level still the psyche's own healing process is activated. Ms Urban is giving a relationship. As the female ego strengthens, so Ruthie's relationship to the male also improves – in the figure, as we have seen, of her father, but also in certain powerful positive projections onto men such as those that girls do make at this age. We can trace that also in a dream. Her father is showing her mother a series of cards with numbers on them. Her mother complains that she cannot tell them apart. Ms Urban comments, rightly, that there is a difference between a single mass of confusion and a plurality of distinct thoughts and feelings. Her father now stands for that differentiation – and that is how, archetypally, it is. That was why it was better for him to set boundaries than for her mother to do it. The mother represents her roots in the un-bounded reaches of the unconscious. It is important that she should not be too rational or too disciplinary either. The father is the point outside. Both are needed. At about this time there are the strikingly powerful transferences onto the teacher and the doctor.

It is at this point that Ms Urban interprets the response to the teacher in terms of the transference to herself, the analyst. But as Ruthie describes her feelings they seem to me to be manifestly those of a daughter who longs to know a *father*, how he ticks, what he thinks about things, what has gone wrong with a relationship which is so important to both of them. She 'yearned to talk to him', says Ms Urban, 'to get the problem sorted out'. Later at home there are 'waves of intense pain and episodes of unstoppable crying'. Ruthie denies, in the session, that this represents her distress with her therapist. I agree with her. The transference to a male teacher has a different feeling-tone; it is the development of a different element in the psyche. The teacher carries, at this point, the weight of the father-imago which has been too absent in the past. Nothing can become conscious until it is first projected. The phenomenon of projection is the substance of psychic life, and happens all the time, everywhere. It is true that the relationship to her therapist seemed also, at this time, to be in crisis. But that is another issue.

It was near to the end of the therapy, and Elizabeth Urban announces it as the onset of the negative transference. Now, given the existence of the shared identity, the negative transference is indeed going to appear, but this one is provoked; and that is quite different. Finding it necessary to change a session, she found it *un*-necessary to tell Ruthie why! Ruthie felt betrayed and was very cross. Transference, whether negative or positive, comes *outwards* from within. This goes the other way – inwards from without. It is strengthened, no doubt, by transference elements from the mother-relationship, but the hurt and dismay are the natural response to a loved and trusted friend who suddenly puts herself in a position of arbitrary power. Power is intrinsically arbitrary, takes no account of the other and is to that extent unrelated.

(Even the boundaries set by the father would not be arbitrary.) Therapists have far too much power anyway. I do not like the story of the father who puts his son on the top of a wall, stretches his arms out wide so that he can jump, then steps sharply aside! Betrayal comes in its own time. Parents and therapists should not administer it, except by accident, which happens often enough. They are there to provide a place in which it can be discussed. This is bound to include *unintentional* betrayals on their own parts, but the intention is all-important.

Therefore I treat the client with great respect. I suspect Elizabeth Urban does too – usually. It is particularly important with a child, for they have often not been treated with respect. Apart from the professional aspects for which one is paid, I retreat scrupulously from authority. I would probably say in such a case, 'I'm afraid I have to change the time of the session. What other time would suit you?' If pressed I would even say why I had to change it. To cut across such a natural response would perhaps assist the transition from a state of infantile omnipotence to Klein's 'depressive position' (in Jung's terms the grounding of the Puer Aeternus) but life will do this anyway. In adolescence a little inflation (or omnipotence) is desirable. It is a necessary energy. It cuts right across the natural *feeling response* to damage it.

Apart from this issue (which is fundamental between Jung and Klein, whose approaches to *what is natural* are not compatible), there is little in practice that I would have done differently. Elizabeth Urban made a relationship. She tried; she did her best. She distinguished in her own mind between the ego and the self. 'It was Ruthie's ego that sometimes shattered,' she says at one point, 'not her self.' That is an important observation. It is not, as it happens, the self as Jung speaks of it. That *cannot* shatter. Even in the full psychosis it can still be felt in the background, and in her last paragraph Elizabeth Urban is in agreement with that. Neither did it matter, necessarily, if she was baffled. The best work may be done when the therapist is baffled. It gives room for the unconscious to speak. In one dream, two birds fly into Ruthie's room, and settle there. One is above the bed and one above the desk. We may well think that feeling and intellect, the un-conscious world of the bed and the highly conscious world of the desk, are coming into relationship with each other; and it is striking that Ruthie has no fear of either bird

Her violence had been successfully contained. The phobic energy, which filled out the image of the pigeon returned, we may think, as a disgust for red meat – hurled out of the family fridge! It was changed from a threat from without (pigeon), to a horror that the ego *rides* – probably with some delight. Omnipotent, certainly. Alarming, perhaps. But it was dealt with well. One gets the impression of a young woman with an unusually abundant libido, and a matching intellect – a rewarding person to work with. One would like to get her painting, sculpting, singing, or whatever suits her, as well as working at A-levels or degree or whatever she worked at later. Without some measure of putting it into imaginal form, an energy of this sort will not in the end find peace. It is, I believe, probable that she will be back one day.

REFERENCES

Jung, C. G. *Collected Works*. London: Routledge & Kegan Paul.

Lévi-Strauss, Claude (1973) *Honey to Ashes*. London: Cape, p. 373. Quotation from C. Nimuendaju, 'The Tacuna'. *UCPAAE*, Vol. 45, 1952.

Orlinsky, D. E. and Howard K. L. (1986) 'The Psychological Interior of Psychotherapy: Explorations with the Therapy Session Report', in L. S. Greenberg and W. M. Pinsof (Eds), *The Psychotherapeutic Process: A Research Handbook*, pp. 477–562. New York: Guilford.

Stevens, Anthony (1998) *An Intelligent Person's Guide to Psychotherapy*. London: Duckworth.

(c) Kleinian comment

Robert Hinshelwood

This is a work of integration. It is both a claim for 'integration' as a central idea in development; and also an attempt to integrate Jungian and Kleinian ideas. In fact Elizabeth Urban's theme, 'Jungian concepts relevant to integration and repair' (p. 20) takes the clinical phenomenology of a patient's integration as the node around which to integrate certain schools of thought. From Jung she takes the notion of 'self' as the locus of the *experience of wholeness*; and from Klein the notions of splitting and integration. I will make some initial comments on theory; and devote the greater part of my space to Ruthie, the child patient whose case Elizabeth Urban uses as a test for the key role of integration which could bring Jung and Klein into line.

THEORETICAL ISSUES

The 'self'

The chapter starts with the notion of self as used by Fordham, who extended Jung's ideas into a developmental psychology useful in psychotherapeutic work with children and adults. It starts unpromisingly since the important distinction between self and ego for Jungians, does not map so closely onto Kleinian concepts where the distinction is less clear. The self, Urban wrote,

> is characterized by totality and wholeness, and is the source of meaning. Functionally it is an organizer and integrator, bringing together and structuring the inner world. (p. 9).

The ego is then less defined, and some sort of lower order set of mechanisms, largely restricted to conscious experience.

But for Klein the organizer of experience and of the internal world, conscious and unconscious is the ego:

> Klein's emphasis was on the importance of relationships with objects. She tended to use the term 'self', 'ego' and 'subject' interchangeably. The term 'ego' (also

'subject') is used as the complement of 'object'. Whereas 'self', she later contended, '. . . is used to cover the whole of the personality, which includes not only the ego but the instinctual life which Freud called the "id"' (Klein, 1959: 249), the ego is '. . . the organised part of the "self"'. (Hinshelwood 1991: 425)

There is clearly a major divergence: for Klein the organizer is the 'ego', for Urban it is the 'self'.

If we stick to the experience of wholeness, there may be more agreement. For Jung the 'self' is the locus of the experience of being whole. In a comparable passage Freud, after 1920, assigned the notion of completeness to an instinct, the libido; thus,

> Eros, which seeks to force together and to hold together the portions of living substance. (Freud, 1920: 60)

The libido is the drive to bring things together to create patterns and complexity; and contrasts with the drive to dissolve difference and to eliminate pattern and complexity (ashes to ashes, etc.) – the death instinct. Klein focused, like Jung, on the *experience* of these more biological entities, the drives. She recognized, too, that the infant's earliest preoccupation is with its completeness. And Urban links this with just the same early preoccupations that Fordham finds in infants. This is fine so far. Both diverge from Freud, who, generally speaking, was concerned not so much with the state of completeness as such but with the contents of the ego being in conflict (notably the Oedipal conflicts). However, Klein's divergence from Freud was less total than Jung's. In mediating her views with Freud's, she stressed two separate levels: one where the ego is concerned about its own completeness, and one where it is concerned about conflicts within it. The first level, that of completeness of the ego, underlies the second and in some degree determines it. Bion, following Klein, described these as the psychotic and the non-psychotic (or neurotic) levels respectively.

> The non-psychotic personality was concerned with a neurotic problem, that is to say a problem that centred on the resolution of a conflict of ideas and emotions to which the operation of the ego had given rise. But the psychotic personality was concerned with the problem of repair of the ego. (Bion, 1957: 272)

Klein herself was emphatic that there were two levels of function to be attended to, one which underlay the other. She talked about this a lot and continually pressed her audience, readers and students, to understand the primitive levels of the patient's functioning in the material. This doctrine of levels is now so taken for granted by Kleinians that it is little talked of today, and it has less attention paid it than previously. However, Bion's work with schizophrenics tends to point to the necessity for a constant movement between the two levels – he represented this with his symbol Ps $\leftarrow \rightarrow$ D. That is to say, if the ego feels to a degree that it has achieved more completeness, then it is confronted by a neurotic conflict; and psychotic personalities escape from the level of neurotic conflict into a psychotic disintegration of themselves.

Deintegration

Urban carefully describes Fordham's view of deintegration and the contrasting idea of disintegration. Deintegration is linked with Freud's model of narcissism, pictured as an amoeba pushing out a pseudopodium, which nevertheless, does not separate completely from the organism, and subsequent withdrawal of the pseudopodium. Deintegration (and reintegration) might I suppose be compared with the ordinary processes of normal projection and introjection described by Heimann (1952) and elaborated clinically by Money-Kyrle (1956) in the Kleinian framework.

Urban stretches Freud's pseudopodium analogy, describing it as a strain for the amoeba which, under certain pressures, can rupture. This is a moment when the link with the amoeba snaps, and we have 'splitting'. It might equate with projective identification and the loss of parts of the ego – this is disintegration and the subject suffers real pathology.

There is a link made between Fordham's deintegration and disintegration and Klein's two kinds of object-relations, associated with the depressive and paranoid-schizoid positions. In the depressive position when a projection is made into an object, as described by Heimann, we might say that 'A' gives 'B' a piece of her mind – by this we mean that 'A' is angry with 'B', knows she is angry with 'B' and intends that 'B' will actually feel inside him something of that anger. 'A' puts anger into 'B'. but 'A' continues to acknowledge her anger. I regard that as corresponding to Urban's (Fordham's) 'deintegration'.

However in another process, 'A', initially angry, may provoke 'B' to anger with her, by making 'innocent-sounding' remarks: 'Oh, darling, I have a headache tonight', for example, and then she sleeps soundly. Then an initial state in 'A', anger, is transported into 'B' rejecting him, thus leaving him emotionally disturbed rather than her. So, 'A's mental state is lost and, as it were, gained by him. The result is psychoanalytically called 'omnipotence' (see Hinshelwood, 1995), or projective identification. This might coincide with Urban's (Fordham's) disintegration, although I recognize that this is my own interpretation of what Urban is saying . But if it is so, then we have a set of theoretical models that is so similar that Urban is correct to link Jung/Fordham's theory to Klein's.

Depressive position

Urban locates reparative process ('repair' and 'reparation') in the depressive position (as described by Klein). However, her focus is the repair of the self, and this is precisely what the Kleinian view of the depressive position is not. In the depressive position, the repair is of a damaged object. It does not deal with a disintegration of the self; disintegration of the self is a preoccupation of the paranoid-schizoid position.

From a Kleinian point of view, the stress on the repair of the self considerably downplays the object-relations. And this is a major difference from Klein. 'Pining', a word suggested by Klein, and Fordham being about the only person to take up the suggestion, was intended by Klein to indicate the special poignancy of 'feeling for' a damaged loved one. This is an important issue – at least for a Kleinian. In Urban's account of the Jungian view, priority is given to narcissistic concerns – and we move away from the 'feelings for' the object. For Kleinian analysts, patient and therapist cannot stay just with a concern for the state of wholeness of the patient's mind – there has to be a move to a new level, a concern with the state of the object as well. In effect, this would be an emergence from narcissism, into the Kleinian (rather than 'Urbanian') depressive position.

Urban's focus on the drive to completeness, stresses the paranoid-schizoid and potentially psychotic processes. Her emphasis tends to obscure the neurotic level of conflicts, leaving it neglected in the case of Ruthie as I shall discuss later. This leads us to important technical issues, which I will now take up in examining the clinical material.

THE CASE MATERIAL

First a brief comment about the observed baby, Edward. Edward was very distressed – and thus distressing for the baby observation seminar, but 'Nothing external in the observation accounted for the unreachable depth and intensity of his response; he was responding to something internal' (p. 13). From a Kleinian point of view, this assertion seems improbable; unless this 12-month-old baby is completely psychotic; and it is definitely difficult to prove this negative assertion. Rather a Kleinian would expect an experience of *something* external, even if it is an external object whose identity is exaggerated and distorted by unconscious phantasies and their products, internal objects. The baby is then responding to a visible, palpable external object, even though it may be difficult to recognize for an observer. The point of the baby observation seminar is, surely, to display that interaction with an external object and to speculate about the baby's distortions of it. What mother had actually done with Edward, or with his bowl, which he interpreted in terms of a desperate perse-cution, is not clear, since the process of that observation is not given. I mention this in order to ponder whether the particular focus on the 'self' has led Urban to play down the relations with an external object – however distorted. Or, to put this another way, there seems to be an assumption that Edward withdraws narcissistically into a world wholly of hallucination, because such an assumption is required by theory.

Ruthie

Nearly half of Elizabeth Urban's chapter is devoted to an illustrative child psycho-therapy case, which is described with great vividness, sympathy and humanity. The case report, unfortunately, gives no really extended piece of process. As in the observation of Edward, we do not really get enough to see how the stated *impressions* of Ruthie emerged as evidence from the process of her sessions. With that limitation, it is hard to gauge the real impact of the patient's, and the therapist's, unconscious object-relations upon each other. It is possible that the theoretical emphasis on 'self' drew the author away from the immediate object-relations of the encounter. But in general terms, in an object-relation, each party reacts to the other. When the patient conveys distress, then 'the analyst is inevitably disturbed in the sense of affected' (Brenman Pick, 1985: 157). If the therapist is not distressed, or affected, then he is somehow not quite connected. Money-Kyrle (1956) and Rosenfeld (1987) also agree, it is necessary for the analyst to be sufficiently open to the patient's disturbance that the analyst also in a sense becomes a little disturbed.

In Ruthie's case, I think that the therapist is in fact sensitive in that way. The evidence is that she can write a very sensitive account, indicating in fact her emotional openness. However, the author describes herself as visibly portraying a calm and settled mind (p. 20); stating

> I viewed my therapeutic role to be similar to that of Edward's mother: to allow space, to monitor the degree of persecution, and to process the fluctuating states of mind. (p. 20)

I think more is required than simply to 'monitor the persecution', and my own belief would be that the therapist herself *felt* some of the disturbance too. In fact, surely she could only monitor it by feeling disturbed by the 'flap' in the room with her. So, I doubt if this picture of the unflappable therapist is an accurate one. I suspect that the therapist believes that she *should be* calm and collected at all times (and that this is a required version of 'containment', in our contemporary jargon). If my guess were to be accurate then I think this is an example of a therapist's enthusiasm for technique overcoming her sensitivity to her patient.[1]

I make this point for a (very strong) reason. The therapist has reported a case of phobia in which anxiety is overwhelming and all over the place. It is referred to as a 'flap', and one of the patient's methods of coping is to project 'flap' into pigeons in the street in a very concrete way and then avoid them like the plague. In addition, the therapist's formulation is that there is great confusion in Ruthie's mind about whether the flap belongs to herself or her mother – and thus whether her mother is responsible for making her an over-anxious child, or whether she is responsible for causing mother to have more anxiety than mother can cope with.

If this formulation is plausible, we must follow its consequences. A patient who is bothered about uncontainable anxiety, and is confused over where it belongs is, in my view, very likely to re-experience such a situation with the therapist. At one point Ruthie burst out in rage that the therapist

---

1 Not enough is written in my view about the *therapist's* superego, which we all have and which demands of us that we follow a perfect technique.

was just like her mother: I was inconsistent, sometimes I answered questions and sometimes I did not, and session times changed. She exclaimed, 'I never know what to expect from you!' (pp. 18–19)

The problem with mother's flap – inconsistency, and changeableness – is quite clearly recreated in the therapy (and also the school, actually). The therapist might agree with us here, but it does imply that Ruthie is anxious about flaps in the therapist, as in all sorts of people, and reacts to them as she does to pigeons. Even if the therapist is not disturbed, Ruthie will be watchful and suspicious – and that needs understanding and putting into words. It seems to me therefore that an absolutely central aspect of this treatment would be to follow the moment by moment experience that Ruthie has of the state of mind of the therapist.

The therapist's flap, real or projected, must be, continuously, one of the major aspects of Ruthie's experience whilst in her sessions with the therapist. Of course there are differences in the way that therapists of different schools will see the need to interpret the here-and-now transference. But, the therapist explicitly described Ruthie's 'interest in my mind, which she found calm and settled' (p. 18). I wonder what a patient who is preoccupied with who is flapping, makes of an object which is selfconsciously calm. There is a real possibility that the patient will feel that the therapist has lost touch with the patient who is preoccupied with the therapist's flap. In fact, apropos of the incident with the teacher (p. 19) when Ruthie had been stirring up his state of mind with teasing and with high jinks, she felt that next day he retreated and 'became distant and disapproving'. The implication is that if she projects flap into someone they can well move out of touch – just as she herself avoids flapping pigeons. My concern therefore is that the therapist in retreating into her 'calm' technique, may be allowing the patient to repeat her experience of an object that cannot contain flap – and is felt as distant, calm, but out of touch.

Although, I have been fairly categorical about the further need to explore the patient's view of the object's state of mind, we cannot know, from the material provided, that it did not happen. Though the therapist does not highlight the flap in the therapist's mind, it would seem necessary in this therapy to do so with a patient who is overwhelmed by the flap in peoples' minds. My question therefore is whether Elizabeth Urban's theoretical emphasis, on repairing the self, led her to become distant from the patient's concern for her object (i.e. her therapist's mind) or at least in this account of the sessions written for these purposes.

These thoughts lead in a different direction from Urban's technical aim with Ruthie, which appears to be to give Ruthie *an experience of* a calm mind, without interpreting what that calmness means. In my contrasting stance, we interpret the patient's perception of the therapist as explicitly as possible even when one is actually disturbed by the patient, or indeed feeling cut off emotionally from the patient. Incidentally, this is not an easy task, and so no-one should ever be too critical of this area of work!

I found myself concerned with the question: what is the 'flap' about. Urban is exclusively interested in the damage to the patient's mind by there being a flap in it (arising there, or infected from mother and others). Urban's assumption is that the flap can be contained by simply addressing the container (Ruthie's mind). In contrast, I would address my understanding to the contents as well. That understanding *is* the containment. Little in the case report suggests that the therapist is interested in understanding what Ruthie thinks is so flap-worthy. I have the uncomfortable feeling that Elizabeth Urban is once again restricted by her own allegiance to theory. She makes the brisk assertion early on, 'A psychoanalytic understanding of a phobia would usually include sexuality' (p. 14), as if something other than this approach – I presume a Jungian or Fordhamian approach – could dispense with that. It is quite a daring challenge to report the therapy of an adolescent without mentioning sex! But this is in fact what Urban has done. She justifies this:

> Although treatment included the gradual understanding of emotional, cognitive and sexual aspects of what the pigeons represented to Ruthie, in what follows I shall focus on the aspects of the phobia that related to certain states of confusion. (p. 14)

Of course the chapter is angled in a certain direction – towards the disturbance in the sense of self. However, there is an assumption in that statement which I contest. This is that there can be an uncontentious separation of the two levels – the level of self-phenomenology, and the level of the Oedipal phantasies, conflicts and anxieties.[2] In a different (Kleinian) view, for a patient with a neurotic disorder (and maybe some personality disorder, as Ruthie), the understanding of the emotional, cognitive and sexual aspects are just that containing process which the patient could take in to support her sense of wholeness. Therefore, interpretation of the self problems would need to go along hand-in-hand with the interpretation of the object-relations and conflicts.

The exclusion of adolescent sexual material – even for purposes of theoretical exposition – leaves us impoverished in our understanding of the containing process, i.e. in Urban's terms, the self's drive for wholeness. I cannot give a full account of this in the material, since it is not given to us. However, the incident of teasing, and high jinks, with the male teacher at school, cannot, to anyone with ordinary common sense, be without a high sexual content. It must have been for the teacher, and for Ruthie's colleagues at school, even if Ruthie could sustain a complete separation (splitting-off) from her sexual involvement. The teacher's retreat is likely (very likely) to be understood by Ruthie, as his anxiety about her sexuality, and his need to keep distant from contact with it. It may well be that the therapist was alive to this sexual content and did interpret in the transference, how Ruthie brings sexuality to her session, but I would say that this is the very stuff of the process that will contain – or make whole. Understanding the self which is confronted with sexuality

---

2 It may be that once again the impression of contrast, which I have, arises from Urban's need to select according to her theme.

might have featured more prominently in the case presentation. If there really is a rupture in the self caused by the flap over sex, and if the healing of the self must entail a containing of the flap caused by thoughts of sex, then sex cannot be left out of the containing process.

This leads on to another point of technique. A week before, Ruthie had her painful experience of rejection by the teacher, she had a similar problem with her therapist. The therapist cancelled a session and, 'I said I did not intend to tell her why' (p. 18). Ruthie's giggling turned to rage. Again it seems to me that an allegiance to technique (a command somewhere in the therapist's superego perhaps: Do not reveal personal information!) overrides an understanding of what it *meant to Ruthie* that she was not privy to this information. Ruthie, too, has a view about the 'why' of the not-telling. And if not told, her explanation will be based on unconscious phantasies, probably of a sexual kind – that the therapist is excluding Ruthie, to go off and have sex with someone (possibly the teacher whom Ruthie later links with the therapist). Then, to Ruthie's mind, the therapist does not tell Ruthie, because of a supposed embarrassment about sex. Ruthie may then experience the therapist as getting in a flap. And then she is likely to experience the rattled therapist as dealing with the flap by some stonewalling process. For Ruthie, it means that she is left with the flap, does not know what to do with it, and does not any more know if it is her flap or the therapist's (especially if the therapist is now appearing calm about it all). All Ruthie can then do is to regress into a primitive expression of the rage.

All this of course is my surmise, which may be entirely wrong. A construction of a piece of process now, after the session, cannot be tested. However, I have followed it through to try to indicate the intimate connection between two levels, the neurotic level (an object-relationship with a fraught sexual content) and the containing level dependent on the effective wholeness of self. Urban's conclusions therefore lead clinically away from a Kleinian approach.

IN CONCLUSION

How has Urban managed with her integrative intentions? She is to be congratulated on her attempt to draw together different points of view, and conceptual schemes around the fulcrum notion of wholeness and integration. She has succeeded I think in conveying sufficient relatedness between Jung, Freud, Klein and Fordham to make some dialogue between them possible. I have tried to comment on the theoretical and technical difficulties in this spirit. Although I do appreciate her work on bringing together different conceptual systems, it seems to me that the attempt has not been completely successful. The paper is perhaps most successful in helping us to clarify certain differences so well. Perhaps here I shall pick out the two main ones.

First of all is the apparent neglect, in my terms, of the 'flap'. I believe that this may indicate a different emphasis in the Jung/Fordham camp, where structural features of the self are more important than the experienced anxiety. Or to put it another way, you have to repair the container (self) before you can have a conflict or anxiety in it. That sounds sensible enough. However, my position is that the content is so fraught with anxiety that the container ruptures; and thus both must be attended to. In Bion's terms the thought determines the origins and development of the thinker – i.e. the contents (thoughts) are instrumental in influencing the 'thinking apparatus' as well as the other way around. It is a two-way process, requiring attention to the influences in both directions.

Jung and Klein also differ in their appreciation of the self: for Klein it is the ego plus internal objects; whilst for Jung the self is the ego plus archetypes.[3] Their similarity, though, is that the self tends to be seen as *experience* rather than mechanism. That throws Jung and Klein together in a fundamental way.[4] The difference is that with Klein's emphasis on the experiencing ego, words make all the difference. Symbols, being the expression of the organizing ego, they are the medium of understanding, containing and development. Therapy is based in understanding experiences. Whereas with Jung, perhaps the experience of archetypes is a primal one, preverbal. Thus Urban's technical base is in giving Ruth a healing experience that bypasses verbal understanding. Such technical difference points to much further debate.

However, I want to convey a final hesitancy. That is about the method of integrating the sets of concepts. Urban's method, in common with many (the majority of others, perhaps), takes a particular concept found in different conceptual systems and tries to match the conceptual abstraction of one school, with the conceptual abstraction of another. At its best it is grounded in clinical work, and thus depends on clinical phenomenology. However, serious problems with this method of resolving differences have increasingly become obvious. Particularly, clinical phenomena do not all appear the same to different clinicians (as I have demonstrated in my comments on Ruthie). Concepts in one system, manifestly do not mean the same as in another. Over time, the meaning of a concept tends to drift, and does so under semantic 'pressures' that are specific to that theoretical system. So, the same concept in another system will be subject to different pressures. Thus, meaning can drift in completely different directions. I think we can see, in my comments, how the meaning of 'depressive position' has altered under the pressure of Jungian ideas to accommodate the notion of narcissism.

By contrast, another way of comparing concepts is other than in terms of clinical phenomena. We can trace a concept's history back to some common origin for its

3   I am grateful to Robert Withers for this exact formulation of the difference.
4   In fact, Klein's dedication to Abraham's developments of object-relations from 1924 onwards, did take her off on her celebrated divergence from Freud. It is curious to reflect that her mentor, Karl Abraham, trained as a psychoanalyst at Burghölzli, and therefore with Jung and Bleuler. He did not specifically train in Vienna and thus had no direct knowledge of Freud's ideas in practice. There is thus a real possibility that Klein's stress on love, as opposed to the mechanics of libido, has an inheritance in an early Jungian position. It is true of course that Klein's first analyst was Ferenczi, one of Freud's very loyalest supporters. But he too diverged from Freud – and did so along similar lines, stressing the re-humanizing of Freud's physiological psychology (Likierman, 2001).

invention; and then trace the fate of the concept forward again in its two separate (or separating) histories. This kind of 'case history' of a concept is not common, but I believe it may be an approach to integrating conceptual schools which supplements and complements the more traditional, clinically based method.[5] Despite my commitment to clinical work as the base for theoretical thinking, I have come to the conclusion that concepts from different systems vary because of different assumptive frameworks held by the founders of the different schools. We might as well grasp this nettle first of all. Conceptual differences that are non-clinically based, then need to be addressed in terms of assumptive frameworks rather than clinical phenomenology. For instance Freud's theory of ego-libido and narcissism was a major theoretical advance, but it is quite clear that it was motivated (in part, a significant part) by wishing to argue against Jung's non-sexual libido theory. This was at a time when Freud thought Jung was becoming insubordinate. Clinical findings were important insofar as appropriate ones could be found to support Freud in his bid for theoretical supremacy over Jung. When, later, the theory of narcissism resulted in the understanding of psychosis and provided the whole development of object-relations psychoanalysis, its origins in the Freud–Jung rivalry are forgotten. Then as Jungians return to Freud's theory of narcissism, they do so with an unwitting irony.[6] And really we need to revisit these debates with knowledge of the powerful conceptual and semantic tensions which have subsequently moulded them.

REFERENCES

Bion, W. R. (1957) 'Differentiation of the psychotic from the non-psychotic personalities'. *International Journal of Psycho-analysis*, Vol. 38, 266–275. Reprinted in Elizabeth Spillius (Ed.), *Melanie Klein Today*, Vol. 1. London: Routledge, 1988.

Brenman Pick, Irma (1985) 'Working through in the countertransference'. *International Journal of Psycho-analysis*, 66, 273–281. Reprinted in Elizabeth Spillius (Ed.) *Melanie Klein Today*, Vol. 2. London: Routledge, 1988.

Freud, Sigmund (1920) *Beyond the Pleasure Principle*. Standard Edition, Vol. 18. London: Hogarth Press.

Heimann, Paula (1952) 'Certain functions of projection and introjection in early infancy', in Melanie Klein, Paula Heimann, Susan Isaacs and Joan Riviere (Eds), *Developments in Psychoanalysis*. London: Hogarth.

Hinshelwood, Robert (1991) *A Dictionary of Kleinian Thought*. London: Free Association Books.

Hinshelwood, Robert (1995) 'The social relocation of personal identity'. *Philosophy, Psychology, Psychiatry*, Vol, 2, 185–204.

5   My own effort to work out an historic-conceptual methodology of this kind concerned the meanings given to the term 'internal object' from the 1930s onwards (Hinshelwood, 1995).

6   In making his rapprochement with Freud and Klein, Fordham may also have put those Jungian terms with which we started, 'ego' and 'self', under pressure to drift in their meanings.

Klein, Melanie (1959) 'Our adult world and its roots in infancy'. *Writings*, Vol. 3. London: Hogarth.

Likierman, Meira (2001) *Melanie Klein: Her Work in Context*. London: Continuum.

Money-Kyrle, Roger (1956) 'Normal countertransference and some of it deviations'. *International Journal of Psycho-analysis*, Vol. 37, 360–366. Reprinted in Elizabeth Spillius (Ed.), *Melanie Klein Today*, Vol. 2. London: Routledge, 1988.

Rosenfeld, Herbert (1987) *Impasse and Interpretation*. London: Routledge.

(d) Response to commentaries by Julian David and Robert Hinshelwood

Elizabeth Urban

Julian David and Robert Hinshelwood raise points I should like to address in order to explain certain matters and to further clarify Fordham's thinking, which was my original aim in writing in this chapter.

Both object to the way the clinical material is shaped by theory, and both comment on the absence of sexuality in the treatment. Each of these points is to a considerable degree due to the choice of the chapter for this volume, which has proved to have unforeseen limitations. It had originally been written, not for the purposes of this book, but for the 1995 annual conference of the Association of Child Psychotherapists, the purpose of which was to have a Freudian, a Jungian and a Kleinian address the theme of 'Integration and repair in self-destructive children'. I was therefore pressed, as Hinshelwood puts it, 'to select according to [my] theme'. This was to illustrate a Jungian perspective on integration and repair, which to my mind fit easily with the Jungian concept of the self-healing nature of the psyche, one of several distinguishing aspects of Jungian thought. Putting this forward entailed understanding Jung's concept of the self and Fordham's translation of that to infancy and childhood, which I hoped to make clear was not like psychoanalytic concepts of the same term.

It was not my intention to attempt to integrate Fordham's model and Jungian concepts with Kleinian and Freudian ideas, as Hinshelwood mistakenly implies, and nowhere in the chapter do I indicate that this might be the case. I do try to compare and contrast similar concepts, and similar sounding but different concepts in psychoanalysis and analytical psychology. In my attempt to do this, the chapter is top-heavy with theory, and is perhaps bound to create the impression that the treatment was 'theory-driven'. Had this been the case, however, I do not think Ruthie, as sensitive as she was to imposition, would have come back to her therapy, nor stayed with it for as long as she did.

Both David and Hinshelwood make quite salient comments on the absence in the clinical material of Ruthie's sexuality, her relationship with her father, and her parents' relationship. These were important parts of her treatment, but for two reasons were omitted from the chapter. The first was that they did not fall under the theme of integration because Ruthie's anxieties about sexuality and the defences she had against these feelings remained to a significant extent split off. The second reason for omitting this important material was that, when originally writing the paper, I considered it likely that it would be published, which it was in the *Journal of Child Psychotherapy*. That entailed following current codes of ethics in relation to publication, namely that permission be sought from the patient. Ruthie gave this on the explicit understanding that her and her family's anonymity would be preserved, and the implicit understanding that she would read it. She could be persistent and insistent about certain issues (and this was one) and would without difficulty have found the paper, which is the nature of publication. Therefore it would have been inappropriate to include such sensitive, as well as unworked-through, material.

I shall now turn to theoretical issues that have been raised. There is a misconception in certain quarters regarding Fordham. This is based on an over-generalization of the idea that Fordham integrated Jungian and Kleinian thought. It is perhaps upon this misconception that Hinshelwood assumes that I, as a student of Fordham, am attempting this conceptual integration. Fordham was indebted to Klein for developing a way of working with children that made their inner lives available to analysis, and thus enabled Fordham to base his thinking on clinical and observational work. Early in his career he noted conceptual similarities between Jung's archetypes and Klein's unconscious phantasies, and drew extensively on her thoughts on unconscious phantasy and how it operated in infancy in the creation of his model of development. Late in his life Fordham himself stated that 'I was pursuing my own line of discovery all the time. I didn't go along with Melanie Klein's more abstract statements . . .' (Figlio, 1988: 19). In pursuing his own line he was following Jung into areas that differ from Klein and psychoanalysis, as I hope to make clear.

To begin I need to emphasize that in Jungian psychology there are two organizing centres in the personality, the self and the ego. The self in Jungian psychology is, as Hinshelwood understands, more fundamental than the ego, in as much as in Fordham's model the ego arises out of the self. The Jungian concept arose from Jung's long-standing interest in the psychology of spiritual states of mind, not as expressions of infantile states of mind or the defences against them but as irreducible states in their own right. Jung's first reference to what would become his idea of the self was in a paper describing psychic phenomena in which opposites – good and evil, love and hate – were transcended (Jung, 1916). Given his vertex, he related this to certain notions of God, such as those of the early Gnostics and the Hindu concept of Atman, both of which conceive, via non-rational means, an ultimate that transcends opposites. Jung understood these to be expressions of an essential part of mankind, which he terms the self, projected into religion, as well as science and psychology. It represents the intrinsic wholeness of the individual beneath and beyond the conflict of opposites.

Because Fordham found it helpful in his studies on infancy and childhood, he drew upon Jung's concept of the self as a totality (of psyche and soma, conscious and unconscious) to postulate a primary self, a psychosomatic integrate. Fordham's postulate means that the primary state is one of wholeness, and remarks that Klein implies something similar in her concept of splitting, in as much as there is an assumed fundamental wholeness or integratedness prior to early splitting.

Hinshelwood points out that Klein was indeed interested in wholeness, and in his commentary writes that 'she stressed two separate levels: one where the ego is concerned about its own completeness, and one where it is concerned about conflicts in it. The first level, *that of completeness of the ego*, underlies the second and in some degree determines it' (my italics). Here Klein and Fordham appear very close; however, Fordham, drawing upon Jung's concept of the self, has two separate concepts when referring to the two different levels.

Referring to just this, Fordham asks, 'Why is so much attributed to the ego?' (Fordham, 1976: 58). In his presidential address to the Medical Section of the British Psychological Society in 1951, which would have been attended by psychoanalysts, Fordham draws attention to the conceptual usefulness of having two organizers in the personality, self and ego. He examines a description Klein gives of early processes:

> . . . the inside of the ego is felt to be a dangerous and poisonous place in which the loved object would perish. Here we see one of the situations fundamental for 'the loss of the loved object'; the situation, namely, when the ego becomes fully identified with its good internalised objects, and at the same time becomes aware of its own incapacity to protect and preserve them against the internalised persecuting objects and the id. (Fordham, 1958: 45, quoting Klein, 1935: 265)

Fordham's comments convey that the ego, as a concept, is being asked to do too much.

> There is difficulty in picturing the process because the ego is 'a dangerous and poisonous place' where no object can be put. Yet we learn that the objects are there: the internalized persecuting objects. Then we hear the ego is fully identified with its 'good internalised objects' and tries to protect them against the 'internalised persecuting' ones. What is containing what? The ego seems to be containing the objects which are persecuting it from without. Either the ego has two functions and is divided into two parts, or else another concept is needed. What I wish to put forward is this: the self or the image of the whole is as much an object as the good and bad objects or the id' (Fordham, 1958: 45–46).

Fordham thinks Jung's dual concepts of organizers is helpful when studying infancy, because it can explain how the continuity and individuality of the infant self persist despite rapidly fluctuating states of the infant's ego. It is also useful in offering two different perspectives on the same phenomena: one can view instinctual phenomena (the id) as inchoate and disintegrated from the point of view of the ego, but as organized and object-related from the point of view of the (Jungian) self.

Fordham points out that toward the end of her life Klein 'referred to a psychosomatic whole different from, and more embracing than, the ego, the superego, and the id', which was how, from 1947, he regarded the self – as the whole of the personality (Fordham, 1987: 361). Hinshelwood too notes that Klein later contended that '. . . "self" is used to cover the whole of the personality, which includes not only the ego but the instinctual life which Freud called the "id"'. The id and the archetypes are closely linked via Klein's notion of phantasy as 'the mental expression of the activity of the . . . instincts' (Klein, 1952: 58). This can be seen when one juxtaposes the Kleinian statement that, 'Phantasy is (in the first instance), the mental corollary, the psychic representation of instinct (Isaacs, 1952: 83), with Jung's statement that the archetypes 'might suitably be described as the instinct's perception of itself, or as the self-portrait of the instinct' (Jung, 1919: 136). Here it can be seen that Klein's later concept of self = ego + instincts is indeed close to the Jungian idea that self = ego + archetypes.

I think a further step needs to be taken to arrive at self = psyche and soma, 'which can only be supported by inference, since the physical pole of this unity is not and cannot be represented' (Fordham, 1976: 67). I am not clear whether Klein's later concept of self also includes body (that is, whether id = body), although it is certainly intimately related through phantasy and her idea of the concreteness – the bodiliness – of the internal object (Klein, 1935). Fordham certainly included it when postulating a psychosomatic integrate, as did Jung; 'mind and body are presumably a pair of opposites and, as such, the expression of a single entity whose essential nature is not knowable either from its outward, material manifestation or from inner, direct perception' (Jung, 1926: 326).

It is not the case, as Hinshelwood suggests, that Jung and Klein share the idea that 'the self tends to be experience rather than mechanism'. Jung's statement above concerning the unknowable, unexperienceable nature of the self brings this aspect of the concept closer to Bion's notion of 'O'. Because the Jungian self refers to a totality of which the ego is only a part, 'the self is a special case in that a concept of totality is particularly difficult to construct. Indeed it is impossible' (Fordham, 1985: 21). Ultimately the self in Jungian psychology is a mystical concept. Aspects of the self can be perceived in the ego, and developmentally these arise in experience as senses of self, which is what I understand the psychoanalytic concept to refer to when viewing 'self as experience rather than mechanism'. Lastly in relation to this, the self does refer to mechanisms (deintegration and reintegration) and includes the structures that arise from these processes (ego and archetypes).

Hinshelwood takes my distinction between deintegration and splitting, which draws upon an intrapsychic analogy between the self and the amoeba, and extends it into an interpsychic perspective which links deintegration and disintegration. I think this is an interesting link, and describes how a deintegration can relate to an object which processes or digests it so that the experience can be reintegrated and become part of the personality. Deintegrations, which are not processed, need to be defended against, and can result in disintegration (in the ego) and/or splitting in the self (see below).

Fordham made a number of references to similarities between Klein's pair of positions and his pair of processes, the most frequent of which is that both occur throughout life (Fordham, 1989a). He also noted a similarity whereby he saw the paranoid/schizoid position as one of being broken up and objects located 'out there', which he linked to deintegration (experienced from the point of view of the ego), while the depressive position, which could be linked to things coming together, could be associated to (the ego's experience of) reintegration. A clear difference between Klein's two positions and Fordham's deintegration/reintegration is that the latter were postulated by Fordham to account for relating before contents are built up, whereas the processes of projective and introjective identification associated with the paranoid/schizoid and depressive position necessitate contents (Fordham, 1993). Here Fordham is considering that the primary self builds up contents via deintegration and reintegration, processes stimulated by archetypal expectation, a notion which seems to accord with Bion's preconception.

The Jungian model of the psyche as having two centres of organization underlies my theoretical discriminations between other concepts, and if this dual-organizer model is not understood, then the discriminations are muddling. For instance, the distinction I make between disintegration and deintegration is that the former applies to the ego and the latter to the self. As David points out, the self does not disintegrate. Also, I have distinguished repair, which refers to the self, from reparation, which refers to the struggle in the ego when actions of the self brings parts of the self together. Here my use of the 'self' is not, as Hinshelwood infers, in contrast to other, nor referring to a 'sense of self' (narcissism). My use of 'reparation' follows Fordham's understanding of Klein's depressive position, as an aspect of infantile mourning, of which pining is an essential feature. It is this, as Hinshelwood points out, that can lead on to reparation. It was only as Ruthie's self had increased its capacity for deintegration and reintegration, or, to use Hinshelwood's terms, the rupture in the container had been repaired, could the processes involved in reparation come into play. I concluded that there had been repair to Ruthie's self, but that there was unclear evidence that reparation ('the special "feeling for" a damaged loved one') had occurred.

This takes me to the comments on the handling of the case material. Both David and Hinshelwood make valid comments on the absence of attention given to the detail of the dynamics between patient and analyst. Both too refer to their respective traditions, which acknowledge that in any effective treatment the 'personality of both patient and analyst is called into play' (Jung, quoted in Fordham, 1993: 128). That Ruthie had an impact upon me is briefly described when, at the beginning of treatment, I discovered I could only come up with non-sense when she asked me to repeat what I had said. It was this that prompted my thinking about confused, as well as terrifyingly anxious states of mind. I also noted that muddle was certainly evident to both of us when we discussed Ruthie's dream of phoning me while she was in my house and I was in the house of a good friend.

I think Hinshelwood mistakes Ruthie's impression that I was calm with my own 'self-consciously' being so, as if I were aiming toward a 'corrective' experience. When Ruthie commented on my calmness it tended to arouse my anxiety as I anticipated that I would be attacked for it. Over time I came to consider that Ruthie was ascribing to me (and possibly to her go-with-the-flow sister) her sense of her own evolving capacity to feel contained. I think it was invested in us because, if she experienced it, she anticipated her maternal object and/or an envious part of herself would attack it.

It was this worry about being attacked that drew my attention to the absence of anger in the transference. That Ruthie was full of remorseless rage was evident in the violent attacks on her parents and ruthless demands on her mother, and I questioned whether her rage contributed to her anxiety while a defensive confusion kept her from knowing about her own destructiveness. When Ruthie attacked me for being inconsistent and just like her mother, it was the first time she had feelingfully expressed anger and criticism towards me. I was therefore attentive to what followed, namely, intense pain and unstoppable crying. Although it was experienced not in relation to me, but the teacher (who may have represented a split off 'good part' of Ruthie's experience of me), I viewed her pain and deep crying as pining, that is, 'the special poignancy of "feeling for" a damaged loved one'. Hence I took up what followed in the way I did. However, I think Hinshelwood is very good in his thinking about Ruthie's anxieties about confused states and whose they were, and in retrospect I wish I had done more along the lines he mentions.

Both David and Hinshelwood comment on my withholding from Ruthie the reason I have needed to change a session: that my response was an expression of my over-devotion to my theory of technique. Like most therapists, I refrain from revealing more of myself than is obvious or necessary. I doubt that that general principle is being questioned, and regard both responses as reactions to the strength of the statement that 'I did not intend to tell her . . .'. David views this as the eruption of an arbitrary authority, and Hinshelwood sees it as an expression of my superego. By the time Ruthie demanded to know why I was changing the session time, she was very familiar with my practice and would not have expected me to answer her question. When she pushed the matter, I was being firmer than I had been, or needed to be, before. Although my experience at the time was not marked by the drawing of hard lines in the way the statement 'I did not intend to be . . .' seems to have conveyed, there was an eruption of something new that got enacted. It probably would have been preferable to address Ruthie's need to know more about a Mr Urban/daddy/boundary-keeper/analytic technique/protector inside me who would keep me safe from her invasions. However, to have told her the reason for the change of session, which David suggests, would, I believe, have aroused more confusion and anxiety as that was not the usual practice.

In concluding, I should like to note that I have referred more to Hinshelwood's commentary than to David's. This is because David gives most of his attention to what was absent rather than present in the chapter. I acknowledge that the account of process and Ruthie's sexuality were significant omissions, which I have tried to explain. Hinshelwood, although mistaking my aim to integrate theories, enquires into several areas of theory and technique that I feel have contributed to greater clarifications of differences and similarities between schools of thought. He concludes that it must be grasped that 'concepts from different schools vary because of different assumptive frameworks held by founders of the different schools'. Added to this is that the growing diversification of analytic thought is due to the different assumptive frameworks of individual contributors. This makes the integration of different and developing concepts (even within the same school of analytic thought) so unlikely as to be impossible, but to my mind increases the importance of being aware of differences and similarities in order to deepen our analytic identities within a diverse yet common tradition, and to work toward tolerance in the shared aim of understanding the mind and how to lend meaning to mental suffering.

REFERENCES

Figlio, K. (1988) 'Michael Fordham in discussion with Karl Figlio'. *Free Associations*, Vol. 12, 631–641.

Fordham, M. (1958) *The Objective Psyche*. London: Routledge & Kegan Paul.

Fordham, M. (1976) *The Self and Autism*. London: Heinemann Medical.

Fordham, M. (1985) *Explorations into the Self*. London: Academic Press.

Fordham, M. (1987) 'Actions of the self', in P. Young-Eisendrath and J. Hall (Eds), *The Book of the Self*. New York: New York University Press.

Fordham, M. (1989a) 'The infant's reach'. *Psychological Perspectives*, Vol. 21, 64

Fordham, M. (1989b) 'Some historical reflections'. *Journal of Analytical Psychology*, Vol. 34, 3.

Fordham, M. (1993) 'Notes for the formulation of a model of infant development'. *Journal of Analytical Psychology*, Vol. 38, 5–12.

Fordham, M. (1994) *Children as Individuals*. London: Free Association Books.

Isaacs, S. (1952) 'The nature and function of phantasy'. *International Journal of Psycho-Analysis*, Vol. 29, 67–121.

Jung, C. G. (1916) 'The transcendent function'. *Collected Works*, Vol. 6. London: Routledge & Kegan Paul.

Jung, C. G. (1919) 'Instincts and the unconscious'. *Collected Works*, Vol. 8. London: Routledge & Kegan Paul.

Jung, C. G. (1926) 'Spirit and life'. *Collected Works*, Vol. 8. London: Routledge & Kegan Paul.

Klein, M. (1935) 'A contribution to the psychogenesis of manic-depressive states', in *Love, Guilt and Reparation and Other Works, 1921–1945*. London: Hogarth Press, 1981.

Klein, M. (1952) 'The mutual influences in the development of ego and id', in *Envy and Gratitude and Other Works, 1946–1963*. London: Hogarth Press, 1984.

The status of developmental theory

Introduction

For over a century now, work with the formative experiences of early life has been the bedrock of psychoanalysis, and more recently of the developmental school of analytical psychology. In this chapter Christopher Hauke and JoAnn Culbert-Koehn approach this phenomenon from contrasting perspectives.

Hauke argues that developmental theory is ultimately grounded in an outmoded appeal to nineteenth-century biological and evolutionary theory (see Stevens, present volume, for a contemporary evolutionary view of the archetypes). Hauke situates developmental theories within a specific cultural context, which has been categorized elsewhere as modern as opposed to postmodern (Foucault, 1973; Hauke, 2000). If their influence is not critically reassessed, he argues, these theories can lead us to prioritize confirmatory clinical material without even realizing we are doing so. This in turn can lead to an impoverishment of analytic practice, and a justifiable mistrust of analytic theory among the unconvinced. He does, however, argue for the therapeutic value of a developmental approach that treats its reconstructions as one possible narrative among many rather than literal truth.

Culbert-Koehn argues that recent research indicates there are two distinct types of memory – verbal and behavioural memory. The former is fluid and subject to revision in the light of current events, the latter the result of 'burned in' traumas that may have occurred preverbally. Both types of memory she claims can be valuable in analytic work. Verbal memory can yield a narrative account that may be therapeutic, but she agrees that the 'truth' of the events described can never be reconstructed with certainty. Behavioural memory, however, leaves an indelible stamp on the organism, and interpreting such behaviour can lead to a more reliable reconstruction of the original events. She illustrates the therapeutic effect of such interpretations with three cases that proved intractable to more conventional (Jungian) analysis.

Although the two authors do not respond directly to one another in this chapter, their contrasting positions clearly reiterate controversial themes raised in the opening chapter and developed elsewhere in this book.

REFERENCES

Foucault, Michel (1973) *The Order of Things*. New York: Vintage Books.
Hauke, Christopher (2000) *Jung and the Postmodern*, Routledge: London.

(a) Uneasy ghosts: theories of the child and the crisis in psychoanalysis

Christopher Hauke

> it is only possible to come to a right understanding and appreciation of a contemporary psychological problem when we can reach a point outside our own time from which to observe it.
>
> (C. G. Jung, 1945)

No-one can doubt that analysis and analytical psychotherapy are in crisis at the present time: referrals are down and there is fresh internecine strife stemming from the BCP/UKCP split. There is growing and widespread competition from rival theoretical approaches, and short-term help from counsellors of all sorts is often preferred – and not only for financial reasons. There is a steady flow of applicants to 'trainings' which range from one year part-time counselling courses to the four- or five-year 'full' analytic training. But it is by no means certain that the public will then be rushing into treatment with these newly qualified people. On the one hand there are more and more people being referred to counsellors – in GP practices, colleges, workplaces and so on – presumably suffering a degree of emotional stress, disappointment in relationships, unhappiness with their state of mind – in general, the sort of maladies that analytic psychotherapy says it can treat. On the other hand, folk are less and less likely to seek treatment that is broadly based on the theories of Freudian psychoanalysis. Gone are the days of the 1940s when the British Institute of Psycho-analysis had around four hundred would-be patients on their waiting list while they hurried to get analysts qualified. Given the way that Jungians in the UK have pursued their own legitimation crisis by absorbing many of the psychoanalytic ideas from which Jung distanced himself, Jungian therapists also suffer from this discrimination. How has this arisen? After all, did not the whole business of one-to-one therapy based around talking to a trained practitioner, which is now widespread, start – for the twentieth century at least – from precisely the same psychoanalytic roots that are now being marginalized and often dismissed? In such an age of 'psychological man' or 'therapeutic man' how come psychoanalysis is so unpopular?

This chapter intends to unravel part of the answer. The title is inspired by two sources and gives a clue to my approach. In the book *A Most Dangerous Method*

(1994), John Kerr likens the history of psychoanalysis to a 'gruesome ghost story, where the ghost who finally devours all the people in the end is not a being but a theory – and a way of listening' (Kerr, 1994: 15). So part of what I will be looking into is the devouring theory – or *theories* – underpinning psychoanalytical thinking. The word 'uneasy' conveys how, over recent years, some psychoanalytic theories have been experienced with a sense of discomfort by many. This includes not only analysts themselves but also several thinkers and writers on science and culture. The word comes from the title of one of Freud's famous texts: *Das Unbehagen in der Kultur* (*The Uneasiness Inherent in Culture*). You probably know this book better by its badly translated English title, *Civilisation and its Discontents*. There is clearly an uneasiness in contemporary life, as we live it in the industrialized West, that the practice of psychotherapy speaks to and where it is badly needed. But in addition – and sometimes countering the help that psychoanalytic practice might offer for such 'uneasiness' – there is another, separate uneasiness in the *culture of psychoanalysis* itself, where many of its premises and theoretical assumptions are regarded as invalid, unproven, easy to criticize, and, above all, pretty useless in practice.

I first wrote a paper dealing with the way psychoanalysis and Jungian analysis regard images of the child and infant, and how they are theorized and used in practice, which I delivered at a Jung Studies Day at the Centre for Psychoanalytic Studies, University of Kent, in November 1994. I called it *The Child: Development, Archetype and Analytic Practice*. After failing to get it published in the UK, it was accepted by the *San Francisco Jung Institute Library Journal* and published there in 1996. When I submitted it to a British journal, one of the British readers said that she found the ideas in it 'challenging'. We all know what that euphemism means. I mention this by way of introducing this present chapter which I regard as a continuation of some of the ideas in the first one, and a recapitulation of other ideas it contained. I also want to provide a couple of new angles for thinking about how, on the one hand, *psychoanalytic discourse* is embedded in contemporary culture while, on the other hand, psychoanalytic *practice* is sometimes way off the mark.

I begin by discussing the way that Freud's theorizing about the aetiology of neurosis, the unconscious, infant experience and development, and the part it plays in adult pathology – ideas which are embedded intact in so many contemporary psychoanalytical assumptions – stem from the evolutionary biology which was popular in late nineteenth-century German thought. I find it astonishing that no matter how often we acknowledge the cliché that Freud's vision was a singular product of late Victorian bourgeois society, such a view remains restricted to comments about the repressed sexuality of his time rather than constituting a far broader position from which to launch a radical critique of the bedrock of psychoanalytic theory. My view is that psychoanalysis requires – in its present crisis more than ever before – an historical examination of what underpins its theories in an effort to mine the 'pure gold' of contemporary practice – not, indeed, as Freud would have seen it, but more in an effort to discover what makes the contemporary treatments psychoanalysis inspired still so relevant for many today. I am indebted to Frank Sulloway's research published in *Freud: Biologist of the Mind. Beyond the*

Psychoanalytic Legend (1979/1992) but, unlike him, I am a practitioner as well as a researcher, and so I want to think not only about the dubious hypotheses from which psychoanalytic theories sprang, but also about what is valid and what *works* in analytic psychotherapy today despite its peculiar origins.

I follow this with a brief examination of a text by Michael Fordham. Fordham is responsible for keeping Jungian analysis on the map in the UK by developing a way of theorizing about the psychoanalytic concepts of infant libidinal- and ego-development, which brings these concepts alongside Jung's theories of archetypes, ego and self, and individuation. In examining Fordham's text I will be pointing out assumptions imported from classical psychoanalysis and the way these both reveal and disguise their origins in evolutionary biology.

Finally, I intend to tackle the gap between psychoanalytic discourse and analytic practice by looking at the way certain theoretical positions within psychoanalysis are in fact embedded in various discourses elsewhere in our culture. By discourses I mean the way people talk and think – and arrange their thinking – according to frames and perspectives that are in themselves invisible. For this I will refer briefly to historical research on the discourses of child-care previous to the nineteenth century. I make no claims about the direction of influence between psychoanalytic assumptions and their appearance in cultural discourses outside analytic practice itself, but I do wish to make this point: psychoanalytic theorizing – and especially that portion of it that concerns the 'child' – is now, and has always been, historically *embedded* in Western culture. Therefore, our focus at this critical time in its history should be *the untangling of what we have inherited so we can examine more clearly the effectiveness of analytical psychotherapy in the present day, without the burden of being forced to include and account for ideas that, frankly, are well past their sell-by date.* One the one hand, this may be seen as an extension of the same analytic spirit that seeks to heal through both discriminating and linking past and present; on the other hand, perhaps what is required is an 'exorcism' of certain theories that, like ghosts, are haunting contemporary practice.

FREUD THE SOCIOBIOLOGIST

What *are* those psychoanalytic ideas we should consider abandoning? To answer this we need to become familiar with the intellectual atmosphere within which Freud gave first breath to his ideas, and then to note which of these ideas still comprise our basic working assumptions today. By knowing the source of these ideas – and I am thinking here of sexual libido, libidinal stages of development, the Oedipus, fixation, regression, and the aetiological significance of early development, to name a few – we will be in a better position to assess which of them describe the focus and the work of psychotherapy as we find it today and which are, at best, irrelevant and, at worst, positively misleading.

Most now agree that psychoanalysis arose at a time in Western European history at the peak of the Enlightenment's aim to comprehend the processes of nature through Western scientific rationality alone. The self-examination of civilized Europe, or the study of 'Man' as it was then called, began in the second half of the nineteenth century by relying, for the main part, on the established *biological* science of its day. This epistemology was enhanced and accelerated by the radical new theories of *evolution* introduced by Charles Darwin. Thus, anticipating psychoanalysis and psychology by some fifty years, the study of Man was initiated under the paradigm of evolutionary biology – and the laws of biogenetics.

There are a number of general ways in which the Darwinian legacy was a direct influence upon Freud's psychoanalytic ideas. The 'fundamental biogenetic law' advanced by Ernst Haeckel as early as 1866 states that 'ontogeny recapitulates phylogeny' – in other words, the development of the human from fetus to adulthood (ontogeny) provides a brief recapitulation of the evolutionary development of the entire history of the race (phylogeny). As Sulloway notes, this has been the least emphasized 'a priori biological influence in all of psychoanalytic theory' (Sulloway, 1979/1992: 259). By the end of the century, the popularity of the idea was so widespread that the American psychologist and evolutionary theorist James Baldwin could conclude at the end of his book *Mental Development in the Child and the Race* (1895), 'the embryology of society is open to study in the nursery' (Sulloway, 1979/1992: 156). In Freud's own library is a book by a colleague of Darwin's – George Romanes' *Mental Evolution in Man* (1888) – which is annotated throughout in Freud's own hand (Sulloway, 1979/1992: 247fn) but strangely, Freud makes no reference to this book in any of his published writings.

A second influence stemming from Darwin's theory of evolution is the emphasis on how competition for the survival of species entailed conflict and a struggle for existence. Struggle and conflict as a mental paradigm was established early on in psychoanalytic theorizing to the extent that 'Freud never relinquished his belief that the ultimate causes of neurosis lie in the conflict between instincts as a whole and the demands and restrictions that human civilization has placed upon them' (Sulloway, 1979/1992: 257). A third general influence is the idea of *historical truth: the past as a key to the present*. Both Darwin and Freud found meaning in the seemingly trivial: for Darwin the significance of redundant physiological parts such as the appendix in adults and the gill-slits and tail in early embryological development, and for Freud the significance of dream symbols, symptom formations and slips of the tongue, all of which were subjected to an historical approach. As Freud wrote in *Studies in Hysteria* (1895): 'All these [neurotic] sensations and innervations belong to the field of "The Expression of the Emotions", which, as Darwin [1872] has taught us, consist of actions which originally had a meaning and served a purpose' (SE, 2: 181). Both linguistic usage and hysterical symptoms – like the redundant bits of anatomy for Darwin – were viewed as arising from a common phylogenetic root.

Fourthly, common to both Freud and Darwin is their shared emphasis on the *irrational* in Man. This theme – which may be seen as a reaction against the long prevailing Enlightenment emphasis on human rationality – goes back to the previous century and Schopenhauer who not only influenced Darwin, but also Hartmann upon whose conception of the unconscious Freud was to base his own theories. The irrational aspects of Man that were to predominate in Darwin's and Freud's thinking were the *instincts and especially sexuality*.

Lastly, three of Freud's fundamental mechanisms of pathological development – *fixation*, *regression*, and *the significance of early experience* – have their sources elsewhere in materialist, i.e. non-psychological, bio-evolutionary theories. These are of particular significance to the way in which the 'child' in particular is conceived within analytic theory even today. Anatomical fixations, known as 'arrests in development' were well established in mid-nineteenth-century medical pathology and embryology. Writing about *instinctual* fixations, Darwin 'paid close attention . . . to the way in which instincts, inhibited or otherwise altered by new habits, might help to account for evolutionary change' (Sulloway, 1979/1992: 265). In turn this led to firmer theories of instinctual fixation such as 'imprinting' evidenced by the 'following' behaviour of very young ducklings towards their initial carer even if it is a human. Familiar with the anatomical–evolutionary notions of fixations, Freud extended the idea to psychoanalysis asserting that 'in the case of every particular sexual trend . . . some portions of it have stayed behind at earlier stages of its development, even though other portions may have reached their final goal . . . we propose to describe the lagging behind of a part trend at an earlier stage as a *fixation* – a fixation, that is, of the instinct' (*Introductory Lectures on Psycho-Analysis*, 1916, SE 16:340). The concept of *regression* owes much to the English neurologist Hughlings Jackson who conceived the human mind in terms of a hierarchical series of functional levels, the lower ones having been superseded in course of human evolution (1884). Senility, neurological disease and insanity were viewed as a general reversal of this evolutionary process and Jackson referred to these as 'dissolutions' in mental functioning. Acknowledging Jackson's contribution, Freud took up the idea of 'dissolutions' and later applied it to his conceptions of the neuroses when he wrote to Abraham in 1907 of 'the general pathological view that illness implies a regression in development'.

What this brief survey of the biogenetic sources of Freud's psychoanalytic formulations reveals is twofold: namely, that his concepts about psychological development and the pathology of neuroses originated neither from the clinical treatment of adults nor the general observation of infants and children, but subsequent material from these sources *were* later used to *justify* his a priori bio-evolutionary hypotheses. I will offer a concise example which still remains critical to the psychoanalytic perspective today – the Freud/Abraham oral, anal, and genital 'stages' of libidinal- and ego-development.

Freud's emphasis is clear in 1916 when he says of the courses of ego and libidinal development: 'both of them are at bottom heritages, abbreviated recapitulations, of the development which all mankind has passed through from its primeval days over long periods of time' (Freud, 1916: 354). Freud's initial groundbreaking model of the child's pregenital psychosexual development had from the beginning clearly less to do with observed phenomena in real human infants, than with placing instinctual development within an established phylogenetic frame. This overarching project becomes even clearer when we discover that the oral, anal, genital sequence itself derives from Haeckel's notion of the primeval gastraea. This gastraea (from the Greek *gaster*, 'stomach') is a simple marine sponge and is viewed as a critical point in the evolution of animal life – a basic form from which higher animals are descended. Haeckel had noted that in the earliest stages of embryological development, multicellular animal organisms follow a common pattern. As Sulloway says in *Freud, Biologist of the Mind*, 'Specifically (Haeckel) maintained that the fertilized zygote invaginates to create a primitive stomach, a mouth, and, later, an anal orifice', (Sulloway, 1979/1992: 261). Wilhelm Bölsche, with his particular interest in the evolution of sexuality, seized upon Haeckel's idea to depict sexual sensitivity as having been 'gradually dispersed from the original "skin" of the preinvaginated gastraea to the later-evolved . . . organs of sexuality' (Sulloway, 1979/1992: 262), thus completing the phylogenetic sequence: oral dominance, followed by anal, and the later development of the genital. True sexual reproduction was originally 'a sort of higher eating' in Bölsche's characterization. This view perhaps influenced Freud's observation of the suckling infant enough to make him equate the baby's facial expression during feeding to the look of sexual enjoyment and satiation in the adult (in Freud, 1905: 182). In constructing a theory of ego and libidinal development which claimed that adult psychopathology arose from the clash between instinctual urges and repressive social norms, Freud was employing materialist biological ideas to grasp the unobservable psyche. For example, the gill-slits observed on the embryos of a range of animals including humans, are a physical and *observable* phylogenetic recapitulation. Freud postulated a parallel in the theoretical 'oral phase' which is an *unobservable* phenomenon, only indirectly inferable from the behaviour of infants, but one which fits however with theories of phylogenetic recapitulation. It was out of this theoretical exigency that the child was originally prioritized in the psychoanalytic canon. This view of the child as the carrier of development differs from the child-in-relationship-with-its-environment that is the emphasis today, but the contemporary twist should not obscure the phylogenetic, evolutionist origins of the theory. For instance, current depth psychological theory prioritizes 'oral' behaviour when in the development of the real infant a range of skills and 'priorities' are proceeding simultaneously, such as grasping, recognition, memory, imitation, stimulation and quiescence and so on. Daniel Stern's *The Interpersonal World of the Infant* (1985) provides important evidence and discussion of this issue.

It was Freud's excessive emphasis on the instinctual, and particularly the sexual, that led C. G. Jung to break away and develop his own theories. Later, Abraham developed Freud's instinct theory with what became the classical notion of oral, anal and genital stages as potential fixation points identifiable through the adult pathology encountered in the consulting room. Later still, this model came to be viewed by psychoanalysts as too mechanistic, and by the 1930s Melanie Klein, who had been analysed by Abraham, was developing ideas that would eventually form one basis for object-relations theory. In reviewing the cultural roots of the dominance of the child motif in depth psychology, we have perhaps come upon the point in the development of psychoanalysis when these hypothetical stages of ego development became more firmly established by being linked to flesh and blood infants, mothers and breasts, and eventually to the specific historical mother and the infant the adult once was. I want to follow this survey of the genealogy of psychoanalytic concepts with an up-to-date textual illustration from Michael Fordham, the Jungian analyst who is regarded as having made a significant contribution to Jungian psychoanalysis by the way in which he combined Freudian theoretical assumptions with some of Jung's concepts and then establishing these, or so many believe, through the 'scientific' observation of actual infants and their mothers.

Having heard what I have said so far, it seems fair to ask, 'So what if psycho-analysis derives its theories from nineteenth-century evolutionary biology?' Does this necessarily mean that contemporary thinking is wrong? And, besides, are we really still holding to these particular theories?

To take the first question, perhaps it is not so much that contemporary psycho-analytic thinking is *wrong* but that it constitutes a discourse that no longer *fits our times*. Biogenetic theories formed the discourse of a certain era when ideas of progress, breeding and the survival of the fittest constituted the paradigm for what was thought to govern not only the animal kingdom, but also individual human beings and society in general. As Erich Fromm (1979) has pointed out, Freud's blind spot was the way he mistook bourgeois society for civilized society in general, thus making universalist assumptions from his bio-evolutionary perspective. To a certain extent, Darwinian evolutionary ideas still permeate beliefs around contem-porary individual and civic life where the term 'market forces', for example, is redolent of an economic Darwinism which is used to express the success and failure of businesses, individuals and, indeed, whole nations who are viewed as engaged in a pseudo-evolutionary struggle for limited niches in world trade and profits. When it comes to the extension of Darwinism into human economic activity, there are quite contrasting theories now such as 'chaos theory' and 'complexity theory' which offer alternative perspectives backed up by mathematical evidence (Gleick, 1987)

The persistence of Darwinian views no longer stands as the only, or the dominant way of understanding the activity and motivation of individuals and society in general. Despite this, in British politics between 1979 and 1990, the Thatcherite urge to return to Victorian values spoke of attempts to revive the Darwinian discourse of a previous era. But the desperately anachronistic nature of this political move has to be seen in the context of what had been happening to Darwinian evolutionary theory itself since the 1950s. Not only has there been widespread criticism arising from gaps in the fossil record – of which Darwin was aware but hoped, wrongly as it turned out, that future investigation would close – but also criticism of particular cases such as, for example, that of the mammalian eye. Indeed, it has been so difficult to explain the existence of the eye in evolutionary terms that, in 1860, Darwin himself wrote, 'To this day the eye makes me shudder' (Hitching, 1982: 67). Without going into detail, there is a big question mark over how the eye could have 'evolved' gradually through natural selection as, without its complete function of vision, it is hard to see how earlier mutations or 'part eyes' could offer any survival advantage to the species who developed them (Hitching, 1982).

Thus, when it comes to psychoanalytic theories of human psychology that derive from bio-evolutionary premises, I would argue for a *questioning of the theory and the discourse from which it arises* rather than the tendency we find in psychoanalysts who persist in amassing confirming 'evidence' in clinical material and family dynamics, or, worse still, blunder ahead as if the issue was of little consequence. When questioned about the popularity of psychoanalytic explanations despite the lack of valid evidence, philosophers of science tell us that, as with all scientific theories, invalidity alone is not enough to negate the persistence of a theory – it may only be abandoned when *a better theory comes along to take its place.*

I, for one, have little use for concepts of orality, anality and genitality, either as stages in development or as points of fixation or regression. Equally, along with many other child developmental psychologists, I see no evidence for an Oedipal stage or the Oedipal dynamics as Freud described them. In this I seem to be in agreement with C .G. Jung who also thought of libidinal stages and the Oedipal crisis as superfluous concepts in analytic psychotherapy. This brings me to the second question: are we still really holding on to such theories? Well, clearly we are in a general sense, but it is also interesting to notice how the same bio-evolutionary premises lie *disguised* within contemporary theorizing in psychoanalysis and analytical psychology.

MICHAEL FORDHAM AND THE UNEASY THEORIZING OF THE CHILD

In a chapter of his book *Jungian Psychotherapy* called 'The analysis of childhood and its limits' (Fordham, 1978/1986: 124–137), the Jungian analyst Michael Fordham demonstrates the persistence of bio-evolutionary assumptions when he discusses the work of reconstruction in the analysis of an adult male patient. Freud originally conceived analysis as a process of restoring the repressed memories of past trauma to consciousness, thereby removing the neurotic or hysterical symptoms purely through insight. The crudity of this idea has long been abandoned in contemporary analysis and instead we find emphasis being placed on recalling apparent infantile memories in general. As Fordham puts it, 'It is often useful and important to go on until the infantile situations are clear . . . and . . . to keep a track on the age at which they took place, *bearing in mind what is probable at any particular age.* Thus, by relating the present to the past the patient's ego is strengthened' (Fordham, 1978/1986:125; italics added). Fordham's 'bearing in mind what is probable at any particular age' already indicates an a-priori schema arranged according to stages of development. Furthermore, if memories are not available Fordham recommends, 'the additional method of reconstruction *to fill in the gaps*' (Fordham, 1978/1986: 125–126; italics added). Here, the hidden discourse involves a geological metaphor:

like Darwin's fossil record, which formed the basis for evolutionary theory, there are gaps that need filling intellectually with hypotheses that will close them.

Fordham offers the clinical example of a fifty-year-old man who, in analysis, seemed remarkably undiscriminating about the interpretations Fordham offered him and, for whom, as Fordham puts it, 'any intervention seemed to be "swallowed" under compulsion' (Fordham, 1978/1986: 126). The reconstruction commences with: 'On the basis of this observation and his use of food to allay anxiety I suggested that his feeding in infancy might have been important to him and that his way of swallowing interpretations might be an indication of how he was fed as an infant' (Fordham, 1978/1986). Fordham's apparently neutral 'bearing in mind what is probable' has imposed and prioritized an oral stage on the reconstructed grid of the past. A theoretical assumption also evident in Fordham's reconstruction is Abraham's oral-sadistic sub-stage, which involves aggressive feeding impulses. Fordham writes, 'I also suggested that perhaps his mother had used breast feeding to keep him quiet . . . [This] reconstruction . . . also made his predominant lack of verbal aggression more understandable. . . . If he had been fed not so much when he was hungry as when he made a noise or used other methods of expressing his aggression, then the development of his aggression would have been inhibited and bound up inside him, as appeared to be the case in the transference' (Fordham, 1978/1986).

Then, still referring to his patient's verbal style in the analytic sessions, Fordham goes on to hypothesize how this *also* has its source in the 'anal stage' of the man's infancy. Fordham writes, 'there was another aspect: in response to my interpretations he would produce a mass of associations *as if he were under compulsion to do so*. I reconstructed this in terms of his mother's demand that he produce excreta during toilet training' (Fordham 1978/1986: 127, emphasis added). Fordham is then clearly delighted to report that the 'incredulous' patient promptly wrote to his mother who 'replied in a letter which confirmed in detail the main points of my reconstruction: he had been given daily doses of castor oil and suppositories from time to time so as to help the regular functioning of his bowels' (Fordham 1978/1986). Fordham claims that by making such links with the past using memories and reconstructions he helps the patient to understand what is happening in the transference relationship.

There might well be other ways of understanding the patient's way of relating verbally. For instance, when writing this I made the slip of typing 'following' instead of 'swallowing'. This leads me to reflect that, instead of the feeding metaphor that becomes concretized in Fordham's example, another image which is still rooted in biology – that of *imprinting* – could equally be used to 'explain' the patient's behaviour. The image is one of the patient following Fordham's interpretations like the duckling trailing behind its all-important carer. I do not prefer such an 'explanation' and have no urge to extend it at all, but merely offer it as an example of the plasticity of such theorizing.

Concluding his discussion, Fordham claims to have offered, 'an example of developing a theory out of the patient's material and not imposing one.' (Fordham 1978/1986). His reasoning – which stems from Fordham's holding flexible views about which regimes of breast-feeding are preferable for emotional development – goes thus: 'If I had thought that demand feeding, in the sense of not feeding by the clock, was always desirable, and then proceeded with that theory, the development of the analysis would have been jeopardized. It must have been, however, that his mother was not able to distinguish a hungry cry from the energetic crying of a baby needing to be aggressive . . . 'Demand feeding' would then have been misused . . . to keep him quiet and so smothered his aggression' (Fordham 1978/1986). This is the reason Fordham gives for claiming he has not imposed a theory but has 'developed' one out of the patient's material.

I would challenge this claim for theoretical neutrality on a number of levels. For a start, the text assumes that infants' experiences of their mothers' care persists into adulthood in such a way that aspects of the way they relate to an analyst as an adult can be attributed to the mother's care in a cause-and-effect manner. This is a metaphorical version of the old ontogeny-recapitulates-phylogeny discourse, or style of thinking. In this case, the adult patient's behaviour – 'ontogeny' – repeats the experiences of infancy – 'phylogeny' – where the evidence cited comes not from the phylogenetic, fossil record as it did for nineteenth-century biogenetics, but from the more recent historical 'past' as reconstructed or reported by the mother herself. (Incidentally, Freud gave strict warnings about seeking such corroboration as such 'evidence' can so easily go against the hypothesis that is being claimed.)

Secondly, what is also being imposed on the material in this reconstruction is a high degree of *selectivity* and *prioritizing* of the wide range of actions that go between an infant and its mother. Although psychoanalytic reconstructions often involve a wider selection, in this case the focus places entire importance on the experiences of feeding and defecation. Other frequent and relevant aspects of infant–mother interaction such as styles of play, holding, gaze, and stimulation are not prioritized (cf. Stern, 1985, 1990). Lastly, then, such granting of importance to oral and anal experiences reveals how this style of reconstruction is not neutral at all, but is in fact embedded in the earliest assumptions of psychoanalytic thinking – the theoretical point of view that derives from bio-evolutionary discourse of the last century.

This is not to say that Fordham's reconstruction was not helpful in the case he discusses. I am sure it was, and that this style is useful in a number of cases. But I also know that such techniques can alienate a patient and be unhelpful – especially when an analyst has little sense of the background to such methods. What I object to most is the way that it is claimed there is no theory being imposed when, in fact, there is a considerable weight of theoretical assumptions pressing down on the material. Those who are critical of psychoanalytic theory and methods are right to point out the danger in analysts not taking responsibility for the views they inherit from the Freudian past. Whether this arises through an insufficiently critical attitude that renders such inherited views invisible, or whether, as is often the case, psycho-analysis persists in justifying its theories using 'evidence' derived from more and more novel sources rather than frankly questioning the theories themselves – either way analysis needs to get its house in order. There are too many ghosts disturbing contemporary analytic practice.

HISTORICAL DISCOURSE AND ALTERNATIVES TO 'THE CHILD'

Where Michael Fordham is quite correct when he asserts that a degree of healing may be achieved for the patient by linking the past to the present. Nowadays this point of view has been formulated along the lines of creating a narrative, a life-story or the patient's personal myth as ways of describing a main feature of analytic psychotherapy (cf. Hillman, 1983; Covington, 1995; Hewison, 1995). Far from abandoning the need to link the present to the past, I think we should be honouring this aspect of Freud's genius by paying greater attention to what we select as significant in this instead of being driven by what earlier psychoanalytic formu-lations deemed relevant. As I pointed out in my previous paper (Hauke, 1996), over the years, the frontiers of what constitutes the relevant past for psychoanalysis have been pushed back beyond early infancy to babyhood and even the womb. This has been due not only to the influence of individual theorists such as Klein, Bowlby, Winnicott, Piontelli and Fordham, but also to changing social and political influences. For instance, after the Second World War, the critical function of women as carers of their own offspring was emphasized, not just in terms of individual child health but, indeed, as vital for the survival of the Western world itself. *The International Labour Review* of 1954 carried an article by Baers entitled 'Women workers and their responsibilities' in which he claimed the child's normal development is dependent on the mother's full-time role in child-rearing, and that 'anything that hinders women in the fulfilment of this mission must be regarded as contrary to human progress' (in Clarke and Clarke, 1976: 23). We need hardly look further for confirmation of Beatrice Gottlieb's statement in her book, *The Family in the Western World: From the Black Death to the Industrial Age* (1993), where she writes: 'ideas about the treatment of children always seem to be exaggerated versions of fundamental beliefs. Children play a special role in our view of our destiny and are a distillation of what we believe most deeply about ourselves' (Gottlieb, 1993: 169).

Gottlieb's historical survey of children and the family takes her up to the dawn of the industrial age in 1800, and so contains views and attitudes towards infancy that contrast with the middle and end of that century in which evolutionary theory and psychoanalysis emerged. It is interesting, therefore, to ponder about the discourse of infancy in the pre-psychoanalytic era as a way of assessing ideas around the child in contemporary practice. The point being made is that infancy, child-care, and the family are socially constructed and not the 'natural' phenomena that psychoanalysis so often assumes.

In the pre-industrial period of Western society, swaddling of babies was common practice and Gottlieb suggests a sub-text to the practice of swaddling is the sense of the baby as alien and not fully human. Swaddling therefore served to keep the baby in an upright position as he or she would be when grown, and it also discour-aged and avoided a crawling stage which, for the times, was equally viewed as too animalistic. I would add that, despite contemporary parents' expectations and need for greater wage-earning and leisure time, swaddling is not common practice these days, not because it is not convenient – it would be! – but because most of us have abandoned the idea of the infant as an animal that needs humanizing. At least this belief no longer forms a dominant part of the contemporary discourse of the 'infant'.

When it came to beliefs around the feeding of babies, actual nutrition was not the only thing taken in through female milk: long before the psychoanalytic era and formulations like those of Michael Fordham's, it was the belief that *character was transmitted* through breast milk. This was such an important issue that the widespread employment of wet nurses to suckle infants was brought under bureaucratic control in Paris as early as 1350 and had long been part of the French bureaucracy by 1800. This move was not only to ensure that the women had a good supply of healthy milk, but, just as importantly, to confirm that they also had good moral character and a stable disposition – not so they would be a good caretaker, but because the milk was believed to transmit personality (Gottlieb, 1993: 145–146). Vasari reports how Michelangelo joked that his calling as a sculptor lay in the fact that he had been nursed by a stone-cutter's wife, from whose milk 'I sucked in the hammer and chisels I use for my statues' (Gottlieb, 1993: 146).

The barely hidden patriarchal assumption here brings in a further element of the discourse of infancy and feeding. There was a fear connected with nursing and one which probably threatened men more than women. Nursing was viewed as a process in which the animal-like infant drained the nurse/mother of vital forces; breast milk was regarded as a 'form of blood' – specifically menstrual blood – which had first fed the child in the womb and then fed it after birth. Nursing was a lowly job and thus breast-feeding suited a lower-class, more animal-like creature for the eighteenth century, urban, bourgeois family. (Elsewhere in the countryside mothers had far less choice.)

Due to high infant mortality, the wet-nurse system, and the fact that men – who tended to dominate the written word – were seldom involved with young children, infancy is poorly recorded up to the start of the nineteenth century. It is fascinating how this changes with the more prosperous conditions of Victorian times and the improvement in infant survival. Without such social and economic shifts we would not have seen Darwin producing a detailed diary over three years of the mental and behavioural development of his first son, William. In response to the growing interest of child studies in the nineteenth century, Darwin published this in 1877 in the new journal, *Mind*, as 'A biographical sketch of an infant'.

But it was Darwin's observations on infant emotions that were to especially influence Freud. Darwin's idea that the fears of childhood did not derive from the child's experience but were the result of 'the inherited effects of real dangers and abject superstitions during ancient times' was to influence Freud's idea of 'instinctive knowledge' – 'knowledge that shapes much that is fundamental in the overall pattern of Freudian psychosexual development' (Sulloway, 1979/1992: 245–247). The roots of Fordham's ideas about the influence of archetypes in infant development may be seen in Freud writing in 1914 where he calls archetypes 'hereditary schema': 'Whenever experiences fail to fit in with the hereditary schema, they become remodelled in the imagination. . . . It is precisely such cases that are calculated to convince us of the existence of the schema. We are often able to see the schema triumphing over the experience of the individual' (Freud, 1914/1918: 119).

However, as we have seen above, Fordham differs from Jung in that he does not regard the baby as being mainly in touch with the collective unconscious – where lie the archetypes or Freud's schema – but as mainly 'engaged in a dynamic interaction with another person' (Astor, 1995: 12). Fordham's type of psychoanalytic theorizing about the child, then, contains elements of more than one discourse stemming from different historical era. Not only is there a nineteenth-century evolutionary aspect, but there is also a psychoanalytic version of the even earlier idea that character and personality are transmitted through the mother's or nurse's milk.

CONCLUSION: FORECLOSING OTHER DISCOURSES

To summarize, what I have offered is an illustration of the way that earlier discourses of Western culture are embedded in psychoanalytic theorizing and especially in the theories around early life and infancy. What I am suggesting is that not only are these theories the most obvious targets for criticism of the psychoanalytic method, but, for us as practising psychotherapists, they are perhaps the theories which are least necessary. To substantiate this I will conclude with a brief description of what I think constitutes a more helpful frame for psychoanalytic theory and one which is more responsive as a discourse for, and within, contemporary Western culture. You must forgive me for not having worked this out fully yet! I think I know what we should abandon, and I think I know what we should keep, but I do not know what we need to add or develop. So, thus far, I employ Occam's razor.

Forgive me for stating the obvious but, from the patients I see, and those I hear about, and from my observations in general about all sorts of 'helping professions', it strikes me that psychotherapy is concerned with how we all relate to each other. It is about how we get on with each other, *and, of course, how we get on with ourselves*, in our daily lives. It is therefore very much a social as well as a psychological understanding and change that is attended to and fostered in the work of therapy. This then includes much of what is talked about in therapy: our relationships with friends, spouses and parents, the relationships we experienced as children ourselves, and also our relationships with aspects of the world, its politics, values and mores with which we agree and disagree but which all affect us deeply and as invisibly – and unconsciously – as the social air we breathe.

Contemporary culture for many in the West differs vastly from earlier times due to the great improvement in material security we now experience. Although there are exceptions – and for the poor and homeless psychoanalysis is quite irrelevant as a priority – our food supply and shelter are secure enough to have allowed us the luxury of turning our concerns elsewhere. Some thinkers explain the rise in popularity of psychoanalytic thinking precisely upon this change in social circumstances. More specifically, it is said, now the hostility of nature and the risk of survival have been mainly overcome, the focus in the industrialized West has turned upon *ourselves and each other: what remains for humanity is the puzzle of nature that is our relationship with each other and with our inner fantasies.* 'L'enfer c'est les autres.' It is *other people* and our relationships with them that is the stuff of therapy today. It is our inner and outer, social and psychological, intercourse and discourse, that seems to be the true concern of psychotherapy.

Therefore, this is not just a 'culture of narcissism' as sometimes suggested. It is more a sort of 'culture of socialism' if you like! But a 'culture of relationship' carries less baggage. It therefore needs to include far more attention to, and eventually new theorizing about, our social relationships according to a discourse that resonates with contemporary life. This would require far more of a focus on our experience of each other in the here and now and far less of an emphasis on *explanations* of such experiences.

In psychotherapy, as in the wider culture, people are invariably comforted by explanations. But the way in which these pseudo-explanations are delivered within a culture of the 'expert' – the one who 'knows' – runs the risk of producing an iatrogenic effect upon the quality of human relationships in general. Removing the division between those who claim expert knowledge and those who seek information about their own lives is a major task for the start of the twenty-first century. Let us keep the spirit of story-telling and narrative-making in psychotherapy by all means, but let us seriously question discourses derived from previous eras which, in the hands of a few, attempt to impose a way of thinking instead of opening up new avenues. To do otherwise – if I may generate a final metaphor of the 'child' – would be like raising a child in the 1990s according to the strict, narrow mores of over a century earlier. Once grown, we should not be surprised to find before us an adult who is not only poorly equipped for the pace and flexibility of contemporary social relationships, but one who also burns with resentment that the vision of the world delivered through such an upbringing has robbed them of all relationship with the culture they experience all around them – and, above all, that this clinging to the past and extreme lack of foresight has also *deprived contemporary culture of what such an individual might have to offer.*

Perhaps psychoanalysis suffers from such a deprivation and disadvantage today.

REFERENCES

Astor, J. (1995) *Innovations in Analytical Psychology.* London: Routledge.
Clarke, A. M. and Clarke, A. D. B. (1976) *Early Experience, Myth and Evidence.* Somerset: Open Books.
Covington, C. (1995) 'No story, no analysis? The role of narrative in interpretation'. *Journal of Analytical Psychology*, Vol. 40, no. 3, 405–416.

Fordham, M. (1986) *Jungian Psychotherapy. A Study in Analytical Psychology*, London: Karnac. (Originally published in 1978, by John Wiley, Chichester, UK.)

Freud, S. (1916) *Introductory Lectures*, 1916–1917, Standard Edition, Vol. 16 (The Standard Edition of the Complete Psychological Works of Sigmund Freud (24 volumes), edited by James Strachey. London: Hogarth Press and the Institute of Psycho-Analysis, 1953–1964)

Freud, S. (1895) (with J. Breuer) *Studies in Hysteria*, Standard Edition, Vol. 2. London: Hogarth Press.

Freud, S. (1930) *Civilisation and Its Discontents*, Standard Edition, Vol. 21. London: Hogarth Press.

Freud, S. (1905) *Three Essays on the Theory of Sexuality*, Standard Edition, Vol. 7. London: Hogarth Press.

Freud, S. (1914/1918) Standard Edition, Vol. 17. London: Hogarth Press.

Fromm, E. (1979) *The Greatness and Limitations of Freud's Thought*. New York: Mentor, The New American Library Inc.

Gleick, James (1988) *Chaos. Making a New Science*. Harmondsworth, UK: Penguin.

Gottlieb, B. (1993) *The Family in the Western World: From the Black Death to the Industrial Age*. Oxford: Oxford University Press.

Hauke, C. (1996), 'The Child: Development, archetype and analytic practice'. *The San Francisco Jung Institute Library Journal*, Vol.15, no.1, 17–38.

Hewison, D. (1995) 'Case history, case story: an enquiry into the hermeneutics of C. G. Jung'. *Journal of Analytical Psychology*, Vol. 40, no. 3, 383–404.

Hillman, J. (1983) *Healing Fiction*. Barrytown, NY: Station Hill Press.

Hitching, F. (1982) *The Neck of the Giraffe. Darwin, Evolution, and the New Biology*. New York: Meridian, The New American Library Inc.

Hughlings Jackson, J. (1884) 'Evolution and dissolution of the nervous system'. Reprinted in *Selected Writings of John Hughlings Jackson* (1931) 2 vols. Edited by James Taylor. London: Hodder & Stoughton; reprint edition, New York: Basic Books, 1958.

Kerr, J. (1994) *A Most Dangerous Method. The Story of Jung, Freud, & Sabina Spielrein*. London: Sinclair-Stevenson.

Stern, D. (1985) *The Interpersonal World of the Infant: A view from Psychoanalysis and Developmental Psychology*. New York: Basic Books.

Stern, D. (1990) *Diary of a Baby*. London: Fontana.

Sulloway, Frank J. (1979/1992) *Freud, Biologist of the Mind. Beyond the Psychoanalytic Legend*. Cambridge, MA: Harvard University Press.

(b) Jung, Jungians and the idea of birth trauma

JoAnn Culbert-Koehn

My mother died at the moment I was born, and so for my whole life there was nothing standing between myself and eternity; at my back was always a bleak, black wind. I could not have known at the beginning of my life that this would be so; I only came to know this in the middle of my life, just at the time when I was no longer young and realized that I had less of some of the things I used to have in abundance and more of some of the things I had scarcely at all. And this realization of loss and gain made me look backward and forward: at my beginning was this woman whose face I had never seen, but at my end was nothing, no one between me and the black room of the world. (Kincaid, 1997: 3)

In this selection from *The Autobiography of My Mother*, Jamaica Kincaid's description of a traumatic beginning is intense and painful to read. I present it because it so captures the way that this kind of early trauma can leave a dark, indelible imprint.

The Carib narrator of this story is named Xuela. The story is told in the first person, almost like a diary, giving it a special poignancy and immediacy. If I imagine Xuela coming to me as a patient, my attitude would be that something seriously disturbing and overwhelming had happened at the very beginning of her life, something very real with profound emotional consequences. I would not be shy about asking questions, because it is my experience that patients with severe trauma at the beginning usually have been searching for someone to take their deep distress seriously for a long time. Such patients often come with somatic symptoms and palpable anxiety or depression. Only when the analyst is receptive to the idea that something traumatic has most likely occurred can the patient reclaim the necessary traumatic feelings – usually loss, terror and catastrophic anxiety.

Many patients have in place a complicated set of inner voices imploring them not to be vulnerable in the therapeutic relationship or any other relationship where such painful feelings might be experienced. A patient whom I have seen now for two years comes to mind. Her mother was killed in a car accident when the patient was nine, leaving four young children, my patient being the oldest. The two older girls were told not to cry because it would upset the younger children, and none of the children attended the funeral.

This patient entered treatment while making a career change at midlife. Despite a satisfying marriage and two young children, she felt increasing emotional deadness and suffered back pain. For most of the first year in treatment, the mother's death was mourned with great intensity, but not without significant interference from different sectors of the personality, including the patient's fear that having such feelings would disturb her father and ruin their relationship as well as be destructive to her husband and children. There was also a 1950s-style housewife inside the patient who tried to keep her from contact with me as the person advocating a fuller feeling life. In this situation the work proceeded quite rapidly, but that is often not the case. My patient was frequently astounded that so much grief could be stored away waiting for a receptive other and enough ego strength within herself and the therapist to face it. I think my understanding that both the storing and facing of this much grief was indeed possible facilitated the process.

In this chapter I want to advocate for the importance of Jungian analysts paying attention to early traumatic events in patients' stories. In particular I am going to use examples from prenatal and perinatal trauma, because it is what I have studied most. I think work in this area is particularly important with certain patients and can have a very freeing effect. Patients have reported a feeling imaged as being released from an internal prison (Paul, 1997).

I am first going to present examples from current literature on trauma which have affected my thinking. (An exhaustive annotated bibliography on birth trauma from the psychoanalytic perspective can be found in Lynda Share's *If Someone Speaks, It Gets Lighter* (Share, 1994).) Next I will give examples from my consulting room of birth trauma and my own way of working with it. Finally I will make observations about Jung's relationship to birth trauma and the mother complex, suggesting implications for contemporary Jungians.

In reviewing the literature on infant memory, Lynda Share states:

> Recent and very significant research data in neurobiology, child psychiatry and experimental psychology, as well as anecdotal reports, lend support to the possibility that the earliest affective and perceptual experiences/traumas can be stored in the unconscious, the conscious, or both, and are capable of retrieval in infancy, early childhood, and even adulthood. Additionally, researchers have tentatively located a place (the thalamoamygdala circuits) where such memories of affective experience may be stored and processed. (Share, 1994: 142)

Share links Freud's ideas about types of memory with Lenore Terr's recent work on trauma (Terr, 1988). Share states that there are two types of memories getting clinical attention. 'Burned-in' behavioural memory is one type of memory, which can be considered analogous to Freud's perceptual memory. Terr's verbal memory is a second type, analogous to Freud's memory image.

Share points out that those authors such as Spence, Kris and Bowling, who purport the impossibility of reconstructing specific infant memories are referring to 'verbal memory'. This kind of memory comes from a verbal child age of three or older. Verbal memory becomes modified, distorted, and overlain with current experience over time and does not lend itself to veridical reconstruction.

Share suggests that both types of memory are important in our work. 'Using reconstructive *and* narrative approaches in working with these two types of respective memories, we could reach the human experience of our patients at the beginning while at the same time understanding the variations and developments that change such experience over time' (Share, 1994: 143).

Reconstruction is more possible from behavioural memory, which will be reenacted and felt in the somatic countertransference. Behavioural memories will also present in dreams, according to Share. The narrative approach is more applicable to our work with verbal memory.

A vivid example of the storage of infant trauma in behavioural memory comes from Engel and his colleagues' longitudinal study of Monica (Engel *et al.* 1985). Monica was born with a congenital abnormality of her oesophagus. She regurgitated feedings and choked, and an oesophageal fistula was performed on the third day of her life. For the first two years, Monica's feedings were conducted by having her lie flat on her back with a feeding tube inserted into her stomach. No physical holding or contact with the baby occurred during the two years of fistula feeding.

Engel and colleagues were subsequently able to observe Monica's feeding behaviour as a mother. The enduring somatic/behavioural memory of Monica's unusual experience was most remarkable: she bottle-fed each of her infants in a manner similar to the way in which she had been fed, with minimal physical contact.

> Monica attempted to hold her first child on the first day of life but relinquished the position within a couple of minutes, saying that the weight of the baby fatigued her arms. . . . She had difficulty maintaining contact with the babies during feeding; she smoked or drank coffee, watched television, or talked to others while feeding. Once the babies were old enough to hold their own bottles, Monica seldom, if ever, held the bottles during their feedings. This despite the fact that as a child she had continuously observed her own mother feed her four younger siblings in a face-to-face, enfolded position and that her husband, mother, and sister all encouraged her to hold her own babies in an enfolded, face-to-face position. (Share, 1994: 147–149)

The stunning way that Monica's early experience was stored and physically reenacted with her own baby impressed me.

Another very physical example that shows a memory (this one prenatal) stored and dramatically reenacted is from Alessandra Piontelli's young patient Tina Vera (Piontelli, 1992). Piontelli, a child psychoanalyst writing in Milan, tells us of her treatment of little Tina Vera. This is an example that combines a difficult prenatal experience and a life-and-death birth crisis which is constantly recreated in the home environment and in the relationship with the analyst.

Tina Vera started analysis with Dr Piontelli when she was two years and three months old. Piontelli describes her crawling on the ground like a snake or lizard.

She was unable to walk and could hardly stand, but 'numerous and thorough neurological investigations had excluded a neurological cause' (Piontelli, 1992: 197).

Tina Vera was a wanted child. According to her mother, the pregnancy proceeded in a normal way until the fifth month, when she noted an absence of movement. This inactivity was different from her first child, and the mother began to worry. Ultrasound showed no abnormality. When the ninth month of pregnancy elapsed, Tina Vera's birth was induced. During the delivery, Tina Vera was saved from death by the quick intervention of a midwife. The umbilical cord was doubled and tightly knotted around the baby's neck. A cord in a tightly knotted position is not visible on ultrasound because it merges with other soft tissue in the region (Piontelli. 1992: 198).

Dr Piontelli says that Tina Vera's birth must have been extremely traumatic. Once outside, the baby's neck remained swollen for months, her face and eyes infused with blood. She spent the first five months of life inert and asleep. At five months of age she seemed to wake up and then screamed nonstop as if terrified.

Dr Piontelli describes her analytic experience with Tina Vera:

> What immediately struck me in analysis was how Tina Vera seemed constantly to relive her past imprisonment and entanglement inside the womb. Particularly at the beginning of her analysis: she came to her sessions with a long heavy chain tightly doubled around her neck – a chain given to her by her parents. Tina Vera would pass from her mother's hand to mine without any interruption. She also always came to her sessions holding an object or toy which she pressed against her navel.
>
> Once inside the playroom, she would often continue to hold on to some rope-like object such as the belt of my overall or particularly the cord of my curtain, which she used for all sorts of complicated windings around her face and her neck. For a long time Tina Vera never used any toy except the string and the Sellotape. . . . At the end of each session Tina Vera left either holding my hand as before or the curtain cord till she reached her mother's hands without a break. (Piontelli, 1992: 199)

Although Tina Vera's traumatic birth and manner of communication may seem extreme, the replication and communication of *in utero* birth trauma, as well as the desire to establish an unbroken connection with the analyst, are very much present in the material of many birth-traumatized analysands, both children and adults.

A third example comes from Michael Paul's paper, 'A mental atlas of the process of psychological birth' (Paul, 1988). One of Dr Paul's patients dreamed of feeling very small and unprotected after birth, like a shrimp without a shell. The patient had had a difficult birth, and Dr Paul's experience in the countertransference was of this patient verbally beating against him. I have noted patients doing this before breaks – asking repetitive questions in an extremely aggressive and invasive way – beating against me in a way that feels like trying to get inside my body to avoid the pain of separation.

With Dr Paul's patient it was possible to reconstruct that her mother had developed secondary inertia that resulted in caesarean section. During each of her menstrual periods this patient would beat verbally at Dr Paul and then call him at home. He surmised and interpreted that her menstrual periods were experienced as if she were giving birth to a damaged baby, which had been pounding against the uterine wall again and again, attempting to emerge. Dr Paul was a biologist before training as an analyst. He points out that each birth is nothing less than a major stage in evolution which required millennia in the history of phylogeny to occur. In a human birth, the transition from inside a watery environment to an outside gaseous one occurs in a matter of seconds (Paul, 1988: 561).

After providing us with a very vivid description of physical birth, Paul goes on to describe psychological birth:

> The experience of psychic movement toward psychological birth is attended by what seems to be severe mental pain. Terror and severe intense anxiety are frequently described. 'I can't make ends meet,' 'I'm under extreme pressure,' 'I'm up against a wall,' 'I've gotten in over my head,' are frequent references to the instigation of the shift to the outside. (Paul, 1988: 560)

At the time I first read Michael Paul's article, I had recently written my ideas about birth trauma being re-experienced by some candidates exiting from the 'womb of training' (Culbert-Koehn, 1991). I was so excited by Paul's paper that I called to speak with him about it and to ask if he still believed in the ideas he had written about. I remember his enthusiasm when he said it had now been ten years since the publication and that he was even more sure of what he had written. It is now ten years since I wrote my first paper in this area, and I feel increased conviction that it is important for Jungians to study prenatal and perinatal trauma. I am grateful to my patients for the hard work we have done together and their generosity in allowing me to share the material from my consulting room that follows here.

I have chosen three examples, two previously reported and one more recent. Beth suffered prenatal trauma. Mark represents an example of prenatal trauma as well as difficult birth and difficulty bonding. Gretchen had a seemingly normal birth but difficulty in the perinatal period. All three patients had previous Jungian analysis in which they did not feel their 'childhood trauma' was taken seriously. One patient, in fact, was referred to me by her analyst because he was aware that I do 'early childhood work', which he does not. In the Los Angeles Jungian community in which I was trained, working with the personal transference was thought of as a stage to be gotten through in order to get to the archetypal layers of the psyche.

At the time of the session that follows, Beth, in her late thirties, had been in treatment with me for several years. When she began treatment she was suffering from anxiety and various psychosomatic problems. She felt overwhelmed with responsibilities that left little time for herself. Her mother had cancer while pregnant with Beth and underwent radiation treatment during that time. Beth often felt things were 'coming at her', that the world was not safe. She had never had a safe place to be a baby or little girl. These themes dominated the treatment.

Recently Beth and her husband moved into a new home. The previous home was smaller, cosier, near the ocean and womb-like. The new home felt larger, lighter, more out in the world, part of a more established neighbourhood. The session after the move, Beth lay on the couch sobbing, holding her head, contracted in pain. She said, 'I hate the new house and the new bedroom. There are no curtains and too many windows. The light is streaming in, and I feel bombarded and exposed. My husband likes the new windows with no curtains and the bright carpet. I'll never feel comfortable. I can't get comfortable'. As Beth talked I felt her fear that I would not hear her or comprehend her terror. The verbal crescendo and despair were building, and, based on information from previous sessions, I said quietly, 'Do you think this might have to do with your experience in the womb with your mother's cancer and radiation pouring in?' Beth's hands came down from her head as the agony began to subside. She cried then very quietly. We could begin to talk about the pain.

While at the time of the session reported Beth could acknowledge the possible validity of my interpretation and seemed to be calmed in the session, she was still unable to think of her prenatal history on her own. In subsequent years, she has been able to integrate more of her terror and vulnerability, which has allowed her to bring to mind and use her knowledge about her prenatal life.

Next I wish to describe part of an hour with my patient Greg, including a dream which conveys the agonizing rawness of psychic change and rebirth. Greg suffered a difficult, toxic prenatal experience, a caesarean birth, and maternal abandonment following the birth.

Greg began one midweek session by saying he was really upset and feeling abandoned, by God and his parents. He said, 'I feel abandoned when I leave Bakersfield to drive to L.A. and when I leave you to drive home. I feel panic and shame.' Greg said he felt panic when he left Lancaster to go to his job in San Francisco. Then he said, 'I'm separating from another job now in a cosmic way [meaning big]. I feel extremely raw.' He mentioned he had brought his 'turtle dream' from some weeks ago and wanted us to look at it again. He told me the dream as follows:

> I am in a swimming pool with Rachel [his wife]. I suddenly spy a dim figure far below. I feel some sense of panic. Then I realize it's a huge sea turtle, and we're at an aquarium. The sea turtle comes to the surface. We get it out of the water and take it to a pen. Rachel peels the shell off. I'm horrified and say, 'Do you need to do that?' I'm afraid the animal is so exposed it will die. Rachel ignores me. Suddenly the turtle's muscles go through an incredible molting process. They swell, exfoliate and drop off, leaving a core smaller animal which acts like a sea lion cub, though not just like one.

The dream continues:

Now a man comes out with a shell on his head. He meets with Rachel in a small, closed room. I'm outside and envy him. Now I'm off at a wildlife preserve with a biologist woman of my age. She's like Jane Goodall. We discuss being on a parallel path – we met over the same event that we got to in different ways. She's very unconventional and is passionate about not being normal. I feel defensive about her implication that I would follow her around. Finally we're at a large table and someone pushes a hot beverage in front of me. I block it because I'm afraid it will spill on me. Before this I ate some chili. It's clear I'm going to be fed, and I am hungry.

Greg said it was amazing how this dream described the analysis, but what was upsetting to him was that at the time he had the dream it had had a lot of beauty about it. He felt encouraged then but felt now that he was naive about the sense of rawness and loss of defences that the dream implied.

I commented, 'The living experience of the dream is excruciating,' and he agreed.

Greg said he had had another turtle dream in which he was holding a turtle with a shell that had battle scars. There was some kind of renewal, a new animal in an old shell. He said this dream had also been very encouraging to him, but again he just felt despair and hopelessness now. He said he felt some relief in talking to me, but when the hour was over it would be very hard to leave and face his anxiety alone. He said he felt bitter and enraged.

I said, 'It's hard to bear the pain of the analysis. You are enraged and disappointed that the birth of a new self is so fraught with violent feelings.'

Greg agreed that this was true, and the hour concluded. This session contains feelings of panic, envy, rage and shame, leading to isolation. A potential step forward (leaving his job) stirs up in Greg feelings of panic and rawness. Here the tension and terror are not somaticized, but the feelings are symbolized in his dream, which is at once beautiful and horrifying. There is reference to a link between feelings and musculature (the turtle's muscles swell, exfoliate, and drop off), but again, Greg is able to dream this.

This hour brings up many questions. Is the intense rawness, the peeling away of the shell, a reference to his caesarean birth as well as to his current experience in the transference? Can Greg tolerate the pain of the analysis? As he says so poignantly, the dream images have a certain beauty, but the living experience of trying to birth a more authentic self is excruciating. In the dream he envies the man with the shell on his head, which was perhaps Greg's former state. He encounters a Jane Goodall-like woman, perhaps the analyst, who is at home in the wildlife preserve and who is unconventional and passionate in relation to her more primitive self. He is afraid the beverage will be too hot and spill on him. Is this a reference to his experience of the toxic womb, which can indeed feel fiery to the fetus, as well as to his current fears in the transference? The dream ends on a hopeful and alive note ('It's clear I'm going to be fed, and I'm hungry').

When I previously wrote about this session (Culbert-Koehn, 1999), I used it to demonstrate the conjunction of psychological birth with feelings of turbulence and intrapsychic violence. Together with Beth's hour, this work demonstrates how at a time of potential going forward (Beth to a new home and Greg to a new job), certain sectors of the psyche want to retreat and avoid the pain of separation and change. Of course, there could be many interpretations of this material, but I see in these hours a pessimism and pull toward staying in the dark, of the womb, associated with a painful birth trauma imprint.

The third hour presents an example of a patient beginning to relate to an earlier aspect of herself. Gretchen is reporting a new symptom to me, anxiety about falling asleep and floating away. This session occurs just before a two-week break in the analysis. Anxiety related to difficult early beginnings often presents strongly in sessions preceding analytic breaks.

Gretchen spent the first part of the hour talking about her autistic son and trying to get him an appointment with a specialist. The boy cannot tolerate waiting rooms, which she tried to explain to the receptionist and doctor with no luck. I thought maybe this was not the right doctor for her son and wondered also what part of herself Gretchen had not found the right space for with me. She also talked about her husband going away on a work project for a month. She seemed to be preparing herself. It seemed hard for her to say she would miss him. I noted that I would also be away the following week.

Gretchen began to talk in a new way about a 'sleep problem' that she had not mentioned before, that as she goes to sleep at night she feels as though she might float off into space. It is very frightening to her, this 'floating into space feeling'. She said she had it as a kid all the time.

I said I wondered if it felt, at times in her childhood and now, that she was not really tethered *here*, on this earth, that maybe at birth and in relationship to her mother she never felt securely attached. I wondered whether, when I go away, like next week, it brings up the floating-off feeling.

Gretchen became very thoughtful and sad then and said how often, when she was away at school, she felt her mother might die, how panicked she felt a lot of the time. She said when she went away to camp she felt terrible pain. She said, 'I guess you could call it separation anxiety.'

I suggested that maybe that did not really capture how wrenched away from her mother's body she felt. Gretchen said she tried to tell her aunt about missing her mother once on a visit away from home and that the aunt had laughed.

I said that the laughing hurt her and did not help. Gretchen said she thought that no-one understood, even past therapists. I said I thought it had taken her a while before she could tell me, and she could not yet know whether I would understand. Nevertheless, she was trying to tell me because it was quite awful to be alone with such painful feelings.

Gretchen continued her camp story. Her mom always packed her lovely lunches, packed so nicely. Once she made her one for the camp bus, but Gretchen was so upset about leaving her mother that she could not eat most of the lunch. When she got to camp, she did not want to part with the lunch. 'The last bits of my mom,' she said wistfully. 'I hid it under the bed.' She kept it for days, and then the camp counsellor found it and took it away. Gretchen said the counsellor gave her a dirty look.

I said how painful that must have been, and that again, no one seemed to see how lonely she felt. I wondered if she might not be afraid that I would humiliate her or just not understand what it was like to have such feelings.

Gretchen said, 'I was just inconsolable when I was separated from my mother.'

I said, 'And no one seemed to want to see.' Gretchen said that she was having a memory then about one day when the police had come up to the end of her street. She imagined they were coming to tell her that her mother was dead. She said that she had these fears many times, sometimes daily. She thought if her mother died, she would go insane, that she just could not go on being.

I acknowledged how terrifying this had been for her. Based on previous material as well as this session, I wondered if perhaps this was a very early memory, that at times when she was a baby her mother had been so depressed that she had been dead for the 'baby Gretchen', which made her feel insanely frustrated, as if she could not get through and could not go on, insanely terrified with no-one to help her.

Gretchen looked shocked at this, but then she began for the first time in the treatment to describe the loneliness of her infancy and the lack of bonding with her mother and also how devastated her mom had been by her dad's affairs. Gretchen said she was just traumatized: 'There just wasn't a magnetic attraction to *me*. It's the untetheredness you talked about earlier.'

'No place for you to land in her mind,' I said.

'Yes,' Gretchen said. '"I always feel insecure, afraid I will float away, a lack of weight inside, unheld.'

And there the hour ended.

In all three of these examples I offer some interpretations but usually in a tentative manner. I think of what I offer verbally as a guess about another's state of mind. I am open to the patient's verbal comments as well as the material that follows to see how what I have suggested gets received. I may also ask directly, if the patient changes the subject, 'What did you just do with what I said to you?' or 'Where did what I just said to you go?'

So why have I written about birth trauma? Certainly not to suggest that all subsequent behavior is determined by one's birth. I have written previously that I do not think that anyone's personality is so uncomplicated that any one trauma or memory explains everything (Culbert-Koehn, 1997b). What I have observed is that the events around one's birth, or the days immediately following birth, leave a profound imprint and tend to be re-experienced at times of separation and transition. When the events are not experienced consciously, they have a dark, pessimistic, agitating, stifling, debilitating, sometimes terrifying impact. These earliest memories often have both physical and psychological correlates and frequently carry a kind of life-and-death urgency which Wilfred Bion has described as 'catastrophic anxiety'. They can erupt in ways that may preclude personal exploration or further growth and development.

I have also written about a birth complex (Culbert-Koehn, 1997a). The birth complex, like other complexes (mother, father, Oedipal), will be stronger in some patients than others. In this paper I have put together three examples from literature and three from my practice, all quite visceral, to suggest that we not throw away the idea of trauma but rather improve our way of working with it.

As Christopher Hauke tells us elsewhere in this volume, 'Freud originally conceived of analysis as a process of restoring the repressed memories of past trauma to consciousness, thereby removing the neurotic or hysterical symptoms purely through insight'. I doubt that any among us would advocate that insight alone would mitigate the effects of severe trauma. What may be necessary is the re-experiencing of the painful affects in the presence of an other, possibly an analyst, over time. Literature subsequent to Freud also suggests the importance of contacting and working with those sectors of the personality opposed to change, to the vulnerability of feeling life, and to contact with the analyst (Rosenfeld, 1988; Kalsched, 1996).

Jung's view of birth trauma was ambivalent. In one passage he calls birth trauma 'a famous obvious truism' (Jung, 1969: 516). Elsewhere he writes that '. . . therapy must support the regression and continue to do so until the "prenatal" stage is reached' (Jung, 1967: 329). He also states that, 'The so-called oedipus complex with its famous incest tendency changes at this [prenatal] level into a "Jonah-and-the-whale" complex, which has any number of variants. . . .' (Jung, 1967: 419).

This ambivalence about birth trauma seems related to ambivalences about working in the transference. Warren Steinberg points out Jung's contradictory views (Steinberg, 1990). In 1933 Jung said, for example, 'A transference is always a hindrance; it is never an advantage. You cure in spite of the transference, not because of it' (Jung, 1980: 151). In 1946 by contrast he stated, 'It is probably no exaggeration to say that almost all cases requiring lengthy treatment gravitate round the phenomenon of transference, and that the success or failure of the treatment appears to be bound up with it in a very fundamental way' (Jung, 1954: 164).

I think Jung's ambivalence about working with deep mother wounding and working in the transference still affects our discourse as depth psychologists and can contribute to splits within the Jungian community.

My own view of trauma takes Freud's early view of trauma in 'Project for a scientific psychology' (Freud, 1986: 306–307). There he views trauma simply as overstimulation to the existing psychic apparatus. I have taken this now into a Jungian–Bionian context as I work. When a trauma occurs there is stimulation without the ego strength to make sense or integrate it. From a Jungian perspective, in severe trauma overwhelming feelings, even archetypal energies, are released. From a Bionian perspective, the overstimulating affect may be expelled (as in projective identification), frozen somewhere in the psyche, lodged in a body symptom, or acted out until an other, in some cases an analyst, can find the lump of undigested traumatic feeling and help metabolize the experience.

I often think of a six-year-old girl who, when upset, told her mother, 'I need a different mommy. Your brain and my brain are just different. We have different brains, and there is no way your brain can help my brain.'

When people come to our offices, I think they are looking for another brain, another heart, another spirit that can help them grow. Sometimes this will involve the integration of past traumas; sometimes it will involve birthing as yet unborn psychic potential; sometimes this will involve mediating parts of mother and father or other archetypes that have not yet been incarnated (Edinger, 1962).

I think that the heritage passed on to us by Jung and Freud is a rich one. I agree with Christopher Hauke that we need to be aware of what we have taken in from them, that our forefathers not simply be 'ghosts' that haunt and inhibit us. Hauke suggests that depth analysis may not be forever popular or profitable, and I believe, as Jung and Freud experienced, that there will always be hatred of the unconscious. I suggest that Jung and Freud are lively fathers with whom we can have active inner discourse. We need plenty of room in our minds for new data about our theories, our patients' minds and lives, and our own psyches. We will need different therapists and different forms of psychotherapy for different patients. But for me, to para-phrase Donald Meltzer, the practice of depth psychotherapy continues to be among the most interesting conversations on this earth.

REFERENCES

Culbert-Koehn, J. (1991) 'Birth trauma and training', in M. Mattoon (Ed.), *Personal and Archetypal Dynamics in the Analytical Relationship*. Proceedings of the International Association for Analytical Psychology Congress, Paris, 1989, Einsiedeln, Switzerland: Daimon.

Culbert-Koehn, J. (1997a) 'Analysis of hard and soft: Tustin's contribution to a Jungian study of opposites', in J. Mitrani and T. Mitrani (Eds), *Encounters with Autistic States: A Memorial Tribute to Frances Tustin*. Northvale, NJ: Jason Aronson.

Culbert-Koehn, J. (1997b) 'Prenatal and perinatal influences in contemporary Jungian analysis', in M. Mattoon (Ed.), *Open Questions in Analytical Psychology*. Proceedings of the International Congress for Analytical Psychology, Zurich, 1995, Einsiedeln, Switzerland: Daimon.

Culbert-Koehn, J. (1999) 'Birth, violence and the millennium'. *International Journal of Prenatal and Perinatal Psychology and Medicine*, Vol. II, no. 4, 427–436.

Edinger, E. (1962) 'On the relation between personal and archetypal factors in psychological development'. Unpublished paper.

Engel, G., Reichman, F., Harway, V. and Wilson, D. (1985) 'Monica: Infant-feeding behavior of a mother gastric fistula-fed as an infant – a thirty-year longitudinal study of enduring effects', in E. Anthony and G. Pollack (Eds), *Parental Influences in Health and Disease*. Boston, MA: Little Brown.

Freud, S. (1986) 'Project for a scientific psychology', in *The Complete Works of Sigmund Freud*, Vol. 1. London: Hogarth Press.

Jung, C. G. (1954) 'Psychology of the transference'. *Collected Works*, Vol. 16. New York: Pantheon Books.

Jung, C. G. (1967) 'The dual mother'. *Collected Works*, Vol. 5. Princeton, NJ: Princeton University Press.

Jung, C. G. (1969) 'Psychological commentary on "The Tibetan Book of the Dead".' *Collected Works*, Vol. 11. Princeton, NJ: Princeton University Press.

Jung, C. G. (1980) 'Lecture V'. *Collected Works*, Vol. 18. Princeton, NJ: Princeton University Press.

Kalsched, D. (1996) *The Inner World of Trauma: Archetypal Defenses of the Personal Spirit.* London: Routledge.

Kincaid, J. (1997) *The Autobiography of My Mother*, New York: Plume Books.

Paul, M. (1988) 'A mental atlas of the process of psychological birth', in J. Grotstein (Ed.), *Do I Dare Disturb the Universe?* London: Karnac.

Paul, M. (1997) 'Primordial development of the penitential transference', in *Before We Were Young: An Exploration of Primordial States of Mind*. London: Free Association Books.

Piontelli, A. (1992) *From Fetus to Child*. London: Tavistock.

Rosenfeld, H. (1988) 'A clinical approach to the psychoanalytic theory of the life and death instincts: An investigation into the aggressive aspects of narcissism', in E.B. Spillius (Ed.), *Melanie Klein Today*, Vol. 1. London: Routledge.

Share, L. (1994) *If Someone Speaks, It Gets Lighter: Dreams and the Reconstruction of Infant Trauma*. Hillsdale, NJ: The Analytic Press.

Steinberg, W. (1990) *Circle of Care: Clinical Issues in Jungian Therapy*. Toronto: Inner City Books.

Terr, L. (1988) 'What happens to early memories of trauma?'. *Journal of American Child and Adolescent Psychology*, Vol. 27, 96–104.

Transference, countertransference and beyond

Introduction

This chapter continues some of the themes opened up by the previous two and returned to in the final chapter. In it Barry Proner takes the position that the proper focus of analytic work is the here and now of the transference/countertransference relationship. Verena Kast on the other hand argues that at times in an analysis new symbols can arise which prove pivotal to the client's development, and that these can in effect transcend the transference.

Doubtless, some of this difference of opinion hinges on discrepancies in the authors' definitions of transference. Kast acknowledges that Jung's dialogic view of the analytic relationship makes it difficult to identify what is objectively real within the analytic relationship. She nevertheless clearly conceives of transference as a distorting influence on that relationship. Proner on the other hand refers to transference constituting as well as distorting relationships. His definition is therefore broader than hers and includes both real and ph/fantasy elements. Despite these considerations, however, there remain real differences in their methods.

Proner argues that his approach is compatible with Jung's but like many 'London-based Jungians' he has clearly been more influenced by Kleinian ideas than the 'Zurich-based' Kast. He believes in 'waiting for the material to unfold' and recommends the analyst revealing a minimum of information about himself. In this way he can develop into the patient's 'external phantasy object'. If the analyst does give information about himself, Proner claims this is likely to interrupt that process. Analysis in Proner's view is therefore an asymmetrical relationship. It is also an abstinent one for the analyst. The analyst should reflect on his countertransference feelings in order to discover their meaning – not reveal them. Proner believes that revealing them is more likely to be in order to relieve the analyst than to further the analytic process.

In contrast, Kast believes that the analyst is inevitably personally involved in the unfolding analytic process whether he reveals things about himself or not. Even withholding information says something about the analyst. For this reason the process may sometimes be interrupted if the analyst withholds personal information and enhanced if he reveals it.

This makes analysis for Kast a more equal relationship, where both partners mutually influence each other, and fantasies can sometimes be shared. On the other hand she would agree with Proner that the analyst must not prematurely offer personal material in an attempt to defend against the experience of being drawn into the patient's inner world. While Proner talks of the analyst as an external phantasy object, she talks about complexes getting constellated in the analytic relationship in this connection. There are clear similarities between these two formulations.

These similarities and differences of approach can be seen most clearly with reference to Kast's case. Both would recommend avoiding being drawn in to quickly gratifying Kast's client's wish for 'the story'. But Kast did offer a story once she had experientially understood how the patient was positioning her in the transference and she had fed this information back to her. Kast acted this way partly out of compassion for her own position as a real person in pain as a result of the real relationship with her client. She could justify her action analytically on the utilitarian basis that it resulted in a turning point in her client's development.

Proner has a more ascetic view of the analytic task. For him the terrible pressure to produce a story to save the life of the analysis is best understood in terms of Kast's patient's attempt to push unbearable anxiety into the analyst. He would therefore recommend interpreting this anxiety (perhaps in terms of the patient's fear of death) rather than relieving it by offering the story requested. Offering such a story, he argues, could result in the avoidance of material related to that fear.

(a) Transcending the transference

Verena Kast

THEORETICAL SECTION

The goal of analysis

In my view the activation of the unconscious within an analytic relationship is at the core of Jungian therapy. This is an activation that can enable individuals to deal more creatively with both their problems and their own disposition. It can also form part of their individuation process. But if the ego complex is not sufficiently coherent, that coherence must be developed before it can be effective.

Symbols are activated in a therapeutic relationship when the analyst shows an interest in the analysand's total personality – in his uniqueness, potentials and inhibitions. Once these symbols have emerged from the unconscious, they may be perceived as meaningful. They can then be shaped and eventually understood.

The goal of therapy is the assimilation of developmental impulses awakening in the psyche. This helps the individual to deal more competently with both self and others. Greater understanding of even the darker aspects of the self can then ensue. As a result projections may also become easier to recognize. The overall goal is increased autonomy, increased ability to relate, and increased authenticity.

The activation of the unconscious takes place within an analytic relationship, in an 'I – Thou' partnership. In such a concentrated encounter, old patterns of relating occur, but new ones can also arise and develop. The analytic relationship is distinguished from everyday ones in that greater attention is paid to the impact of the unconscious, and to transference and countertransference.

Transference, countertransference and the analytic relationship

In talking about transference, countertransference and the analytic relationship I will refer to Jung's well-known diagram (Jung, 1954), which I have transformed as Figure 1 (Kast, 1992).

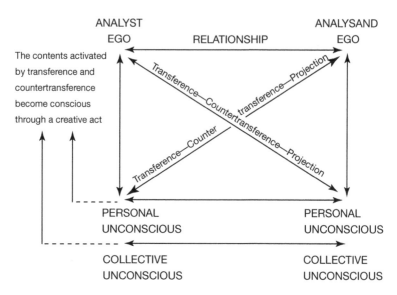

The contents activated by transference and countertransference become conscious through a creative act

Figure 1

A relationship takes place between the analyst's and the analysand's egos. In my view, this includes all those areas of the encounter where the analyst is perceived as a real person and in this capacity enters into contact with the analysand (see also Jacoby, 1984). Transference can be understood as the distortion of perception in relationships; earlier patterns of relating (complexes) are transferred onto the analyst or analytic situation. But transference is usually a compromise between the original complex content and defences enacted in the specific relationship with each analyst. Transference on this view is not only the repetition of biographical experiences; it is also the analysand's plausible version of the analytic couple's communal reality. This means that a person shows different aspects of their biography and complexes to the individual analyst, who responds to that in a specific way. Archetypal images may be transferred in addition to these complexes and past experiences.

I define countertransference as the analyst's emotional reaction to the analysand, and, in particular, to situations of transference. Countertransference and transference do interact. But there is even more: a mysterious relationship or fusion seems to exist between the unconscious of the analyst and the unconscious of the analysand. This mutual unconscious can be sensed in analysis as the atmosphere of the relationship (Stein, 1995). This might help explain the factor of 'contagion' when, for instance, the analyst physically senses the analysand's unperceived and unexpressed fear. This unconscious relationship is a prerequisite for what we call countertransference and, at best, is an opportunity for the analysand to participate in the analyst's self-regulation, assuming that this functions!

These unconscious processes, and perhaps each person's unconscious identity, make it possible for the analyst to consciously perceive both archetypal and complex constellations. This can eventually lead to the establishment of the transcendent function. Part of this process may involve the analyst finding an image – be it archetypal or personal – to express the emotional situation constellated within the therapeutic relationship. In this way a significant symbolic situation can be made conscious through the analyst's creative act. This means in the best case that the psyche of the analysand opens itself to a creative attitude. In such situations, the analysand feels understood and more competent at dealing creatively with life and its difficulties.

Countertransference is a compromise between the images and emotions the analyst perceives, his or her defence mechanisms and reality sense. It has features that are specific to each particular analytic relationship. The analytical dialogue has a special tension within it as a result. The world of the analysand should be seen as true to life as possible – but the analyst focuses on some aspects of this life more than others. In psychoanalysis this issue has been discussed for the last twenty years. Gill talked about the analyst as 'participant observer', Hoffmann as 'participant constructivist' (Thomä, 1999). This is close to Jung's view of the analytical relationship as an interaction of two psychic systems (Jung, 1935/1971).

The analyst is a human being, with a particular view of life and humanity, and a particular experience of being brought up as a man or woman in a specific social situation. All this forms part of the therapeutic interaction. Countertransference reactions are therefore not merely a response to the analysand's projective identifications. Whether they take the form of an emotion, phantasy, or image, they arise in answer to a specific activated complex-constellation (Kast, 1997: 21ff), which influences both – analyst and analysand. Because of this they refer to a communal unconscious, and are therefore a co-production.

American Ego-Psychologists speak in a similar vein about an 'enactment', originating between analysand and analyst (Chused, 1991). This enactment takes the form of a symbolic interaction between analysand and analyst with an unconscious meaning for both of them, which has to be expressed for conscious understanding to occur. If we consider this discussion there is an evident change in the view of the analytical relationship. There is less focus on transference and countertransference as mirror images of one another that are difficult to disentangle. Instead the analytical relationship is seen as a mutual production – an encounter that establishes itself again and again. This relationship itself is the new centre of interest.

Although it is now accepted that there are aspects of reality in this encounter, and that we have to deal with this, no one knows exactly how to do this. How far should we bring in our position as analyst? What supports the analytical process in this context? What inhibits it? And what helps us understand the unconscious better in these circumstances? Very few people are willing to share their experiences with these problems. This leaves us unsure of how to deal with a countertransference that is regarded as a co-production. Helmut Thomä, a senior Freudian psychoanalyst with a great reputation, proposes allowing the analysand some access to the analyst's emotions, ideas and behaviour – providing this is a part of the analysand's reality

(Helmut, 1999). But although this idea is intellectually convincing, it is not easy to transfer to analytical reality.

It is evident, however, that the idea of the analyst as an objective mirror is very much subverted here. With this goes the analyst's power to define what is realistic or unrealistic, good or bad, transference or not, as well as what constitutes a distorted perception. The paradigm of the anonymous analyst thus changes to that of the analyst as participant constructivist. The anonymous analyst no longer exists. Our speech and our silence like our emotional reaction or lack of it, always reveal something about us. This in turn has an effect on the relationship. Thus the idea that the analyst could be 'objective' is exposed as an idealization of the analyst – albeit one that is often maintained by the analysand.

The previous view – that of regarding everything that occurs in the analytical situation as a transference repetition connected to the analyst – lead to an important asymmetry in the relationship, as Balint pointed out as early as 1968 (Balint, 1968, 1970). If the frame of interpretation is always the relationship to the analyst, he becomes a very important, omnipresent object. The analysand is not allowed to feel, think or experience anything unconnected to the analyst. So the weakness of the analysand is overemphasized, and his or her strengths correspondingly neglected. As a result the analytical process with the 'objective' analyst is not sufficiently oriented towards the analysand's resources.

In my view the analyst's task is to allow the analysand to make a new start in the analytical relationship and to find him – or herself. It is up to both of them to let this happen. These considerations lead to a re-evaluation of one of the most important interventions in the analytical process – the interpretation. Jungians who take Jung's dialogic (I do not mean dialectic!) view of the analytic relationship seriously speak of a communal space of fantasy, where fantasies are exchanged. And this exchange can lead in the end to a mutual interpretation giving the analysand a new under-standing of himself and his life – or a new perspective on his future life.

The extent to which Jung really regarded analysis as an encounter in this sense can be deduced from a sentence he used in a letter to James Kirsch written in 1934: 'In the deepest sense we all dream not *out of ourselves*, but out of what is lying *between us and the other*' (Jung, 1973).

The above discussion between Freudians and neo-Freudians sounds familiar to those of us who have taken Jung's diagram and ensuing comments on the nature of the analytic relationship seriously. Nevertheless, it is my impression from the literature that we Jungians have tended to neglect a systematic exploration of these issues. And even when we have discussed or mentioned them (Jacoby, 1984), there is a lack of verbatim clinical material to refer to. Naturally we may not wish to publish our interventions, for fear of showing too much of ourselves, or being too personal. Some of us have certainly experienced an analysis in which analysts shared much too much personal material. But we have an interesting and very important clinical issue here, and I guess Jungians have quite an experience in what Freudians would today call 'enactment'. It is up to us to reflect on this, discuss it and utilize it.

It is a pity then, that some of us have been so willing to adopt the Freudian or Kleinian approach to transference/countertransference issues, and have neglected ideas in our own theory. It is natural that such concepts with their huge impact on clinical work should be studied from different perspectives. It is also natural that we should attempt to find the interventions that help most. But why is our theory – which nowadays seems to be so very 'postmodern' – almost unknown?

The individuation process is the core theoretical piece of Jungian therapy. It is linked to the transcendent function, to symbol formation, and finally to the creative resources of the human being. Individuation establishes itself within the analytical encounter. So symbol formation and the understanding of the unconscious remain essential to our clinical work. I maintain that this cannot always be reduced to transference/countertransference considerations.

CLINICAL SECTION

Despite suggesting that we should focus more on the analytic encounter, there are still situations that are best understood in terms of transference/countertransference. I will give a clinical example that illustrates how I work with this situation in practice.

Turning points in analysis

I speak of turning points when a new formation of symbols becomes possible. When symbols appear that formerly could not be perceived, they encourage different emotions and foster new behaviour, insights, and hopes. The appearance of new symbols in analysis, which often occurs after long periods of 'fiddling around', has to do with special situations of transference and countertransference that are conducive to deeper understanding. The theoretical key to understanding this connection is concealed in the concept of complexes.

I understand complexes as generalized, internalized, episodic relationship patterns which always imply an emotionally toned collision between a significant other and the ego as it is at any given time. These complexes can be formed throughout life, but for the most part originate in childhood. They can easily be transferred, notably onto the analytic relationship (Kast, 1997). When a complex is expressed through the activity of fantasy; it can become a turning point in the journey from captivity to liberation. Within this fantasy lies the energy necessary for the individual's continued development. Complexes that are unconscious, or not understood emotionally can often be experienced collusively in the transference/ countertransference (Riedel, 1989; Heisig, 1999). One characteristic of the experience of a complex episode is the feeling of being separated or even abandoned by the significant other in a situation where bonding would be required. In dealing with complex constellations therefore it is important to re-establish the experience of 'we together' in the area of the complex.

Collusive transference/countertransference and the formation of symbols

Collusive transference/countertransference usually occurs when the behaviour of the analyst has been polarized by the behaviour of the analysand. Even if the analyst is aware of this process, initial behaviour patterns cannot be changed. A relationship pattern repeats stereotypically. Since a complex represents the harmful collision between a significant other and the ego as it was at that time, it can easily become split within the analytic relationship. The analyst then behaves like the person to whom the child related, and the analysand behaves as he or she did in the original complex situation. These roles can also be reversed. Such situations in analysis are 'complex', they follow a stereotypical course; they are emotionally charged and lead to no results. Both the analyst and the analysand fend them off, since both feel under intense pressure. Each is caught in a collusive transference/countertransference situation.

I would like to propose the following hypothesis. Before new symbols can be formed, and the complex expressed through imagination, the complex constellation must be recognized as a reflection of the childhood relationship situation including its emotions. The role models involved must be recognized as inner aspects of the analysand, and to a certain extent of the analyst as well. Often, it takes the analyst's experience to bring all this out.

It is possible to regard a complex involving transference/countertransference as a process of symbolization, and the analytic situation as the symbol formed. But that situation must then be understood emotionally; otherwise the energy inherent in the complex remains mired in a somewhat childish tug-of-war of transference/countertransference. Collusive transference/countertransference must therefore be acknowledged. But often quite a bit of involvement is needed before this can happen. Once truly understood though (that is once the analysand and his life-story are acknowledged) the analyst is better able to understand his own behaviour in the unique situation. New symbols can then be formed and perceived. However, a great deal of empathy and sensitivity is necessary to understand oneself in these circumstances.

Clinical example

I will present a therapeutic situation in which a turning point in analysis occurred. This involved a collusive transference/countertransference with its origins in a childhood 'complex-situation'. The corresponding symbol formation is clearly perceived as a developmental focal point, which is repeated in the therapeutic relationship. In the process, I hope to show how this transference/countertransference repetition is transcended by the activation of new symbols within the therapeutic relationship. In this sense new elements within that relationship completed, rather than competed with, transferential elements.

The analysand was a woman of 48, a teacher of literature at a college and mother of two grown-up children. Her presenting problem was that she felt 'easily overwhelmed, nervous, depressed, without breath, alone, and in despair'. She feared that life would lose its order and she would be unable to restore it. In addition she felt her creativity was being blocked and this hindered her work as a teacher greatly.

After about half a year of analysis, in the 23rd hour, she started the analytic encounter by asking: 'Supposing you are accused of murdering someone. But if you can tell a really good story, you can save yourself. Which story would you tell?' She added, 'You are only accused of murder, you didn't actually do it.' She then turned to me expectantly.

I felt an immense pressure, to invent a good story to save my life, or at least my life in this analysis. First I got paralysed and said: 'This is an unexpected task – a bit special. I have to think about it, I have to understand your question better. It sounds a bit like a complex.' I left open whose complex it was, although a complex had clearly been constellated between us.

Thinking about the situation, I remembered a key complex-situation we had been working on, two months earlier.

The analysand's narrative to illustrate the key complex-situation: 'You have to tell the best story.'

'My father liked a kind of "entertaining conversation". One evening I was sitting with my three elder brothers and my father at the table. I was perhaps six – not yet at school. [She was the youngest and the only girl. At the time the family was living at the Bodensee]. Father said: 'Imagine you are on the opposite shore of the Bodensee, it is night and the last ferry boat has left – how do you manage to come home?' Each of the brothers had an idea – there was an atmosphere of great competition. Finally I was asked as the last one – I wanted to tell them something special, but the brothers had already taken all the options that came into my mind. Father was asking very insistently. I was getting more and more stressed and anxious. He did not help by asking questions or offering an idea. I had no solution and started to cry. The brothers and my father laughed at me – I felt hostile, helpless and greatly ashamed. Then I remembered the Grimm's fairy tale of the three little men in the woods. I identified with the girl who has to go and fetch strawberries in the winter. She helps the little men, is a most helpful maid, removing snow and giving them her hard bread. In return she gets everything she needs – she becomes very special. I felt much better, but I did not mention my fantasy.'

In this narrative the clash between the adult and child can easily be seen, as can the related emotions and a more archetypal fantasy whose purpose seems to be to evade the complex constellated. The father and the brothers are experienced as entertaining, but demanding, overstraining, not empathic, excluding and devaluing. The girl is isolated, and wants badly to relate to the demand, which seems to be almost impossible. She collapses, cries and feels ashamed. The fairy tale comes into her mind: she identifies with the helpful maid, and in everyday life too she tries to be extremely helpful.

This complex narrative – and I am sure it is a generalized episode – gives one explanation for her being so easily overwhelmed. The complex is represented as an 'episodic memory'. The complex holder is not only identified with the child but also with the father. Unconsciously my analysand is identified with this aspect of the complex. She loves entertaining by discussing virtual situations. She also likes to exclude others, she is demanding – and this also on the subjective level – towards herself. Consciously, however, she is identified with the girl, especially with strategies of reparation, and of being helpful. She easily bursts into tears and she is in despair.

The complex-constellation in the analytic relationship

We agreed that the complex 'you have to tell the best story' was being constellated in the analytical relationship. But what we had to understand was the meaning of being accused of murder and of the need to produce a good story – on pain of death. We talked about the wish to kill and the fear of killing. We found a deep aggression towards the father and the brothers behind the anxiety connected to the complex-situation, which could not be expressed in that situation. But I decided not to talk about hidden aggression towards me. She seemed far more anxious than aggressive. We also talked about being unjustly accused of destructiveness, and not being able to defend oneself. But defending oneself seemed beside the point – at least at this point in the analysis. It was far more important to save oneself with 'the good story'. The good story could have helped the child to avoid the destructive reaction, and also to avoid the compensatory strategy of being helpful.

The question for our analytic situation was, 'Can we find "the story" together to avoid destructiveness?' The analysand could not manage this. 'You don't have the story?', she asked.

Me: 'I am feeling like the girl of your entertaining complex, without breath, I feel an enormous pressure to have *the* story.'

I started to think about a story but at the same time felt a defensive reaction on my part. Surely she had to tell the story by herself. 'But is that correct and helpful?', I wondered as I reflected on my reaction. 'Shouldn't it be more of a co-production, out of an experience of "we together"?' I was still unable to make any decision about this, when she said, 'I can see you don't like the situation. You are caught in your system. You are ambivalent. One side of you would like to invent the story, but your analytic rules do not allow you to do so.'

I told her she was correct about the ambivalence: I was thinking about inventing a story, but I did not believe it would help. Only she could find the story, but I would try to help her. She agreed that I could find *a* story, and that she could find *the* story.

Then, for hours nothing substantially changed. She brought no dreams and no problems except the desperate need to find the story – and I had to produce it. I had communicated to her at length how it felt for me to be in the position of the girl of her 'narrative complex', and in the position of the father as well, asking *her* to invent a really good story. I had a lot of empathy with her – as a child – and as an adult woman having to find the good story in order not to be accused of the most evil thing you can do, even if you have not done it.

In the 29th hour I also felt empathy with me. I had to find the story, but I was not allowed to do so. And if we together did not find it – the analytic process could be killed.

Out of this new empathy with me in my situation, Sheherezade suddenly came into my mind. She told 1001 stories about love and death, to keep the interest of the king, who wanted to kill her because he had been deceived and disappointed by a woman he loved.

'Our situation reminds me of Sheherezade (1001 Nights) – saving her life by telling fairy tales every night. But she had the possibility of telling 1001 stories – she did not have to tell *the* story,' I said.

'Sheherezade – that's it. Not the helpful maiden – the courageous and loving Sheherezade,' she exclaimed.

The pressure was gone: not *the* story, but different stories. And she started, 'By the way, I have to tell you a wonderful story . . .' She told me how she seduced the extremely mean head of her school into being very generous with her students by telling him that they loved his generosity so much. She started to write the papers she had to write. She started to write stories. She felt relieved about having lost the idea of finding *the* story, and being allowed to invent thousands of stories – to save her life. And she became more and more conscious of how she identified with the father aspect of her complex. She was not making people tell her stories – she told them stories, being very pleased when she got a good story in return. Sheherezade as a symbol became very important in her life – not only as storyteller, but also as a courageous clever woman who was able to help herself.

Obviously Sheherezade could have come into my mind much earlier, as a kind of archetypal countertransference. But she did not appear earlier. This might have to do with my reluctance to construct a grandiose inner world from archetypal images and the emotions connected with them. But in addition such a construction would have avoided the complexes constellated both in concrete everyday life and the concrete analytical relationship. So perhaps she also did not appear in my thoughts – because it was not the right moment. After all, the analytic encounter is a co-production, a process of co-creativity, in which both partners influence each other. Perhaps that mutual influence had to be actually lived through before Sheherezade could meaningfully emerge.

REFERENCES

Balint, Michael (1968, 1970) *Therapeutische Aspekte der Regression.* Stuttgart: Klett.

Chused, J. F. (1991) 'The evocative power of enactments'. *JAPA*, Vol. 42, 1083–1106.

Heisig, Daniela (1999) *Wandlungsprozesse durch therapeutische Beziehung. Die Konstellation und Neuorganisation von Komplexmustern.* Giessen: Psychosozialverlag.

Jacoby, Mario (1984) *The Analytic Encounter. Transference and Human Relationship.* Toronto: Inner City Books.

Jung, Carl Gustav (1935/1971) 'Was ist Psychotherapie'. GW 16, Olten: Walter, pp. 21–30.

Jung, Carl Gustav (1954) 'Psychology of the transference'. *Collected Works*, Vol. 16, para 422. London: Routledge & Kegan Paul.

Jung, Carl Gustav (1973) Letter of 29.9.1934 to James Kirsch. *Letters*, Vol. 1, p. 172. London: Routledge.

Kast, Verena (1992) *The Dynamics of Symbols. Fundamentals of Jungian Psychotherapy.* New York: Fromm International.

Kast, Verena (1997) *Father–Daughter, Mother–Son. Freeing Ourselves from the Complexes that Bind Us.* Shaftesbury, UK: Element Books.

Riedel, Ingrid (1989) 'Symbol formation in the analytic relationship', in Proceedings of the Eleventh International Congress for Analytical Psychology. Einsiedeln: Daimon, pp. 55–73.

Stein, Murray (Ed.) (1995) *The Interactive Field in Analysis.* Wilmette, IL: Chiron, Clinical Series.

Thomä, Helmut (1999) 'Theorie und Praxis von Übertragung und Gegenübertragung im psychoanalytischen Pluralismus'. *Psyche*, Vol. 9, no. 10, 820–872.

(b) Working in the transference

Barry Proner

My aim in this contribution will be to try to show that the use of the transference as a central philosophical and emotional orientation in analysis is not only appropriate, but that it is compatible with Jungian perspectives. Jung himself considered the transference, notwithstanding his unconcealed anxiety about methodically analysing the transference himself, to be 'the alpha and the omega of analysis' (Fordham, 1974). He asserted that 'Thanks to this personal feeling Freud was able to discover wherein lay the therapeutic effect of psychoanalysis' (Jung (1913) quoted in Fordham, 1974). As in many other areas Jung was 'ahead of his time' when he considered that transference entailed much more than just the sexual area, as was thought by Freud at the time. Jung said that there are 'moral, social and ethical components', a view that seems nearer to Melanie Klein's much later conception of the transference as the *total situation* than to Freud's view in that period. He observed, for example, that the patient may bargain with the analyst like a child who wishes to get special favours from his parents, or may seek out 'special adventures' which the analyst must not prevent since they may contain value for the patient. 'We have to let the patient and his impulses take the lead' (Jung (1913) quoted in Fordham, 1974). He saw the sexual fantasies as analogies related to empathy, adaptation and 'the urge towards individualization'. Jung saw that both negative and positive transference furthered individualization (Jung (1914) quoted in Fordham, 1974.)

Michael Fordham noted that Jung described transference as having 'biological value' as 'a bridge across which the patient can get away from his family into reality'. Jung also thought that the infantile elements of the transference represented a 'powerful hindrance to the progress of the treatment, because the patient assimilates the analyst to his father and mother' and the more he does this so much more will transference do him harm (Jung (1913) quoted in Fordham, 1974). Fordham observed that although Jung credited Freud with the discovery that the transference itself is the therapeutic factor in analysis, it appears to have been Jung's view, while the Freudians at that time seem to have believed that improvement lay in making unconscious contents conscious. Fordham wrote:

> Jung went along with Freud in recognizing the incestuous, erotic and infantile characteristics of transference, as well as accepting its resistance phenomena.

Where he went beyond psychoanalysis is in his emphasis on the goal-seeking and therapeutic function of transference in which the real personality of the analyst became highly significant. His emphasis on transference as a potentially therapeutic situation and on the real personality of the analyst seems to have been his own particular contribution. The idea that once the projections have been recognized and resolved, a bridge to reality can be made with the aim of attaining moral autonomy, defined, even in 1913, as the 'urge towards individualization', is characteristic and central in the development of his thesis. The social and religious, moral and ethical meanings of transference are also much more important to Jung than to Freud.

It seems to me that a consideration of the importance of the transference/countertransference 'situation' in the analytic process would be served by first thinking about some of the aims of analysis. Then I would like to say something about how the transference/countertransference may be used in the furtherance of these aims. (I consider the two, transference and countertransference, to be interdependent parts of the same process, but I will refer to the process only as 'the transference' henceforth.)

In my view, analysis provides a type of emotional relationship that cannot be found elsewhere. It is an experience of extra-ordinary intimacy and meaning, expressly of a non-enacted and non-erotic kind. Significantly, it is in the context of the relationship itself that new developments take place in the psyche (and, accordingly in the brain).

This relational model of the analytic process is analogous to an early mother–infant couple, in which existing infantile parts of the psyche, including the propensity to form archetypal images, are brought to the fore and primitive emotional experiences and defence systems and their attendant imagery are re-experienced and re-worked in the relations between the patient and the analyst. Thus it is by means of the relationship that the opportunities exist for the alleviation of mental disturbance, the recovery of lost parts of the self, and progressive emotional growth and development. I submit that these are amongst the foremost aims of analysis and are inextricably linked with the analysis of the transference.

In the early days of psychoanalysis, Freud thought the therapeutic action of psychoanalysis to be in the uncovering of unconscious conflicts and educating the patient to them. This 'suggestion' method offered the patient intellectual knowledge but not psychic change. It was replaced when Freud recognized the importance of transference phenomena, first as resistance, then necessity, and then as therapeutic instrument. At first the salutary effect of the transference was believed to lie in the induction in the patient of strong positive emotional ties to the analyst. The dangers of this practice were soon realized. The analyst was 'omnipotently' controlling the patient, and the patient the analyst. Negative and erotic transference material appeared. The 'insights' were again short-lived.

Once understood, this impasse led many analysts to investigate the process whereby lasting psychic change takes place. The analysis of the nature of the transference, its unconscious roots, its reflections in symptoms, in dreams, in the vicissitudes of emotional life and consequently the ego (especially the in the area of symbolization and thinking) – all seen in the 'here and now' – ultimately took its place at the centre of the procedure. Meaning and feeling lay at the centre of the transference, in the drama that is always taking place in the inner world.

This was a major advance. The analyst was no longer an 'omnipotent' and 'omniscient' figure but rather someone who reverberated emotionally at a very deep level whilst remaining aware of the dangers of unconsciously taking part in the internal drama. (Racker described this latter as 'identifying with the inner object'.) The countertransference and its manifestations became an important area of study in itself. Racker, Heimann, Money-Kyrle, Fordham and many others gave much attention to the various forms that countertransference may take and how it may be worked with to think about the transference. Bion advanced the thinking about the analyst's position in his thoughts on memory, desire and understanding as qualities to be eschewed in the approach to an analytic session.

Refraining from the imposition of one's own views and the projections of one's own emotional life into the patient was of the highest priority. The impulse to reassure, advise, praise, or otherwise gratify was noted as counterproductive. Humility and modesty were essential qualities of the analyst. Freud referred to the comment of the seventeenth-century surgeon, Ambroise Paré, 'Je le pansai, Dieu le guérit'. (I have dressed his wounds, God healed him.) For a Jungian analyst, the self, with its integrating and life-affirming qualities, is an ally in the analytic process.

Two further developments that have established their place in modern trans-ference analysis stem directly from Melanie Klein. First is the observation that the unconscious relations being played out in the transference are not merely the replaying of long-past emotional life, but living, present experiences taking place in the inner world and changing all the time. Secondly, this came to be best understood through the interplay of projection and introjection between the patient and his objects, notably in the action of projective identification. In James Strachey's phrase, the analyst is an 'external phantasy object' (Strachey (1934) quoted in Caper, 1991: 20).

I shall offer two clinical vignettes that I hope will illustrate some of these points.

Patient 1: Mrs X is an intelligent and highly successful businesswoman in her fifties who had recently separated from her husband of twenty-five years. She was referred by a colleague who works as a counsellor in a general practitioner's surgery, ostensibly because of nervous states at work that had resulted in various somatic complaints. She told me that she had suffered from a range of severe phobias all her life, which now interfered with her daily activities. She also told me that she felt unloved and unloving all her life, apart from the love she feels for her now-grown daughter. Mrs X described her relationships with her parents as cold and lacking emotional understanding. She has one sister who believes herself to be possessed by the devil and has regular exorcisms. It was evident quite early on that, amongst other difficulties, my patient had little capacity for recognizing or naming her own feelings.

She agreed readily to attend three times weekly and decided to use the couch when I offered it. Soon she was talking quite freely and trustingly, seemingly taking to the process like a duck to water. She developed mainly positive feelings towards me particularly after my first interpretation of a dream, which she found very moving. Soon she was reporting dreams regularly and freely telling me of the events taking place in her mind and in her external world. In fact what appeared to be the case was that she felt listened to and understood – virtually for the first time in her life.

She felt 'supported' and strengthened very early on. In the first year of her analysis, she became divorced, her mother died, she moved house and she left her long-term job as a business executive to start a freelance consultancy.

The patient found surprisingly soon that her states of panic when driving on motorways and when going across bridges, into lifts and tall buildings, to name only a few, diminished in frequency and intensity. She felt that I understood her and that I was emotionally available for her. All of this contributed to corresponding feelings in me that I was an effective and appreciated analyst who therefore needed to take care not to encourage a split in her feelings between her 'bad' parents and myself.

These apparent changes in her proved to be superficial, as was my hubris, and belied deep insecurities in the patient. At times she requested, because of an important meeting at work or another equally 'serious' reason, a change in the time of her session, or needed to cancel one of her sessions. With every disturbance of the analytic framework the patient suffered serious depression and emotional setbacks. My own feelings of being a good analyst soon evaporated. Breaks, especially the longer ones, were traumatic. We came to see that the more important element was not the 'correctness' of my interpretations but the question of her overriding need for me to be there for her, keeping the framework steady. Her word for it was that she felt 'supported'. When I was there and analysis was uninterrupted, she felt that 'God's in His heaven/All's right with the world'. In my absences, the very opposite experience prevailed. Through this material, her dreams and my thinking about my own feelings in being either a wonderful or a terrible analyst (either way being neither a real nor an ordinary analyst), we found that she suffered such profound rage and such disappointment that I could be absent or 'unreliable' that she 'wiped me out' and lost me in internal as well as in external reality, at those times. Yet it was the emotional experience of an analytic relationship that she could in reality genuinely depend upon, even when she was angry and disappointed in the relationship, that enabled her, perhaps for the first time in her life, to relinquish her 'self-reliance' that had always obviated the need for emotionally significant relationships. This led to her beginning to be able to bear her dependency on good objects, to acknowledge their importance and to mourn her losses, If I were to link all this too quickly and too 'knowingly' with her early emotional needs and deprivations, she would have viewed this as yet another 'understanding' interpretation but it would have been one of many that did not offer the possibility of real psychic change.

Patient 2: here is an example of the projective identification process, and how it can facilitate the analyst in his understanding.

My patient, Miss Y, in five-times-weekly analysis, was silent for the first few minutes on a Monday morning. She said she had had a lot to say but now nothing will come. After a while she said that over the weekend she had had a horrible telephone conversation with her former husband, who has been psychotic and alcoholic. He has obtained her telephone number from a mutual friend. She had not heard from him in a long time. He was drunk and very aggressive, pleading and arguing with her to come back to him. He said that she broke her marriage vow that she would stay with him forever.

My patient fell silent for a long time. I asked her what she was thinking, She said, 'Nothing. I have no thoughts.' I asked her what she was feeling. She replied, 'Peaceful.' She wept silently. I began to feel helpless and useless. I felt sleepy. Although she felt 'peaceful,' I now felt that I had abandoned her and was leaving her in something terrible. Yet I did not want to say something just to break the silence and 'make her feel better'. I felt it was important for her to take responsibility for the state she was in and for us to see what came out of it. This led me to say after a short while that she felt quite helpless and that she wanted me to know what it was like to be faced with someone in distress and to be unable to help. I said that her feeling of helplessness made her lose her thoughts.

She replied with a number of thoughts about her husband and her original family, whom she left 'in a mess that [she] could not clear up' to go and live in another country. She felt terribly guilty and bad. But now she thinks that her husband, like her family, must take responsibility for his own difficulties, rather than her taking them on. (She has done that with others all her life.) She added that she feels now that they must take responsibility for the wish to make things better for themselves, rather than her carrying that wish for them.

The concept of the transference has changed greatly from what was first seen by Freud as an impediment to analysis (as for example when a patient threw her arms around him), then as resistance to be analysed, only to evolve much later, into the central tool of analysis. Jung expressed varied and ambivalent feelings about the analysis of transference phenomena, and seemed to feel in awe of its power. He often asserted the view that the transference should be resolved so that analyst and patient can get on with the 'real' relationship and work on individuation. In the early days of psychoanalysis and analytical psychology, 'patients' were seen mainly to be transferring the person of the external object, the actual figure, onto subsequent relationships. A major change in the concept was inaugurated by James Strachey, who observed that it was not the external objects that were transferred but their inner world counterparts, the internal objects, and that this conditioned patients' views of the world. He suggested that understanding the way these inner objects are constructed enables the analyst to promote inner change. Later, Melanie Klein, whose interest and studies throughout her working life were in the area of early emotional experience, soon after her elaboration of the concept of projective identification described something she called 'the transference situation'. She wrote,

'It is my experience that in unravelling the details of the transference it is essential to think in terms of *total situations* transferred from the past into the present, as well as emotions, defences, and object-relations' (Klein, 1952) Betty Joseph (1985, 1985) wrote,

> She went on to describe how for many years transference had been understood in terms of direct references to the analyst and how only later had it been realized that, for example, such things as reports about everyday life, etc. gave a clue to the unconscious anxieties stirred up in the transference situation. It seems to me that the notion of total situations is fundamental to our understanding and our use of the transference today. . . . By definition it must include everything that the patient brings into the relationship. What he brings in can best be gauged by our focusing our attention on what is going on within the relationship, how he is using the analyst, alongside and beyond what he is saying. Much of our understanding of the transference comes through our understanding of how our patients act on us to feel things for many varied reasons; how they try to draw us into their defensive systems; how they unconsciously act out with us in the transference, trying to get us to act out with them; how they convey aspects of their inner world built up from infancy – elaborated in childhood, experiences often beyond the use of words, which we can often only capture through the feelings aroused in us, through our counter-transference, used in the broad sense of the word.

The author is telling us that to a very great extent the transference is now thought about and interpreted through the workings of projective identification. Everything that occurs verbally and non-verbally – action, inaction, the order and style in which the patient presents what he presents, the symbolic content of the words – in short the total situation, is taken into account in the analyst's reflections. Bion and others identified and refined various forms of projective identification, not only defensive or 'pathological' but also 'normal projective identification' for communication. The latter form promotes 'healthy' emotional development when the communications are adequately received and transformed into a form that can be 'thought about'. It is related to, but not identical to, the process of deintegration and reintegration of the 'archetypes' in emotional development.

These various forms of projective identification can be seen from earliest infancy as well as in the analytic process. Studies in infant observation have contributed materially to our understanding of their operation.

There is an important distinction between 'analysing the transference' and 'working in the transference', in my view. The former is a method in which, along with placing emphasis on a number of different areas as part of the analytic process, transference is spotted and perhaps interpreted or referred to, or perhaps just made a mental note of. Working in the transference, by contrast, refers to the use of the transference as the central orientation in the analytic method, a practice that is predicated upon the belief that virtually all the material brought to the analytic session, whether verbal or non-verbal, whether dreams or free associations, communicates something about the ongoing inner relationship between the patient and the analyst. Incidentally, the relationship between the patient and the analyst is not viewed as of greater importance than other relationships, past and present, but the idea is that the analysis of that relationship 'gathers in the transference' from relations in the external and internal worlds into a 'place' where it can be thought about. It is the meaningful relationship in the consulting room, in the 'here and now'.

I am aware that my remarks about transference work may well seem to apply strictly to four- or five-times-weekly analysis, in which there is greater containment of the emotional experience of the patient than in less frequent psychotherapeutic work. I believe that these same principles apply whatever the frequency of the work, although this may dictate the nature of the interpretations.

Much consideration is given to how and when one interprets the transference, which requires skill and forbearance as well as courage and conviction. The subject of interpretation is a very large one that requires much consideration. One works somewhat differently with patients who come less frequently than with those who come for daily analysis. In the first case, the transference often has to be kept in mind to a greater extent, rather than necessarily interpreted openly or in the same way. Undoubtedly one also works differently with different patients and these variations should be given careful thought. Nevertheless the same basic principles apply.

One thing I have found, though, is that with supervision, analysts who thought they could only work once or twice weekly with patients may discover in themselves and in their patients' material that they both want to work more frequently. Anxiety, for both the analyst and the patient, about working so closely and with such emotional intensity is very often the inhibiting factor when on the surface, reasons such as time and money have been given by the patient and accepted readily by the analyst.

Those who work 'in the transference' place considerable importance on waiting for the material to unfold and avoid doing anything that may change the direction of it. This means that the analyst does not begin or structure the session. The patient has a minimum of information about the reality of the analyst's life and background, and about his internal life directly, except that very deep aspects of himself are engaged in his relation to the patient. There must be, moreover, an absence of social or any other contact between the patient and the analyst outside the session. The method also entails special handling by the analyst of all things that arise in the session, whether they are questions that the patient asks (and the way in which he does it), requests, actions, attempts at physical contact, as well as the analyst's private emotional responses. Everything that arises has potentially great meaning in the transference relationship and can potentially inform the analyst as to 'what is going on' in inner object relations.

This method seeks to avoid stimulation through anything other than the inevitable person of the analyst, such as painting or other means of expression, or bringing things to the room. (This is different in the case of child analysis, for special reasons. For one thing, young children are less verbally adept and may use the toys and other materials provided in the way that an adult may use verbal association.) Physical contact of any sort whatsoever with patients may have vast repercussions in unconscious life. So have any actions into which the analyst may be drawn. One patient tried to persuade me to buy her husband's nearly new car at a knockdown price. Another offered gifts. Still another invited me to use his film star friends' ski house in Switzerland. As will be apparent, the analyst who works in this way, 'in the transference', leads a working life of deprivation and self-denial, in a sense. It is also a deeply enriching and rewarding one. The relationship he is offering the patient is very quickly understood as unlike any other, and clearly not a social or a parental one. It is asymmetrical in the absence of all personal information about the analyst. The analyst does not spontaneously say anything that comes to mind, unlike the patient. That does not by any means connote that it is lacking in meaning and intimacy. It is quite the contrary and patients are not slow to understand this. Neither, need it, in my experience, exclude spontaneous warmth and humour.

This rather rigorous and disciplined approach has as its basis what is called 'the analytic attitude' which has been accused of being cold, unfeeling or 'inhuman'. Caper writes,

> While it may seem that the analyst's lack of responsibility for whether or not his interpretations heal the patient is a rather cold and inhuman attitude, and perhaps even an irresponsible one, I would argue that precisely the opposite is true – that only by resisting the urge to achieve a cure with an interpretation can the analyst discharge his primary responsibility to the patient, which is not to heal him, but to help him recover himself.
>
> In the long term, this approach brings great relief to patients, even, or rather especially, to more disturbed ones. I believe that this sense of relief arises from the patient's gradual recognition of the analyst's single-minded, even-handed focus on the business at hand, which is to see what is active in the patient's unconscious at the moment, and why. The effect of this is to relieve the patient of a profound anxiety that his inner world cannot be explored realistically, in a balanced way, without evasion, splitting, or the need to fix it immediately. (Caper, 1991)

Caper also addresses the question of the transference relationship versus the 'real' relationship, to which Jung referred so often and which patients not infrequently feel is lacking in their analysis.

> While the healthy part of even disturbed patients feels relief and gratitude at the analyst's ability to bear the patient's projections (as manifested by his ability to do more than calmly interpret all aspects of his patient's unconscious), a disturbed part of even healthy patients feels that the analyst's exclusive commitment to even-handed interpretation is nothing more than pointless, artificial device. This part of the patient seems to regard transference figures that act out their roles as external phantasy objects as absolutely real, and the

real figure of the analyst as artificial. . . . What leads the patient to feel the analytic relationship is artificial is, paradoxically, the analyst's very insistence on being real – his careful avoidance of the manifold collusions with the patient's unconscious phantasies that the patient expects of him in his role as an external phantasy object. . . . It is therefore quite important to keep in mind, when the patient feels that one is being 'real' and empathic, that one may be unwittingly colluding with the patient's perverse attack on the analyst's, and his own, reality sense.

What is Jungian about this perspective on the transference? I believe, along with Jung in 1913, that the transference relationship has a prospective and developmental function. Might we be permitted, even, to say that the transference is an 'archetype'? It would seem to me to have all the characteristics. As such, it is a function of the self, Let us remember that Jung said that the transference showed all the stages of individuation.

One of Melanie Klein's contributions to the Freudian metapsychology was her introduction of the concept of an inner world in which 'something is always going on'. Informed by the primitive perspectives of early life, the inner world is as 'real' a world as the outer one. It is 'inner reality'. It is seen metaphorically as a 'space', where relations are continually taking place between the subject and his/her objects. These inner figures are effectively archetypal in their quality and their impact. Jung, too, saw the unconscious as a world of figures, quite in distinction to the psycho-analytic thinking of the day. He seemed to understand that what took place there was not mere 'fantasy' but rather a level of reality that governs our thinking and our behaviour. Both Jung and Klein 'told stories' as Michael Fordham said on a number of occasions.

The tension between negative and positive transference phenomena constitutes a balancing of opposites that is always present. It is one of the fulcrums of analytic work in this way. It was expressed by the psychoanalyst W. R. Bion in his formu-lation that the 'paranoid-schizoid' and the 'depressive' positions are always in dynamic tension and that is where the enormous energy of vital life forces is. One of Bion's major formulations is that there is, in one way or another, an inner relationship between what he called the 'contained' and the 'container', the self and the other. It is in this relationship that unbearable states of mind are made suitable for thought; they are made bearable. They have 'names'. In the absence of a good 'container–contained' relationship, there is 'nameless dread'. Catastrophic anxieties expand infinitely into space. This can be seen in dreams, for instance. In the infant's mind, originally, the 'container' is in the mother's capacity for thinking about her baby's experience and the 'contained' is the emotional life of the subject, the baby. This has numerous permutations and ramifications. For one thing, it provides, retrospectively, meaning to the therapeutic effect of the analytic relation-ship. The 'container–contained' relationship is also a concept of Jung's although expressed in different language and a different context. The present idea is perhaps closer to Jung's metaphor of the *vas*, the alchemist's vessel in which transformations take place. As with many of Jung's ideas, here was a profound concept that contained the basis of something that was to be described later on in terms of object relations by clinicians with an interest in emotional development. Projective identification is another of those concepts that can be found in Jung in another form or other words, yet which show his emotional understanding of the later (in this case Kleinian) concept.

What about symbols? In my view, symbols arise within, and may perhaps most effectively be integrated into emotional life through, the analysis of the profoundly meaningful 'I–thou' relationship. Symbols are present not only in a patient's dreams; they exist perhaps ubiquitously, in all the material of the session, and in all of the analysis. Dreams are taken as part of the whole analytic picture, in the context of the anxieties and the defence systems that are of most immediate relevance. Dreams, therefore, are understood in the transference at least as much as the transference is to be understood in the dream.

I would like to discuss what is and what is not very different in the approach of Verena Kast and my own. She works with borderline patients who have difficulties in symbolizing. We seem to agree that what is to be analysed is unconscious mental life and that 'the activation of the unconscious' takes place in a relationship. However, we place very different emphases on the nature of the unconscious mental life to be analysed, and how to do it. We see the material very differently. For instance I do not 'find images' *per se*, generally confining my interventions to the interpretation of the unconscious emotional world of the relationship, often through understandings that derive from the affects and bodily experiences of infancy. This is a 'developmental' rather than a 'symbolic' model, but no less archetypal in its roots. In fact, transference and countertransference might be considered to be archetypes.

I do not feel that transference is 'the distortion of perception in relationships'. It is true that transference can distort relationships, but it is also the essence of relationships, without which they would not exist.

I believe that symbols do not have to be given to the patient. They emerge spontaneously in the analytic relationship. In this sense the analyst analyses what is there, and 'giving symbols' is mainly done through putting unconscious conflicts, anxieties and defences into words. I see the task of the analyst as no less interventionist, but I place much more emphasis on the process, the interaction, than on the content. The danger in the attitude of 'giving symbols' and on 'the analyst's creative act' is of the analyst presuming omniscience and omnipotence. This is no less so when the analyst desires that something should take place, for example that 'the best case' should occur, or even that the patient should have symbols. The 'activation of symbols' is but one possible development, often one which occurs when the patient feels deeply understood over time in both their positive and negative affects and develops a stronger relation to good internal objects. This means that there are fewer 'explanations' and more of a struggle to find meaning. There is little use of terms such as 'mysterious relationship of fusion' and 'communal unconscious' or 'communal relationship', which suggest the wish to deny separateness and to protect both analyst and patient from the painful realities of separateness and differences.

My view is that Kast misses the point of 'the transference' as the analytic frame of reference when she asserts that 'the analysand is not allowed to feel, to think or to experience something which is not connected with the analyst [and the analyst] becomes a very important, omnipresent object'. In my view the patient, or any human being, is always in relation to an object, a meaningful other, and the analytic process both crystallizes and draws the powerful unconscious affects of that relationship onto the person of the analyst. It can then be understood emotionally and transformed in a way that cannot be done in relation to people outside the 'I–thou' relationship.

It must be admitted that working more or less frequently with patients makes a huge difference in the *way* one can work. If one has the privilege of seeing a patient daily, the affects that are aroused are much more containable and it is therefore possible to work in a more personal way that arouses those affects. Nevertheless, it is also noted that one can work less frequently with patients within the same frame of reference without leaving the patient in too much anxiety.

Kast's clinical illustration brings out the differences in our theory and method quite clearly. If I were with this patient, I might focus my attempts at understanding on the process of the interaction. The analyst 'felt immense pressure to invent a good story to save [her patient's] life' and 'got paralysed'. This was valuable information for the understanding of the emotional relationship. As I see it, the patient seems to be drawing the analyst into an experience of basic and extreme fear and challenging her '*to save [the patient's] life*' through responding to her. She is attempting to make the analyst understand the fear of death that has profoundly disturbed her development. 'Telling a good story' seems to have no less importance than being able to engage the object of her love and hate in a relationship in which her murderous feelings can be contained and transformed. I think that the experience of containment, although never straightforward, is to be found through the experience of having her urgency to communicate her fear and despair understood. To reply only to her conscious need and 'offer a symbol' may instead leave the patient as mis-understood as she has always been. It may serve to allay the analyst's anxiety but be a burden to an already burdened patient.

There is an oft-heard opinion that it should be possible to find all the ideas we need within our own theories. This is not confined to our own group. However, I am more of the opinion of a younger colleague, who experienced the following when she attended a group that was composed of students from the different schools, for a case presentation. Someone she met there told her that he had never met a Jungian before and he wondered why she was there. She answered that she feels the analytic community is like a multicultural society: the individual members do not have to lose their identities when they find they can benefit from what others outside their own group have to offer them.

REFERENCES

Caper, R. (1991) 'A mind of one's own'. London: Routledge. Proceedings of the 37th Congress of the International Psychoanalytical Association, Buenos Aires, July. Reproduced in Controversy Eleven of the present volume.

Fordham, M. (1974) 'Jung's concept of transference', *Journal of Analytical Psychology*, 19, 1.

Joseph, Betty (1985) 'Transference: The total situation', *International Journal of Psycho-analysis*, Vol. 66, 4, 447–54.

Klein, M. (1952) 'The origins of transference'. *International Journal of Psycho-analysis*, Vol. 33, 433–8.

Strachey, J. (1934) 'The nature of the therapeutic action of psychoanalysis'. *International Journal of Psycho-analysis*, Vol. 50, 275–292.

(c) Response to Barry Proner

Verena Kast

These two chapters illustrate different ways of viewing the transference–countertransference. Barry Proner refers mainly to Jung's writings around 1910: myself to the 1930s. Our different views speak for themselves and can stimulate ideas, which seems very important in this field. No one has *the* truth. So we need to try to find theories, which are helpful and consistent in themselves, and which can be readily communicated among colleagues. This is why I think that the clinical vignettes have to be as precise as possible, and should be used to promote understanding rather than used as a basis for criticism.

If I compare Proner's views and my own, it seems to me, that facilitating the development of symbols (by way of the transference–countertransference) is more important than the process of transference–countertransference in itself. Symbols are not only vehicles for the individuation process, but also refer to life-history, and future development. Most importantly, they shape the emotions that are connected with complexes, archetypes and the real analytic relationship. I believe that emotional attunement is a very important part of that relationship, and you cannot find that in a vignette, because it is often only conveyed in the tone of voice. But enabling the patient to deal creatively with problems and with life is the central goal of analysis. This capacity can be furthered through the real analytical relationship with its possibilities of new experiences, new ways of relating and better bonding. This is not only important with borderline patients as Proner argues. Although I have of course worked with such patients, they were never my main group.

I see the analytical relationship more in terms of co-creativity and intersubjectivity than Proner. Naturally the concept of the communal or shared unconscious can be used as a defence to deny separateness. This concept of separateness is archetypal – we have to deal with it. But there are moments of something like intersubjectivity (I know that you know that I know), which I believe can be very important in the analytic process. These are not conscious. This communal unconscious can include the constellation of complexes with the archetypal fields behind, as well as more straightforward shared aspects of the analytic relationship. These 'communal complexes' can be demonstrated via the association test. Proner's use of the concept of projective identification incidentally, seems to be very close to the concept of the collusional transference–countertransference that I allude to. But the concept of the complexes seems to me to afford a better understanding of what is going on in these specific situations.

I do not mean to imply that we should find all the ideas we need within our own theories. I think we should be open to different ideas. But we ought to reflect these in the mirror of our own theory. For me it is important to have a coherent Jungian theory of development, not a system of belief. We need a scientific standpoint; and that means questioning what we believe to be true.

Over the years many colleagues have questioned me about Jung's idea of the analytical relationship as an interaction of two systems. Several have asked me where they can find a discussion about this within our group. It seems crucial to me to admit that such a discussion does not really exist.

Finally I would like to remark that I do not agree with Proner that transference and countertransference are 'archetypes'. For me, it is the need for bonding that is archetypal. Archetypes can be understood as ordering or structuring principles, common to all human beings. They allow us to register emotions and information – usually in images – as having meaningful connections. They also promote meaningful and life-preserving behaviour and action in any given existential situation. Transference and countertransference seem therefore to be best regarded as particular instances of an archetypal need. They relate specifically to the analytical process and are not archetypes in themselves.

The political in analysis

CONTROVERSY FOUR

Introduction

Christopher Hauke

Innovations in any discipline are highly difficult and this may be more true of depth psychology than most. We only have to scan its history of ostracism and exclusion – Jung, Reich, Rank and even, to a certain extent, Klein – to discover a conservatism that has been difficult to surmount throughout the twentieth century. Into this comes Andrew Samuels with his ideas around politics and the psyche – not just another application of analytical psychology but a new way of understanding psyche so that our political feelings, thoughts and behaviour become integral to the perspective of depth psychology. Samuels' article summarizes his views on why politics, political passions and the political psyche constitute valid material in the consulting room. He explains his position at length and offers counter-arguments for several of the objections he anticipates. Offering evidence from clinical situations and international workshops with therapists, his writing is persuasive. It is particularly welcomed by many who have had similar clinical experiences but have been without intellectual back-up for their intuitions in the face of psychotherapy's ongoing – but far from universal, as Samuels' survey points out – bias against political material in the consulting room.

Bob Withers takes up the opposing view – but without following the psychotherapy profession's conventional line of objection: he makes no claim for privileging the 'inner' world over the 'outer' as if all clinical material must necessarily be translated into the dynamics of object relations or archetypes. He simply points out that there are dangers in taking up 'outer world' political material without the therapist being fully aware of their own biases and unconscious processes. This might seem an obvious objection – and, indeed, one which Samuels himself counters – but Withers gives several examples (some from his own direct experience) which will give all readers pause for thought. Thus Withers offers a caveat to Samuels' convincingly expressed opinions that fill out the debate and – in the spirit of this book – move it further forward.

(a) Working directly with political, social and cultural material in the therapy session

Andrew Samuels

The roots of this chapter actually lie in a number of recent political developments with which I have been closely involved. I have carried out a number of consultations with politicians in Britain and the United States designed to explore how useful and effective perspectives derived from psychotherapy might be in the formation of policy and in new thinking about the political process. It is difficult to present psychotherapeutic thinking about politics so that mainline politicians – for example, a Democratic senator or a Labour Party committee – will take it seriously. I have found that issues of gender and sexuality are particularly effective in this regard. Partly this is due to the perennial fascination and excitement carried by such topics. Partly it is due to the feminist politicization of such issues over the past thirty years, which has gradually led to their presence on the agenda of mainstream politics. Partly it is because gender is itself a hybrid notion from a political point of view. On one level, in the social world of lived experience, gender and sexuality are everyday realities, suffused with experiences of power, powerlessness, vulnerability and misunderstanding. Gender has its own socio-economic dimensions and set of electoral significances. But, on another level, gender is also an exceedingly private business as part of a story that people tell themselves and have told to them in attempts to produce, create or discover identities and relationships with others. Gender and sexuality are therefore liminal, sitting on the threshold between internal and external worlds, contributing to and partaking of both.

I have also been involved in the formation of three organizations whose objectives are relevant to the content of this chapter. Psychotherapists and Counsellors for Social Responsibility is a professional organization intended to facilitate the desire of many psychotherapists, analysts and counsellors to intervene as professionals in social and political matters making appropriate use of their knowledge and, it must be admitted, whatever cultural authority they possess. The second organization is a psychotherapy-based think-tank, Antidote. Here, the strategy has been to limit the numbers of mental health professionals involved so as to reduce the chances of psychotherapy reductionism and foster multidisciplinary work in the social policy field. Antidote has undertaken research work in connection with psychological attitudes to money and economic issues generally, and is also involved in work in the area of 'emotional literacy', but expanding the usual remit from personal relationships and family matters to include issues in the public domain. The third organization is a broad front based at St James's Church in London. The St James's Alliance consists of individuals from diverse fields such as politics, economics, ethics, religion, non-governmental organizations, the media and psychotherapy. It attempts to incorporate ethical, spiritual and psychological concerns into the British political agenda and to facilitate a dialogue between non-governmental organizations, single-issue groups and progressive political organizations. It is an experiment in gathering in political energy that is split up and dissipated under current arrangements.

It will be thought that psychotherapists and analysts such as myself are making these moves from on-high and from a detached position, careless of the political issues affecting our own profession. However, all three organizations have been active in and profoundly affected by the acrimonious yet relatively successful campaign waged by elements of the psychotherapy profession to end discrimination against lesbians and gay men as candidates for training in psychoanalytic psycho-therapy and psychoanalysis. When psychotherapists engage in politics they need to do so with a degree of consciousness of the appalling mess in which their own professional politics are usually to be found, as well as irony or even self-mockery as regards the counter-intuitive and slightly mad content of much of what they have to say.

WHAT SHALL WE DO ABOUT POLITICS?

In this chapter I explore how the practice of psychotherapy might be politicized so that therapists and analysts who seek to work with the whole person, including the social and political dimensions of the experiences of their clients, may do so with greater confidence and clarity. I believe this detailed work has not really been done yet. I shall not be focusing much on the external and internal political dynamics of the therapy encounter itself and hardly at all on the aforementioned politics of the profession, though these both remain concerns of mine. Therapy is embedded in politics and culture; therapy has its own politics and culture. These are pretty obvious points by now. Instead, I intend to present some ideas about the relationship of therapy practice to politics. Although these ideas derive from work with individuals, they may be even more pertinent and useful in group analysis and psychotherapy. The group matrix may facilitate the politicization of the practice of therapy rather well (see Brown and Zinkin, 1994: passim; and see endnote 1).

By 'politics' I mean the concerted arrangements and struggles within an institution, or in a single society, or between the countries of the world for the organization and distribution of power, especially economic power. Economic and political power includes control of processes of information and representation to serve the interests of the powerful as well as the use of physical force and possession of vital resources such as land, food, water or oil.

On a more personal level, there is a second kind of politics. Here, political power reflects struggles over agency, meaning the ability to choose freely whether to act and what action to take in a given situation. This is often a feeling-level politics, a politics of subjectivity, a politics to which feminism introduced us.

But politics also refers to a crucial interplay between these two dimensions, between the public and the personal dimensions of power. There are connections between economic power and power as expressed on the domestic, private level. Power is a process or network as much as a stable factor. This version of political power is experienced psychologically: in family organization, gender and race relations, and in religious and artistic assumptions as they affect the lives of individuals.

Where the public and the private, the political and the personal, intersect, I think there is a special role for analysis and psychotherapy in relation to political change and transformation. The tragicomic crisis of our *fin de siècle* civilization incites us to challenge the boundaries that are conventionally accepted as existing between the external world and the internal world, between life and reflection, between extroversion and introversion, between doing and being, between politics and psychology, between the political development of the person and the psychological development of the person, between the fantasies of the political world and the politics of the fantasy world. Subjectivity and intersubjectivity have some political roots; they are not as 'internal' as they seem.

There is little point in working on the orientation of psychotherapy to the world of politics if its own basic theories and practices remained completely unaltered. I support the continuing practice of therapy and analysis with individuals and small groups. This is because I do not agree that analysis and therapy inevitably siphon off rage that might more constructively be deployed in relation to social injustices. In fact, I think that it is the reverse that often happens: experiences in therapy act to fine down generalized rage into a more constructive form, hence rendering emotion more accessible for social action. Even when this is not what happens, the potential remains for a move from private therapy to public action – and I propose to discuss that potential in this chapter.

The idea is to develop a portrayal of the clinical setting as a bridge between psychology or psychotherapy and politics, rather than as the source of an isolation from politics. Critics of the clinical project of depth psychology (e.g. Hillman and Ventura, 1992) have noted the isolation – and this is not a totally wrong observation. But I want us also to see the potential links and to create a truly radical revisioning of clinical work, not a simplistic huffing and puffing aimed at its elimination.

One of the most potent criticisms of therapy and analysis is that the client is encouraged or even required to run away from external concerns – for example, political commitments – and focus exclusively on the 'inner world'. This, it is argued, makes any statement about therapy engaging the whole person an absolute nonsense (see endnote 2). Textbooks of therapy and analysis accentuate the introspection by making it clear that exploration of outer world issues is simply not done in 'proper' therapy and analysis.

Humanistic psychotherapy in its early days seemed to have this kind of vision of therapy in mind but, since the growth of a desire to integrate psychoanalytic thinking, humanistic psychotherapists seem to have adopted a psychoanalytic professional ego-ideal or even superego. When I made this point at the 1997 Professional Conference of the United Kingdom Council for Psychotherapy, the numerous humanistic psychotherapists present clearly knew what I was talking about (Samuels, 1998).

Over a period of time, I sensed that this professional consensus was collapsing and that therapists and analysts were indeed beginning to pay more attention to what could be called the political development of their clients (ibid. pp. 134–137). In my own practice I noticed that many clients seemed to be introducing political themes more often than they had before. Talking to colleagues confirmed that this was also going on in their work, so it was not all due to suggestion on my part. We tended to put it down to the fact that, since the mid-1980s, the pace of political change in the world appeared to have quickened. At times, I still felt that the usual formulation – that such material needs to be understood as symbolic of what is going on in the client – worked pretty well. At other times it turned out that the client had a need to talk about some public issue, maybe to work out what their true feelings and opinions were. But the client might also have learned that you are not supposed to do that in therapy or analysis. For example, during the Gulf War there were certainly some clients who used war imagery to tell me something about their inner state. Yet there were others who were hiding a profound need to talk about the Gulf War behind the flow of regular, ordinary clinical material.

I decided that what was needed was a large-scale investigation, by means of a questionnaire, to see if analysts and therapists were experiencing something similar in significant numbers. I therefore obtained the cooperation of 14 professional organizations with differing theoretical orientations in 7 different countries and sent out 2,000 survey forms. I got a return rate of almost exactly one-third (quite high for a cold-calling survey on which the respondents had to spend some time and write fairly lengthy and thoughtful answers).

In the survey, I asked which themes of a list of fifteen possibles were the most frequently introduced by clients. This produced a worldwide league table as follows: (1) gender issues for women, (2) economic issues (e.g. distribution of wealth, poverty, inflation), (3) violence in society, (4=) national politics, and gender issues for men, (4=) racial or ethnic issues, (6) international politics.

There were some striking departures from the order. For instance, the German analysts placed 'the environment' at the top of the list as the most frequently introduced issue whilst for the British psychoanalysts economic issues came in seventh. This enables us to make all kinds of speculations about whether there is or is not something like a 'national psyche' or, 'collective consciousness', at least as evidenced in the political themes the clients of therapists and analysts bring to their sessions.

I asked the participants how they reacted to, handled or interpreted the material. Seventy-eight per cent of the respondents mentioned that they understood the material as referring in some sense to reality. For many, this was in conjunction with a symbolic interpretation or an exploration of why the client was interested in that particular theme at that particular moment. The replies – thoughtful and extensive – showed considerable struggle by the respondents as they endeavoured to mark out their positions.

I went on to ask if the respondent 'discussed' politics with his or her clients. Of course, I realized the explosive nature of the question and deliberately did not define what might be covered by the word 'discuss'. Worldwide, 56 per cent said they did discuss politics and 44 per cent that they did not. American Jungian analysts do the most discussing (72 per cent) and British psychoanalysts the least (33 per cent). However, it is interesting to note that the implication of the one-third 'yes' of the British psychoanalysts is that 43 of them admit to discussing politics with clients (one-third of the 129 respondents).

I asked the respondents the obvious question: 'Have you ever been/are you politically active?' Sixty-seven per cent said they had been politically active at some time – a figure which unsurprisingly, dropped to 33 per cent at the present time. My intuitive impression, just from talking to colleagues, that a good many of them had been politically active at some time was borne out. The stereotype of a profession composed of introspective, introverted, self-indulgent types was challenged.

So what might it all mean? In the most down-to-earth terms, it could mean that if a person is contemplating analysis or therapy, and if that person is interested in politics (however defined), it would be as well to explore with a potential therapist or analyst what they are likely to do if one brings political material to the consulting room. For the profession is clearly divided about it. Even if everyone who did not return the survey forms abhors politics in the consulting room, there is still a significant minority of practitioners who do not. This other, hitherto unknown group of clinicians sees that involvement in and concern for the world is part of growing up, of individuation, and maybe even part of mental health. The split in the therapy profession is at its most destructive when it is between the public, apolitical, hyperclinical face of the profession – something that has quite rightly been criticized – and a much more politically aware, private face of the profession. Many therapists and analysts seem all too aware that they are citizens too, that they have political histories themselves, that they too struggle to find the balance between inner-looking and outer-looking attitudes. As a British psychoanalyst put it when replying to the questionnaire:

> We are political animals. Everything we are and do takes place within a political framework. It is impossible to divorce this from the inner world of either our patients or ourselves.

The survey on political material brought to the clinical setting was not a scientific instrument, nor even a conventional social scientific instrument. Nevertheless, several eminent social scientists have kindly commented that my methodology not only resembles certain cutting-edge practices in social science ('naturalistic research') and was appropriate to my project. The survey has been published in a leading sociology journal (Samuels, 1994). Hence I hope that discussion of the survey will not only focus on issues of methodology, thereby distracting us from my overall thesis, which is that as psychoanalysis and psychotherapy move into the next century, the range of material suitable for clinical investigation should expand to include political themes and issues. If this were to happen, then we would move one small step nearer to realizing the ideal of an analysis of the whole person. Moreover – and maybe this is the crucial thing – therapists and analysts would also move one small step towards realizing the century-old project of depth psychology to shed light on what Freud referred to as 'the riddles of the world'. (See Samuels, 1993: 209–266 for a fuller account of the survey.)

POLITICIZING THERAPY PRACTICE

When attempting to link psychoanalysis or psychotherapy with political and social issues, we need to establish a two-way street. In one direction travel men and women of the psyche, bringing what they know of human psychology to bear on the crucial political and social issues of the day, such as leadership, the market economy, nationalism, racial prejudice and environmentalism. Going the other way down this street, we try to get at the hidden politics of personal life as broadly conceived and understood: the politics of early experience in the family, gender politics, and the politics of internal imagery, usually regarded as private. The dynamic that feminism worked upon between the personal and the political is also a dynamic between the psychological and the social. It is so complicated that to reduce it in either one direction (all psyche) or the other direction (all sociopolitical), or to assert a banal, holistic synthesis that denies difference between these realms is massively unsatisfactory. There is a very complicated interplay, and this chapter trades off the energy in that interplay. One hope is to develop a new, hybrid language of psychology and politics that will help us to contest conventional notions of what 'politics' is and what 'the political' might be. The aspirations of so many disparate groups of people worldwide – environmentalists, human rights activists, liberation theologians, feminists, pacifists and peacemakers, ethnopoliticians – for a reinvested and resacralized politics would gain the support of the psychological and psychotherapy communities.

It is worthwhile focusing on therapy and on clinical work for two main reasons – first, because the results of the survey show that this is a hot issue for practitioners just now; second, because exploring the politicization of practice might help to answer the awkward question: why has the political world not shown up for its first session with the therapists who are so keen to treat it? Freud, Jung and the great humanistic pioneers like Maslow and Rogers truly wanted to engage with the institutions and problematics of society. But they, and even more their followers, did this in such an on-high, experience-distant, mechanical fashion, with the secret agenda of proving their own theories correct, that the world has been, quite rightly, suspicious. Objecting to psychological reductionism in relation to political and social is reasonable – not resistance. But what if clinical experience were factored in? At the very least, there would be a rhetorical utility. For, without their connection to the clinic, to therapy, why should anyone in the world of politics listen to the psychotherapeutic people at all? What do we have to offer it if does not include something from our therapy work? Therapy is certainly not all that we have to offer, but it is the base.

The professional stakes are very high. In certain sectors of humanistic and transpersonal psychology clinical work is becoming more overtly politicized so that the whole client may be worked with. But this is still very much a minority view in the psychodynamic and psychoanalytic sectors of psychotherapy. Politically speaking, most clinical practice constitutes virgin territory. The stakes are so high because what people like me are trying to do is to change the nature of the field, change the nature of the profession – that which we profess, believe and do. As the survey showed, this attempt is part of a worldwide movement in which the general tendency is to extend the nature of the psychotherapy field so as to embrace the social and political dimensions of experience.

If we do want to treat the whole person, as some of us do, then we have to find detailed ways of making sure that the social and political dimensions of experience are included in the therapy process regularly, reliably, and as a matter of course. We must try to achieve a situation in which the work is political always already – not unusually, not exceptionally, not only when it is done by mavericks, but when it is done in an everyday way by Everytherapist.

The detailed work is not easy to do. About seven years ago a remarkable book appeared entitled *Psychoanalysis and the Nuclear Threat: Clinical and Theoretical Studies* (Levine *et al.*, 1988). All the editors and all the contributors were the most *echt*, kosher psychoanalysts one could find – they were all, in fact, members of the American Psychoanalytic Association. The following passage appears in the editorial introduction:

> In the best of circumstances analysts may assume that considerations of politics are irrelevant to the analytic space. We raise the possibility here that the potential of nuclear weapons for destroying the world intrudes into the safety of that space. We no longer live in the best of circumstances. Thus, the construct of a socially, culturally, and politically neutral analytic setting may be a fantasy, one that embodies the wish that the outside can be ignored, denied, or wished away.

In a basically favourable review of this book, the psychoanalyst and social critic Alexander Gralnick stated:

> Unfortunately, few of the contributors to the theoretical part of the book deal with the many important assumptions and unsettled issues in psychoanalytic

thought and clinical practice that the editors hoped consideration of the nuclear threat would prompt them to discuss. . . . Though bound by traditional concepts, some authors seemed to recognize that psychoanalysts may not be as neutral as they believe themselves to be. . . . These psychoanalysts are plagued by their own resistances and anxieties about the further changes they face and how creative they dare be; they are naturally limited by being at the *earliest stages of* changes we all face, and, like the rest of us, are handicapped *by lack of a needed new language.* (1990: 68; emphases added)

I too, am at the earliest stages of this project, and I, too, am handicapped by the lack of a much-needed new language. These thoughts and speculations are my best shot.

I shall eventually be discussing and proposing the politicization of therapy practice under the following headings:

1 The therapeutic value of political discussion in the session.
2 Exploring the political myth of the person in therapy.
3 The hidden politics of internal, private imagery.
4 Citizen-as-therapist – a therapeutic model for political engagement.
5 Working out a socialized, transpersonal psychology of community.

However, as the project has developed, I have found it useful at the outset to attempt to deal with, or at least discuss, the objections to what is being proposed. In this way, readers are alerted to my own awareness of the radical and often risky nature of these ideas. Moreover, dealing first with the objections resembles good psychoanalytic technique whereby resistance is analysed before content. Of course, the objections are not only resistance and I am convinced that an ongoing engagement with objections (and objectors) to the politicization of therapy practice is enhancing for all sides in the debate.

The first objection is that removing the focus of the clinical enterprise away from the internal world and onto the political world constitutes bad clinical practice. The reply to that objection can be equally assertive. Foreclosure on politics, the privileging and valorizing of the internal over the external, may, as we stagger towards the end of the century, itself constitute bad clinical practice. From today's perspective, maybe I do want or need to do some bad practice as I change my practice. Those who do not or cannot change their practices may, from tomorrow's point of view, be the ones guilty of bad practice. What is or is not 'on' in clinical technique has evolved strikingly over the psychoanalytic century. These matters are not definitively settled.

The second objection concerns the problem of suggestion and undue influence on the part of the therapist. This is a sensitive issue these days, given the moral panic surrounding psychotherapy stemming from the notion of false memory syndrome. Is there a risk that a politicized therapy practitioner will foist his or her own political ideas, principles, and values onto the vulnerable, open-to-suggestion client? Would not that be a shattering objection to the politicization of therapy? In reply, I would ask if we are really supposed to believe that a practitioner who sticks to the way he or she was trained and keeps the political out of the consulting room is thereby devoid of the sin of ever suggesting anything to the client. Many studies show that an enormous amount of influencing by the therapist of the client goes on, and in fact may be essential for some kind of psychological movement to happen. At times, even Freud equates transference and suggestion, making a defensive point which also serves me well: you cannot suggest something into somebody unless they are ready for it, unless it 'tallies' with what is already alive in them. I would use Freud against the objection. Suggestion is going on already. There is no reason to suppose that a politicized practitioner would necessarily be intruding his or her own values more than somebody whose interest was in object-relations, sexuality, aggression, spirituality or the soul.

Of course, there is always a risk of discipleship in the psychotherapy situation as those who have had training therapy know. But I feel confident in saying that there is today a huge amount of uncritically accepted suggestion in clinical practice and that, from a certain point of view, the more 'bounded', 'contained' and 'disciplined' the behaviour of the practitioner, the more suggestion is taking place in his or her practice. I think this is inevitable. The technical rules of analysis are not politically or culturally neutral; they do more than 'facilitate' the unfolding of the self. They have themselves cultured depth psychology in a permanent way, and they have themselves done it to a certain extent by suggestion. On the basis of the replies received to the questionnaire on political material that is brought to the consulting room, it is clear that a good deal of rule-breaking goes on in ordinary therapy and analysis – probably much more than is revealed in supervision, wherein words like 'discussion' are dirty words. If psychotherapists and analysts are already discussing politics with the client, then it is clear that the hygienic sealing of the consulting room from politics is a virginal fantasy on the part of practitioners.

The third objection concerns what is to be done when the therapist is confronted with somebody with political views he or she finds repulsive. Discussing my ideas at a meeting of the British Association of Psychotherapists, I was once asked: 'what would happen if Hitler came into your consulting room?' Well, psychodynamically speaking, I think I have seen quite a few Hitler-types in my consulting room already. Although this point cannot settle the very real worries that working with somebody whose views you find repulsive creates, surely we can agree that, from time to time, every practitioner will meet a version of this problem. Moreover, politics is not the only source of repulsion.

A fourth objection concerns the alleged elitism of what I am proposing. Do I have some kind of fantasy that we are going to send a well-analysed vanguard of the psychopolitical revolution out into the world? Of course I have had that fantasy from time to time but, in a more moderate vein, and in terms of developing an argument about changing the field, I do not for one minute think that a person who has had psychological analysis or therapy is in some kind of elite vanguard. However, as indicated, I do recognize that there is some strength in this objection, and I try to stay conscious of the problem.

The fifth objection is extremely subtle and hence difficult to deal with. This objector claims that he or she is carrying out a political therapy practice already. Sometimes I feel that this is undoubtedly the case. At other times, when I am told that the mere practice of therapy, or even just the making of interpretations, are political acts, I must demur. Similarly, when it is blandly observed that all of inner life obviously involves the outer world, including politics, and there is no point in going on about it, I feel I need to know about the fate of the outer world in therapy done by such an objector. I think it is a sign of the times that many practitioners do not want to admit to working oblivious to the world of politics. The rules of the game are changing. And, as the survey shows, it is clear that many people are trying to work in a more politically attuned way. But the mere recognition that inner and outer are connected cannot constitute a politicization of practice. This is a difficult objection to engage with, being told that politicizing practice is all old hat and that everyone is doing it. It injures the narcissism of the pioneer!

A sixth objection concerns the scope and timing of political work in therapy. I am often asked if these ideas are applicable to every client. Of course, they are not. There is a further question in connection with timing and it is certainly important to wait and see where the client is headed. This is easy to say, but I think there may be a smear in the way this objection is sometimes posed, in that the not-so-secret intent is to characterize political work as inappropriate and likely to be done in a clumsy way. Sometimes, a politicized therapist will mistime or misplace his or her interventions. But therapists often take ideas derived from object-relations or archetypal theory or psychosexuality and make use of them in situations where these ideas turn out to be woefully inappropriate and irrelevant. It happens all the time and it is not meant as damaging to the client. Somehow 'politics' is singled out as more likely to lead to such an abuse of the client.

While there is little doubt that political action outside the therapy entered into by a client can be defensive or resistant, this is surely not always the case. Sometimes, when working with politically active clients, there has come a move from within the client to withdraw from politics for a while – and this is, of course, respected. Nevertheless, we might perhaps question the psychoanalytic (or maybe the bourgeois) depreciation of action in general and political action in particular. Political action is psychologically valid, positive and creative. Not to act would sometimes constitute a special form of repression – a repression supported by the institutions of therapy and analysis themselves.

A seventh objection shows the professional politics of the psychoanalytic world at their worst. Consider this reply written by a senior British psychoanalyst to the questionnaire that asked him how he relates to, deals with and manages overtly political material brought to the clinical situation. This is a highly intelligent and articulate man, but attend carefully to the didactic way in which the party line is delivered:

> Although I believe that the insights of psychoanalysis . . . are highly relevant
> to political and social structure, and am (broadly speaking) committed to a

leftish political set of beliefs, most of the questions you ask seem to me to be based on a very profound misunderstanding of the nature of psychoanalytic treatment, in which the analyst's listening to the patient takes place within the framework of the analyst's theory of transference: everything the patient says has meaning in other contexts and much of what he reports and says will be more or less true and relevant in such contexts, but in the context of the psycho-analytical session, the meaning which it is the analyst's job to apprehend is that concerned with what the patient is communicating to the analyst at that moment about the state of his internal fantasy relationships and fantasy transference relationships to the analyst.

Naturally (indeed very often) the patient will turn to political or Political issues from time to time, but it is not the analyst's job to take these at face value or to discuss them in the ordinary sense with the patient. While my experience suggests some people (even analysts) can get confused on this point, and get caught up in being teachers or counsellors or advisers (or even sympa-thizers or opponents) in the consulting room I think it is absolutely clear that the principles of psychoanalytic treatment (as they were set out by Freud and subsequently developed by psychoanalysts) do not provide a basis for a psychoanalyst qua psychoanalyst to relate to his patient's material except as I set out above.

The point I would make here is that one cannot engage with the political in the consulting room without engaging with the politics of our profession itself.

These seven objections do need to be taken seriously and I think I have taken them seriously. I have tried to suggest where there is some mileage in them, and where I think a firm reply can be made.

THE THERAPEUTIC VALUE OF POLITICAL DISCUSSION

Now I want to move on to the first of my positive proposals concerning the thera-peutic value of political discussion in the session. Here, I will bring in the experiences of important practitioners in other fields who sought to politicize the practices of their own fields.

The German dramatist Bertolt Brecht conceived of the idea of a politicized theatre and developed a whole body of practices to go with that notion. Some of his practices, which constitute a sort of Brechtian clinical theory, are relevant to psychotherapy. For example, consider his well-known idea of the alienation effect, or 'distanciation effect'. Via certain technical theatrical devices, the audience is encouraged to step back and to distance itself from the drama going on on the stage in order to apperceive more clearly what the social, political and economic dynamics of the drama are. The intention is that the audience should not only identify emotionally with the characters in the play but should also try to understand and analyse what it is that those characters are doing. Brecht replaces involvement in theatre with what I would call 'exvolvement'. In psychotherapy practice, it is possible to conceive of a therapeutic situation in which therapist and client get exvolved, without worrying that this could be a transgression of the principle that requires maximum emotional involvement and identification with the issues being processed in the therapy. Brechtian exvolvement serves, in very general terms, as a helpful model for the introduction of political discussion in the session as a therapeutic tool.

Another parallel is even more pertinent, and it concerns certain developments in feminist art practice, in particular what could be described as the framing of the everyday. For example, in 1976 the feminist conceptual artist Mary Kelly produced a work which became notorious, called *Post-Partum Document*. This was a record of her evolving relationship with her son over the first few years of his life. The part that everybody remembers, and on which I will concentrate, is the first room of *Post-Partum Document* in which the only works on show were the faeces – and urine-stained nappy (diaper) liners of this little boy, backed by white vellum, well framed and hung on the walls of the Hayward Gallery in London. The condition of the nappy liner showed how ill or healthy the baby (or his bowels) were at any one moment. Kelly could therefore track and comment upon her 'success' as a mother. The irony and political pointedness were deliberate.

A similar art work was created by Care Elwes in 1979, called *Menstruation 2*. Seated on a clear perspex stool in a clear perspex booth in a white, diaphanous dress with no underwear or sanitary towels during the time of her period, she would allow the menstrual blood to flow, staining the garment, all the while dialoguing with an audience that surrounded this booth about what the wider implications of her female bodily processes were, what they meant to her, and about what the audience thought was going on.

Mentioning these art works is not intended to start a discussion about conceptual and feminist art. But these works worked because the ordinary was framed, whether in the traditional frame of a picture, in which the artist puts a stained nappy liner, or by the frame of the perspex booth in which a bleeding woman stains her garments before spectators and discusses it with them. My argument is that political discussion within the therapy frame will be different from ordinary political discussion in bar, living room or workplace. Just as menstruation, framed in the way I described, ceases to be menstruation and becomes conceptual art and has an impact in the cultural sphere, so, too, a discussion of politics in a therapy situation that, if transcribed, would look ordinary takes on a wholly other significance. Contained within the therapy vessel or frame (itself a therapy term), the ordinary becomes something other, and enters the psychological processes of therapist and client in a way that may be profoundly unsettling, possibly clarifying, and occasionally transformative. If we seek to explore the meaning and relevance of the political for ourselves and our clients, then an espousal of political discussion, in which the therapist has to make all the usual therapist's decisions about his or her degree of involvement, openness and about the timing, is one way to proceed. Perhaps it is necessary to try it to see what happens. For a practitioner reading this who already discusses politics with clients, maybe these thoughts will help to theorize what is presently being done on an intuitive or ethical basis. There are simply no books or articles about the matter.

THE POLITICAL MYTH OF THE PERSON

The next proposal concerns what I call the political myth of the person. Is there such a thing as a person's political development? just as we refer to psychological development generally, or people talk about how they have or have not developed over a lifetime, there might be a way of approaching politics on the personal level that can make use of the idea of development without getting hooked up on linear, normative and mechanistic notions of development.

How does the political person grow and develop? An individual person lives not only her or his life but also the life of the times. Jung told his students that 'when you treat the individual you treat the culture'. Persons cannot be seen in isolation from the society and culture that has played a part in forming them – as much feminist thinking has demonstrated.

Once we see that there is a political person who has developed over time, we can start to track the political history of that person – the way the political events of her or his lifetime have impacted on the forming of their personality. So we have to consider the politics a person has, so to speak, inherited from their family, class, ethnic, religious, and national background, not forgetting the crucial questions of their sex and sexual orientation. Sometimes, people take on their parents' politics; equally often, people reject what their parents stood for. Social class often functions within the unconscious and sometimes I have found that it is the social class issues of the socially mobile client's parents that are truly significant.

But all this is a bit too rational. If there is something inherently political about humans – and most people think there is – then maybe the politics a person has cannot only be explained by social inheritance. Maybe there is an accidental, constitutional, fateful and inexplicable element to think about. Maybe people are just born with different amounts and kinds of political energy in them.

If that is so, then there would be implications both for individuals and for our approach to politics. What will happen if a person with a high level of political energy is born to parents with a low level of it (or vice versa)? What if the two parents have vastly different levels from each other? What is the fate of a person with a high level of political energy born into an age and a culture that does not value such a high level, preferring to reward lower levels of political energy? The answers to such questions shape not only a person's political myth but the shape and flavour of the political scene in their times.

The questions can get much more intimate. Did your parents foster or hinder the flowering of your political energy and your political potential? How did you develop the politics you have at this moment? In which direction are your politics moving, and why? I do not think these questions are presently on either a mainstream or an alternative political agenda. Nor are they on the agenda of many therapists or analysts.

My interest is not in what might be called political maturity. No such universal exists, as evaluations by different commentators of the same groups as 'terrorists' or 'freedom fighters' shows. My interest is in how people got to where they are politically and, above all, in how they themselves think, feel, explain and communicate about how they got to where they are politically – hence my reference to the political myth of the person. From a psychological angle, it often turns out that people are not actually where they thought they were politically, or that they got there by a route they did not know about.

In therapy, we can explore how the client got to where he or she is politically and, above all, how the clients themselves think, feel, explain and communicate about how they got to where they are politically; a subjective narrative of political development. We ask how a person became a Hampstead liberal, not whether being a Hampstead liberal is a good thing in itself – whilst not denying that we have a viewpoint about Hampstead liberals. Moreover, not all Hampstead liberals became Hampstead liberals in the same way. We want to know how Hampstead liberals have experienced their becoming Hampstead liberals.

When a client describes his or her political experiences, in the sense of formative or crucial political experiences, an analyst or therapist would listen with the same mix of literal and metaphorical understanding with which he or she would listen to any kind of clinical material – but with the ideas of political myth and political development in mind as permanent heuristic presences. Sometimes, the most productive path to follow would be to accept the client's account of his or her political history; at other times, what the client may have to say may be understood as image, symbol and metaphor; at other times, as defensive and/or distorted; sometimes, it will be a melange of these ways of understanding; sometimes, a tension or competition may exist between them. In a sense, all of this moves us towards a conception of what could be called the 'psychological citizen'.

The implications for depth psychology of taking in these ideas about political development could be profound. In 1984 I suggested to my fellow members of the training committee of a psychotherapy organization that we should start to explore with candidates something about their political development – its history, roots, antecedents, patterns, vicissitudes and current situation – just as we looked into sexuality, aggression and spiritual or moral development. At that time, the idea was regarded as a bit way out, but more recently it has evoked a favourable response. Similarly, if political and social factors are part of personality and psychological development, should not analysts and therapists explore those areas in initial interviews with prospective clients?

Incidentally, here, as so often, I have found that what looks like new theory is really only a necessary theorization of cutting-edge practice. In the survey, when I asked the respondents to say something about their own political histories and what had influenced their own political development, they tended to cover the same ground as I have covered in this section of the paper, though with very wide linguistic, conceptual and hermeneutic variations.

Why do I refer to political 'development'? Might this not be rather conservative from an intellectual standpoint? There are now numerous books on 'moral development', 'spiritual development', 'religious development'. And 'the development of personality' is a well-researched and much-argued-over field. So the general idea of development seems to be in the *Zeitgeist*. The idea of development is obviously intended to be applied as non-normatively, non-judgementally and non-positivistically as possible, though it will be as well for me to admit immediately that my own personal political beliefs and values will enter the picture and help to bring a kind of hierarchy into play. This is absolutely unavoidable, but I do not believe that my having beliefs and values of my own makes me any less neutral than or different from theorists in the fields of moral, spiritual, religious and personality development who undoubtedly have moral, spiritual, religious and psychological positions of their own to defend and privilege.

THE HIDDEN POLITICS OF PRIVATE, INTERNAL IMAGERY

The image of the parents in bed

My first proposal about the hidden politics of private, internal imagery concerns the primal scene – the image of father and mother together, the image of their intimate relationship, whether in bed or not. I have suggested on several occasions that primal-scene imagery functions as a kind of psychic fingerprint or trademark. Now I want to extend that idea in a political direction, to argue that the kind of image held of the parents' relationship to each other demonstrates, on the intrapsychic level, a person's capacity to sustain conflict constructively in the outer world – a crucial aspect of the person's political capacity. In the image of mother and father in one frame, the scene can be harmonious, disharmonious, one side may dominate the other side, one parent could be damaging the other parent, there will be patterns of exclusion, triumph, defeat, curiosity or total denial. These great and well-known primal-scene themes are markedly political. How they work out in the patient tells us something about that patient's involvement and investment in political culture and his or her capacity to survive therein.

I see the primal scene as a self-generated diagnostic monitoring of the person's psychopolitical state at any moment. The level of political development is encapsulated in the primal scene image. This is why images and assessments of the parental marriage change so much in the course of therapy or analysis. The parental marriage is not what changes in the majority of instances. Nor is it merely an increase in consciousness on the part of the patient which makes the image change. The image changes because the patient's inner and outer political styles and attitudes are changing. And the specificity of the image communicates what the new styles might be. The parents stand for a process as well as for particular attributes and capacities.

The experience of primal scene imagery may be additionally understood as an individual's attempt to function politically, coupling together into a unified whole his or her diverse psychic elements and agencies without losing their special tone and functioning. A sort of universalism versus multiculturalism on an individual level. What does the image of the copulating parents tell us about the political here-and-now of the client? The image of the parents in bed refers to an unconscious, pluralistic engagement by the client with all manner of sociopolitical phenomena and characteristics, many of which appear to him or her as so unlikely to belong together (to be bedfellows) that they are 'opposites', just as mother and father, female and male, passive and active sexual partners are said to be opposites, or 'whites' and 'blacks', or Israelis and Palestinians, or Catholics and Protestants, or rich and poor are regarded as irreconcilable political opposites.

Thus the question of the image of the parents in bed as a harmonious coming together of conflicting opposites can be worked on in more detail, according to the degree and quality of differentiation a person makes between the images of mother and father. For a primal scene only becomes fertile when the elements are distinguishable. In plain language, it is not a stuck image of parental togetherness that we see in a fertile primal scene, but something divided and unstuck, hence vital – but also linked, hence politically imaginable. The psyche (society) is trying to express its multifarious and variegated nature (multiculturalism) – and also its oneness and integration (universalism). Primal scene images can perform this pluralistic job perfectly and the message they carry concerns how well the job is going. Via primal scene imagery, the psyche is expressing the patient's pluralistic capacity to cope with the unity and the diversity of the political situation he or she is in. As Aristotle said, 'Similars do not a state make.'

I do not think that the reproductive heterosexuality of the primal scene should to be taken as excluding people of homosexual orientation. Far from it: I am convinced that the fruitfulness signified in the primal scene, and the problems therein, are completely congruent with homosexual experience. I also think that there is a set of cultural and intellectual assumptions that need to be explicated. Why is it that psychological fecundity, variety and liveliness do not yet get theorized in homosexual terms? Why is psychological maturity still envisaged in a form of complementary wholeness that requires heterosexual imagery for it to work at all? Why do we not refer to a conjunction of similars? One could easily defend the thesis that heterosexual primal scene imagery works quite happily for persons of a homosexual orientation by recourse to metaphor, saying that primal scene heterosexuality refers not to the fact of reproduction but to the symbol of diversity, otherness, conflict, potential. Similarly, one could also point out that, since everyone is the result of a heterosexual union, heterosexual symbolism is simply inevitable and not excluding of a homosexual orientation. But I am dubious about these liberal manoeuvres because they still leave a question mark in my mind concerning the absence of texts replete with homosexual imagery that would perform the psycho-logical and political functions of primal scene imagery. We might begin a search for the homosexual primal scene. Though this idea may sound controversial, it merely involves a recognition that the primal scene is about processes and functions and not about the actual parents. Hence the proposition that there could be a primal scene couched in gay or lesbian imagery will only cause problems to homophobic members of the psychotherapy world. We know by now how much psychoanalytic theory about homosexuality is little more than dressed-up prejudice, marching in step with the moral majority.

Personal narratives of primal scene imagery, and their working through, demonstrate to a considerable extent a person's capacity to sustain political conflict constructively. This general point about politics becomes more pertinent when applied to the professional politics of the field of depth psychology. Stuck parental imagery fits the field's symptoms of intolerance, fantasies of superiority, and diffi-culties with hearing the views of others. If depth psychology's primal scene imagery could be prodded into vigorous motion, perhaps by active ideological dialogue, I would feel more optimistic about its future.

The example I shall soon be giving of these ideas concerning political readings of primal scene imagery is the well-known general problem of not being able to imagine the parents' sexual life at all, or of having a bland and non-erotic image of it. Clearly, denial and repression play important parts in this, but my argument will be that to restrict our understanding to these personal ego-defence mechanisms is to cut ourselves off from the plenitude of collective and public meanings in primal scene imagery.

Before discussing the 'non-primal scene', I want to say something further about why the primal scene is so important for politics. One particular reason for choosing to focus on the primal scene is that we are then invited to address the conventional twinning of man with active and woman with passive sexual behaviour. This twinning both reflects and, I think, inspires many gender divisions. When individ-uals access and work on their primal scene imagery, often in fantasy or via the transference in analysis, it is remarkable that the conventional male/active–female/passive divide does not invariably appear. Quite the reverse. In fact, it often seems as if the unconscious 'intention' of the sexual imagery associated with the primal scene is to challenge that particular definition of the differences between men and women. The challenge to the sexual status quo symbolizes a kind of secret challenge to the political status quo.

From the standpoint of gender politics, this discussion of the political relevance of a primal scene enables us to introduce the mother in a transmogrified and politicized form, as an active player in the sexual game and hence, potentially, as an active player in the political game.

Here, I am reminded of the midrashic story of Lilith. She was, as readers will recall, the first consort of Adam, who was created from the earth at the same time as Adam. She was unwilling to give up her equality and argued with Adam over the position in which they should have intercourse, Lilith insisting on being on top.

'Why should I lie beneath you', she argued, 'when I am your equal, since both of us were created from dust?' But when Lilith saw that Adam was determined to be on top, she called out the magic name of God, rose into the air, and flew away. Eve was then created. Lilith's later career as an evil she-demon who comes secretly to men in the night (hence being responsible for nocturnal emissions) and as a murderer of newborns culminated, after the destruction of the temple, in a relationship with God as a sort of mistress. Lilith's stories are well documented by scholars of mythology. The importance for us is that the woman who demands equality with the man is forced to leave the Garden and gets stigmatized as the personification of evil.

What of the missing primal scene, the inability to imagine the parents' sexual life that I referred to earlier? I regard this non-primal scene as deriving in the first instance from a colossal fear of the consequences of conflict. (Again, sexual conflict symbolizing political conflict.) For, if the bodies of the parents are not in motion, then psychological and sociopolitical differences between them, including asymmetries and inequalities, need not enter consciousness. Over time, consciousness of political problematics impacts on the individual's internal processes, his or her capacity to experience different parts of the self in their own particularity and diversity whilst at the same time sensing that they participate in the whole in a more or less coherent sense of identity. The denied primal scene signifies a loss of faith in the political nature of the human organism and of society itself. Conversely, images of vigorous, mutually satisfying parental intercourse, including, perhaps, some kind of struggle for power, reveal a private engagement with the conflictual dynamics of the public sphere.

In my workshops, I get participants to do the following exercise. I ask them to divide a sheet of paper vertically. In the left-hand column, they are to list (1) their earliest memory (or fantasy of their earliest memory) of their parents' physical intimacy; (2) the same at adolescence; (3) the same today. In the right-hand column, they should list (1) their first political memory or the first time they became aware of political conflict; (2) their politics at adolescence and their general attitude to politics at that time; (3) the same today. The participants are asked to take home the piece of paper with its two columns – primal scene and politics. All they are asked to do is to reflect on what has been written down, scanning the entries in the two columns referring to each point in time and the developmental process revealed by a comparison of the two columns. The feedback has been fascinating; perhaps present readers would like to try the exercise.

Dream imagery

An Italian client dreamt of a beautiful lake with clear deep water. He said this represented his soul and then immediately associated to the pollution on the Italian Adriatic coast. The image of the lake, and the association to coastal pollution, suggested, in the form of one symbol, the client's unconscious capacity for depth and his present state, of which he was all too conscious – a state of being clogged up by 'algae', like the coastal waters of the Adriatic. When disparate psychological themes are thrown together like this, the symbolic image makes a powerful impact on the individual, who cannot ignore it. In this particular instance, the notion that there was possibly a 'solution' for the clogging up of his lake/soul potential, and the idea that being clogged was a state he had gradually got into over time and was not a witch's curse, together with the vision that depth and clarity and beauty were options open to him, were powerful and liberating thoughts for the client to entertain. He made a choice to return to Italy, to tell his father that he was homosexual, and, in his words, to 'get more involved', perhaps in environmental politics.

Returning to the dream of the lake, I would like to suggest an alternative reading, couched in more political terms. I think that this re-reading constitutes a further statement about the political properties of private, internal imagery. The images of the dream can be approached via their individual presence, or via their political presence, or via the movement and tension between the two. In the dream of the lake, the tension between the individual and the political presences of the image was prominent and insistent; after all, the client was Italian. What, the client and I asked together, is the role of pollution in the soul, or even in the world? What is the role of pollution in the achievement of psychological depth? Can the soul remain deep and clear while there is pollution in the world, in one's home waters? Did the lake, with intimations of mystery and isolation, clash with the popular, extroverted tourism of the Adriatic? Eventually, the patient's concern moved onto the social level: who owned the lake? Who should have access to such a scarce resource? Who would protect the lake from pollution? These were his associations. From wholly personal issues, such as the way his problems interfered with the flowering of his potential, we moved to political issues, such as the pollution of natural beauty, not only by industry but also by the mass extroversion of tourism. And we also moved back again from the political level to the personal level, including transference analysis. I do not mean to foreclose on other interpretations, but rather to add in a more 'political' one so that the client's unconsciously taken up political commitments can become clearer.

I think much imagery can be understood in therapy as performing this particular kind of transcendent or bridging function, transcending and bridging the gap between the apparently individual, private, subjective and the apparently collective, social, political. Much of this chapter argues for the general thesis that there is a constant relationship and articulation between the personal/subjective and the public/political dimensions of life. Can we discriminate these separate dimensions in such a way that eventually we can, on a more conscious level, better bring them together? I think we do find that private, internal imagery carries a public and political charge. Moreover, we need to be better placed to make practical, clinical use of the, by now conventional, observation that the external world, particularly its social and power relations, has an effect on our subjective experience.

Applying this approach to imagery to a psychological analysis of the politics of the client, we would try to discriminate the individual and the social aspects of an image and see whether they can be brought to an equal level of consciousness. This process would increase the range of choices available to the client, rather than collapsing them into a solution. In the example, the question of ownership of the lake at first seemed a distant 'political' concern. But gradually the client's social sensitivity came to the fore: he asserted that the lake, like his soul, was not a commodity to be owned by anyone. Then a celebration of his social conscience came to the fore. He addressed the fate of his 'Italian-ness' on a personal, individual level. Finally, as the hidden politics of his imagery continued to pulse, he discovered more collective, cultural and political associations to pollution on the Adriatic. I hope it is clear that the public/political and private/ subjective dimensions were both thoroughly alive.

This interpretive reworking of the imagery onto a sociopolitical level provides the beginnings of a model by which therapists and clients can track moves between individual and social realms and a means of studying conflicts and harmonies between culture and individual as these appear in the session. For individual and culture are not the crude opposites that many, including Freud, have taken them to be. Both terms enjoy the complex interaction produced by their dynamic relationship; the relationship changes the nature of the original 'opposites'. The more deep and personal the experience, the more political and public it may turn out to be.

The politics of imagery now operates, in the external world, at a pace that often precludes rational debate. If we are to avoid being permanently after-the-event – an unending social deferred action or *Nachträglichkeit* – then we have to try to engage with the political dimensions of psychological imagery.

CITIZEN-AS-THERAPIST

My fourth proposal concerns ways in which the client, by modelling his or her thought processes and actions on those of the therapist, can find in the *method* of therapy itself a source of empowerment. Incidentally, the use of the word 'empowerment' does not preclude the recognition that its use may be disempowering. Whoever empowers has power; whoever is empowered lacks power. But this postmodern cliche has its own intellectual and moral limitations – in Hillel's words: 'If I am not for myself, who will be for me? If I am only for myself, what am I? And if not now, when?' Many clients (and therapists too) ask how we can translate our emotional, bodily and imaginative responses to Bosnia, to ecological disaster, to homelessness, to poverty worldwide, into action. How can someone begin to make political use of their private reactions to public events?

There is a sense in which this is the key political theme of our times: the ways in which we might translate passionately held political convictions – shall we call them political dreams? – into practical realities. I think it is possible to take a subjective approach to a political problem, maybe one that has been fashioned out of personal experience, and refashion that response into something that works – actually works – in the corridors of power. From a client's point of view, it is his or her political impotence and the consequent despair, hopelessness and self-disgust which may be addressed.

Virtually everyone reacts to either the political issues of the day or the political dimensions of experience in a private and often heartfelt way; but most of us diffidently assume that our cloistered responses are not really of much use in the objective world of 'real' politics. Even though we all know there is no objectivity when it comes to politics, we behave as if there were, in obedience to an ideology of civic virtue that cannot abide passion in the public sphere. For the powerful fear the dissident fantasies of the radical imagination.

Clinical therapy and analysis ponder the same kind of problem: how to translate the practitioner's private and subjective responses to the client (the 'counter-transference') into something that can, eventually, be fashioned into a useful intervention.

In their widely differing ways, therapists and analysts have, over time, managed to work out how do this – and this is my point. Therapists and analysts have already managed to privilege and valorize their subjectivity, seeing how its very construction within the therapy relationship gives it the potential to provide a basis for useful intervention in the session.

Therapists and analysts already have texts that teach them how to translate their impressions, intuitions, gut responses, bodily reactions, fantasies and dreams about clients into hard-nosed professional treatment approaches. They already have the idea that their subjective responses are precious, valid, relevant, effective – and there is some knowledge about how to do something with those responses.

So, without realizing it perhaps, we – therapists and clients – in the world of psychology and therapy do possibly have something that could be shared with the disempowered, with political activists – or made use of when we ourselves get politically active. For example, most clinicians know that their bodily reactions to the client's material are a highly important pathway to the client's psychic reality. Similarly, it is possible to honour and deploy the bodily reactions citizens have in response to the political world and the culture's social reality. After all, just as client and therapist are in it together, so, too do citizen and political problem inhabit, quite literally, the same space.

All citizens, not just those involved in therapy, could start to function as therapists of the political world, learning to use their bodily and other subjective reactions as organs of political wisdom, helping them to understand the problems of the political more deeply and guiding the course of their actions. It would be another way to speak the political.

The evolution of a kind of political knowledge analogous to the therapeutic encounter would reflect the fact that so many people already possess a therapeutic attitude to the world. Many of us want to participate in nothing less than the resacralization of our culture by becoming therapists of the world. But it is hard to see how to go about it. I certainly did not invent the notion that citizens have bodily and other subjective reactions to the political – we all know of that from our own experience of our own bodies and our own subjectivities in the political world. But it may be a novel contribution to suggest, as I do, that the political, with its problems, its pain, its one-sidedness, may actually be trying to communicate with us, its therapists. Does the political really want therapy? Will it come to its first session? Will the unconscious of the political and the several unconsciousness of us, its therapists, get into good-enough communication?

Here I am trying to do something with what is already known about citizens and the political – but not, as yet, much theorized over. I see this 'therapeutic' way of speaking and doing politics, not as something regrettable, an over-personal, hysterical approach to politics; rather, I see it as one path left open to us in our flattened, controlled, cruel and dying world. What official politics rejects as shadow – and what can undoubtedly still function as shadow – turns out to have value. Is that not a typical pattern of discovery in therapy anyway?

Putting the citizen in the therapist's seat is itself a dramatic and radical move. For, in many psychoanalytic approaches to politics, the citizen is put firmly in the patient's seat, or on the couch: citizen as infant. Then the citizen has to be regarded as having only an infantile transference to politics. It is certainly not as empowering as having a countertransference and it is the therapist's right to speak – the therapist's power – that I want clients to seize hold of and to spread around.

This strategy for empowerment is a further psychological extension of that fundamental feminist insight that the personal realm reflects the political realm, that what we experience in the subjective world can be the basis of progressive action and change in the political world.

I am trying to explore these ideas at public workshops as well as in therapy sessions. At a workshop in New York shortly after the Los Angeles riots of 1985, I asked a largely non-professional audience to imagine themselves as 'therapists' of a 'client' called 'the LA riots' and to record their physical, bodily and fantasy responses to their client (i.e. to track the 'countertransference'). Unexpectedly, just doing the exercise itself created a cathartic effect. Participants eagerly reported how they had often reacted somatically or in other markedly subjective forms to political events. But they feared these responses would not pass muster in everyday political discourse. Their conception of politics was conditioned by the notions of 'objectivity' that I mentioned earlier; they had bought the con trick of the powerful.

When we came to discuss the riots in more rational vein, a whole range of novel, imaginative and practical ideas about urban and ethnic problems came out of the group process of this audience. Moreover, 'the political' was redefined, reframed, revisioned. Most of those present did not believe that there were avenues available in official political culture for what often gets stigmatized as an irrational approach. I think their assessment is right. Utilizing a perspective derived from one hundred years of the practice of therapy, in which so-called irrational responses are honoured and heeded, is a small beginning in creating a new, more psychological approach to the problems of power and politics.

Lest it be thought that only an American audience could manage to do the exercise described just now, let me say that I have found similar reactions in Brazil, working with people in liberation theology, in Leningrad (as it then was) working with young Russian therapists hungry to marry their inner worlds with what was going on around them, and in Britain.

I feel that this kind of politics, this other way of speaking the political, favours participation by those who are presently on the margins of power: women, gay men and lesbians, members of ethnic minorities, those in transgressive families, the physically challenged, the economically disadvantaged, psychiatric patients. These are the people with whom therapists and clients should stand shoulder to shoulder, in the same ethos of unknowing and humility and respect for the wisdom of the other that characterizes all good clinical work.

For those diverse groupings should not be regarded as Marx's hopeless lumpen-proletariat. Rather, they are the last untapped sources of new energies and ideas into the political and social realms. Disempowered people certainly do need the kind of economic and financial transfusions that only politics of the official kind can presently broker. But they also need validation from the profession that makes its living and derives its authority – its power – out of working with the feelings, fantasies, behaviours and embodiments that are banned and marginalized in life in the late modern world. There is a potential in everyone to be a therapist of the world. Throughout our lives, all of us have had private responses to politics. We need to raise to the level of cultural consciousness the kind of politics that people have carried within themselves secretly for so long. The therapy client, armed with therapy's own power to make something useful out of subjectivity, can take his or her place as citizen-as-therapist.

A SOCIALIZED, TRANSPERSONAL PSYCHOLOGY OF COMMUNITY

In contemporary Western politics the buzz word is 'community'. Aside from the politicians, many clients also speak in therapy of a sense of pulling together that used to exist and is now lost. They feel the loss keenly. For other clients, the idea of community is more proactive, referring to a new kind of egalitarian politics based on their belief in what is shared, held in common, faced together. Communitarian thinking will (hopefully) both refresh our ideas of the state and, for many amongst this group of clients, of the power dynamics of the therapeutic relationship.

It is extraordinary that in the many lucid discussions about community that are taking place, there has been little space for a psychological contribution. Communitarian politics requires an overtly socialized psychology and when we try to create one we find that it will have, at some level, to be a transpersonal psychology. Politics is also a transpersonal activity and, like most transpersonal activities, politics points in what can only be described as a spiritual direction. Psychotherapy is not a religion, though it may be the heir to some aspects of conventional religion. The project of factoring the psychological into the political seems to want to be done in quasi-religious language. Perhaps this is because psychotherapy, politics and religion all share, at some level, in the fantasy of providing therapy for the world. The very word 'fantasy' must, I am sure, create problems for some readers. Fantasy is not in itself pathological and there is a necessarily utopian role for fantasy in political discourse.

Sometimes I see psychotherapy as a new monasticism, meaning that just as the monks and nuns kept culture in Europe alive during the so-called 'Dark Ages', so, too, in their often equally rigorous way, the therapists and analysts are keeping something alive in our own age. However, the values that psychotherapy keeps alive are difficult to classify. They do not always have the ring of absolute Truth (though such a possibility is not ruled out); nor are they based on a fixed account of human nature (though that is what is invariably being attempted, time and again). In its discovery of values and value in that which other disciplines might reject, psychotherapy helps to keep something alive in the face of threats ranging from state hegemony, to vicious market forces, to nostalgic longings for a return to a past in which it is assumed that the old certitudes of nation, gender and race would still hold.

We sometimes hear calls for a global ethic or a global sense of responsibility to be placed at the heart of political theory and the political process. My question is: how can this be done without some kind of psychological sensitivity and awareness? Such sensitivity and awareness may not be easily measurable by the sturdy tools of empiricism but reveal themselves in dream, in parental and primal-scene imagery, in an understanding of a person's own political history, development and myth. Hence, clinical work on oneself coexists with political work in one's society.

My working out of a 'clinical' model with which to engage political problematics is intended to make every citizen into a potential therapist of the world. An active role for the citizen-as-therapist is highlighted, and nowhere will this be more apparent than in relation to experts (myself included). People's active, generative, inventive, compassionate potential is not being tapped and, as I see it, in order to tap into that kind of energy we need a reinvention of politics inside and outside the therapy session.

NOTES

1   I have tried to be careful in my use of the words 'politics' or 'the political', 'culture', 'society' and the 'collective'. By 'culture', I mean the assembly, limited in time and space, of the social, material, mental, spiritual, artistic, religious and ritual processes of a relatively stable and sizeable community. I use the words 'society' or 'societal' in the following senses: the means by which relations between individual and others are structured; the institutions that cause differences between individuals to acquire significances beyond those individual differences; whatever promotes learnt forms of behaviour and communication that excite support and approval or condemnation and punishment; relations between organizations and groups. The 'collective' implies what is held in common, ranging from a biological/phylogenetic use of collective to something like the collective atmosphere in a crowded theatre or soccer stadium.

2   I am aware that there are problems with the use of the term 'person'. I think that the need to retain some idea of the person is necessary when we consider the political dimensions

of life. Paradoxically, my speculations about the political person and the political development of the person are part of, not in opposition to, attempts to decentre the habitual focus of psychoanalysis on an individual by evoking the place of the in-between, thus helping to dissolve the logic of inner and outer. Nor am I forgetting the wounded and grieving nature of the late modern or postmodern political person: that is why politics is a matter for therapists.

The present chapter first appeared in *Clinical Counselling in Context*, edited by John Lees, Routledge, 1999.

REFERENCES

Brown, Dennis and Zinkin, Louis (1994) *The Psyche and the World: Developments in Group-Analytic Theory*. London: Routledge.

Gralnick, Alexander (1990) Review of Levine, Howard *et al.* (Eds), Psychoanalysis and the Nuclear Threat: Clinical and Theoretical Studies. *International Journal of Mental Health*, Vol. 20, no. 1, 67–69.

Hillman, James and Ventura, Michael (1992) *We've Had a Hundred Years of Psychotherapy and the World is Getting Worse*. San Francisco, CA: Harper.

Levine, Howard *et al.* (Eds) (1988) *Psychoanalysis and the Nuclear Threat: Clinical and Theoretical Studies*. Hillsdale, NJ: Analytic Press.

Samuels, Andrew (1993). *The Political Psyche*. London: Routledge.

Samuels, Andrew (1994) 'Replies to an international questionnaire on political material brought into the clinical setting by clients of psychotherapists and analysts'. *International Review of Sociology*, Vol. 3, 7–60.

Samuels, Andrew (1998) 'Responsibility', in *Development through Diversity: The Therapist's Use of Self*. London: United Kingdom Council for Psychotherapy.

(b) Politics in practice

Robert Withers

INTRODUCTION

Politics, like sex and religion can be relied on for more than its fair share of controversy. So considering how best to approach political material occurring in the course of analytic therapy seems fitting in a book about analytical controversies, especially since most therapists have probably wondered at one time or another how best to work with their client's political issues. Having said that, in this chapter, I will be arguing against the radical revisioning of therapy in response to such material. I will be making three main points.

Firstly in therapy, as in most walks of life, it is generally advisable to replace a particular practice, only when the old one is demonstrably damaging or counterproductive. It will be my contention, with certain provisos, that this has not been demonstrated with regard to conventional analytical psychotherapy's approach to political material.

Secondly if a practice is replaced, it is up to the innovator to show that the new one will not cause more harm than the one it is replacing. I will be raising various doubts and questions about this in relation to the sanctioning of 'political discussion' in the course of therapy. In particular I will be questioning whether the therapist can become involved in such discussions without the client's individuation process becoming obstructed through the imposition of the therapist's own unconscious material. Underlying this doubt is the assumption that therapy is not an equal relationship, because one person pays another for expert help with their problems. That help, is dependent upon the therapist being able to *listen* to the client – and their own countertransference responses – in a therapeutic way.[1] It is hard to see how this therapeutic listening can be combined with active involvement in political discussion.

Thirdly I will be drawing on my own personal analyses to show what can happen in practice when therapists do get drawn into political discussions with their clients. This in my experience is often far from therapeutic.

1 Freud (1912), Bion (1967) and others have characterized this therapeutic listening as an 'evenly suspended attention' or as an analytic 'reverie', while Fordham (1993), referring to Reik (1949), talks of listening with the 'third ear'.

Proviso

There can be little doubt, however, that over the years analysts of all persuasions have tended to reinterpret their patient's concerns about the 'outside world' in terms of their own particular theoretical preoccupations. So during Melanie Klein's (1961) wartime analysis of Richard, she was interested in the Oedipal aspect of his fear of Hitler invading Britain, not its realistic elements. And when Donald Meltzer (1978) re-examined the case, he did so in the light of his own theoretical preoccupation with the transference, if anything offering even less recognition of Richard's real concerns about the course of the war.

It also seems indisputable that the psyche regularly picks up on, and reacts to, events in the outside world, often without full conscious awareness of this. This seems to have happened for example when the participants in the legendary controversial discussions were locked in battle about the place of hatred and aggression in their psychological theories. On that occasion Donald Winnicott attempted to bring the protagonists to their senses by famously remarking, 'I should like to point out that there is an air raid going on' (Grosskurth, 1985: 321), highlighting (perhaps unconsciously) the connection between the battle in the room and the one going on outside.

It is hard therefore to disagree with Samuels' contention that analytical psychotherapists have often failed to give due weight to both their client's conscious concerns about the outside world and their unconscious reactions to it. I will be arguing, however, that it *is* possible to adequately address those concerns and reactions without the radical revisioning of therapy he advocates. On this view it is the analyst's own preoccupations that have tended to exclude the client's concerns about the world from the consulting room – not something intrinsic to the analytic process. The deliberate politicization of analysis along the lines suggested by Samuels is therefore at best unnecessary, and at worst counter-therapeutic.

I will be using a mixture of recent case material and my own experience as an analytic patient to support these contentions. Initially, however, I wish to touch on Samuels' paradoxical finding that, despite not being involved in a war (at the time of writing), therapists seem, if anything, more willing than ever to discuss politics with their clients. Could this be indicative of anything more than the quickening pace of political change in the world alluded to by Samuels in his article?

The intrusion of the political

For James Hillman (1994) the answer is an emphatic 'yes'. The intrusion of politics into practice is a symptom of psychotherapy's attempt to put an end to itself. The psychotherapy of individuals, he argues, has traditionally been concerned with the self, with ego-strength and with individuation. In this way it has reinforced an alienated post-Cartesian world-view, which sees us as isolated individuals living in a dead material world. He welcomes the intrusion of politics into practice as a return of the world soul to undermine that world-view in its inner sanctum. And he regards the ordinary analytic reluctance to discuss politics as a pathological defence against the threat of that intrusion. He has gone on to give up practising individual therapy which, he now believes, is inimical to his broader project of bringing soul back to the world.

Samuels is familiar with Hillman's arguments, and is clearly sympathetic to his overall project. But he falls short of advocating the end of individual psychotherapy. In fact Samuels' article can be read as an answer to Hillman – an attempt to defend therapy from his attacks by defining the conditions under which therapists and their clients may legitimately involve themselves in political discussions. On a practical level, for example, he argues that the containment of the analytic frame can render such discussions therapeutic. And he backs this up theoretically by proposing that each person could be regarded as possessing an innate political potential. The realization of that potential would then become as much a part of a person's individuation process as the fulfilment of their work or love life, and discussing politics a part of routine analytic work. The following personal experiences, however, seem to highlight some of the dangers inherent in Samuels' proposals.[2]

POLITICS IN PRACTICE

The first analysis

I began my first analytic training with an organization that attempted to integrate psychoanalytic and Jungian ideas, in the early nineteen-eighties. My analyst, who was suffering from age-related ill health, had been a communist in her youth and was still a Marxist sympathizer (as was I). She was on a direct line of analytic descent from Freud, and had set the training up. It soon became apparent, however, that the organization was in the throes of a traumatic power struggle. This struggle directly affected me in various ways, and I was flattered and grateful, but also a little uneasy, about my analyst's frank discussion of the related political issues in therapy with me. These issues were complex, but one important strand concerned the conflict between her Marxist-inspired desire to provide therapy for the people, and the emerging organization's more 'conservative' wish for the 'highest' possible training standards. Thus the frequency of analytic sessions for trainees became a subject of heated debate, for instance. In England these political strands are represented by the colours red and blue respectively.

> One day I dreamed that I was attempting to enter a large department store through a revolving door. There were guards on the door. I managed to evade

2 As regards the apparent increase in political material in analysis, I suspect that this is largely due to the greater general openness to multiple discourses that characterizes much of our postmodern world. In analytic terms this would translate into a lessening of the insistence that 'proper analysis' is *really* about one particular thing, whether that thing is the inner world, the transference, the archetypes or anything else (see Hauke, 2000, and McLeod, 1997).

them and get into the building, but there was still an unpleasant paranoid atmosphere. I went into a lift and found myself naked as it began to descend. Ducking anxiously into a nearby storeroom in the basement I found some clothes. Some were blue and some were red. I was unable to make up my mind which to put on, but to my relief found some purple ones and left the storeroom in them.

Purple of course is a combination of red and blue, but I am less concerned with the meaning of this dream, than with my analyst's reaction to it. When I related it, she responded by asking if I was mad. I sat up on the couch in some alarm, and obviously terrified she declared that one of us had to be mad. That day someone else had had exactly the same dream and that was not possible. She then proceeded to lapse into a florid paranoid psychotic breakdown. Some months later when she had somewhat recovered she told me it was she who had had the same dream, and also that this had not been her first psychotic episode. Not surprisingly, perhaps, this incident brought about the total collapse of the therapeutic relationship and also undermined my first training experience.

Nowadays all reputable therapeutic organizations insist that their members take part in continuing professional development programmes, which ensures that analyst's work is regularly monitored and helps to prevent the occurrence of such events. Certainly the actual psychotic breakdown of the analyst in a session is extremely rare, and therefore perhaps best dismissed as an unfortunate one-off experience. I have included this incident in the present account, though, because I believe it illustrates a general problem in an extreme form. If the therapist shares her political beliefs with the client, it may encourage him to identify with her position rather than evolve one of his own. The unconscious dynamics underlying that identification will then tend to get enacted, rather than analysed in the exchange of political views. Of course the same process could occur in relation to other emotive topics on which the analyst expresses an opinion. But the passions and judgement that are an intrinsic part of politics make it especially prone to this danger. In this case the unconscious identification with my analyst seems to have somehow produced a shared dream. Perhaps she experienced this as intrusive and conceivably this contributed to pushing her into a psychotic state (Searles, 1959).

If my first analysis illustrates the potential for political discussion to promote an engulfing amalgam of analyst and client, my second illustrates the opposite danger.

The second analysis

My new analyst, a Jungian, was, like my first, a Jewish refugee from the Nazis. I soon found out she had understandable but particularly strong feelings about the interminable Arab–Israeli conflict, which then, as now, was in a state of eruption. Material related to this often entered the sessions. I dreamed at the start of the analysis for instance that:

I was in a desolate wasteland/garden up an old tree picking plums, which I was passing down to Sigmund Freud who was collecting them in a basket. A disembodied voice ordered everyone to leave. The Israeli air force was about to bomb the garden, which would then be concreted over to make way for some sort of commercial development.

I will return to some interpretations of this dream towards the end of the paper. For the moment, however, I will continue with the theme of the intrusion of politics into this analysis.

I sometimes brought my outrage about Israeli rocket attacks on Palestinian refugee camps into sessions. My highly respected analyst, excellent in many other ways, felt compelled to get drawn into political discussions on such occasions. She would 'inform' me for instance of the 'fact' that the Palestinians had sold their lands to Israeli settlers and were deliberately maintaining refugee camps unnecessarily in order to court international sympathy. Perhaps she believed that she was helping me become conscious of things I was unconscious of in this way. But I experienced her as more concerned to force me to adopt her views than understand (the unconscious motivation underlying the expression of) mine. I would leave these sessions feeling angry and cheated.

When I voiced these feelings she responded by wondering about the transference and countertransference. Was I perhaps re-enacting with her an adolescent rebellion I had been unable to have with my father? This felt a bit more like analysis, but in fact arguing about politics with my father had been one of the many pleasures of our relationship. What is more, I felt my differences of opinion with him had been respected in a way they were not with her. Our impasse continued, and I brought this material for a long time looking for some sort of resolution or understanding that never came. But I eventually desisted and resigned myself to potentially excluding important elements from my analysis in the process.

I can see now that I probably unconsciously contributed to this unresolved conflict myself, partly perhaps as a means of avoiding a repetition of the disastrous identification with my first analyst. My second analyst's willingness to get involved in political discussions with me, however, meant that this went completely unanalysed, along with my yearning for fusion, my fear of that yearning, and the work of mourning my first analyst. In addition, her aggressive defence of Zionism meant that I was able to split off and project my own aggression into her. The work of reintegrating it thus got blocked, as we became stuck in a paranoid-schizoid way of relating (over this issue).

Generic dangers

These personal experiences have no doubt contributed to my distrust of political discussions in analytic sessions. But I believe they also illustrate some generic problems and dangers.

The first concern is that Samuels' proposal to politicize analysis could encourage 'reactive' as opposed to 'reflective' analysis out of the countertransference. Both my analysts seem to have enacted their countertransference feelings in their political discussions with me, instead of reflecting on them and using them in the service of the analysis.

Samuels no doubt would argue that such 'reactive analysis' happens already when analysts let slip their views about morality, religion, relationships etc. But of course that does not mean such practices should be condoned. On the contrary they nearly always distort the analytic process, and interfere with the client's individuation. The effects of this can be very hard to acknowledge and work through. Since the judgements that are an inevitable part of political discussion make it especially likely to stir up powerful emotional reactions, underlying unconscious material can easily become obscured. How can therapy be protected from these effects?

The above experiences seem to show that the existence of the analytic frame per se affords absolutely no protection whatsoever.

In addition, in practice the client is likely to feel pressured to adopt the analyst's political views, especially in a training analysis. But even if he reacts against this pressure, he is not really developing his own position.

On a related note, the spectre of the Nazis and of totalitarian communism is not so distant a memory as to rule out the nightmare scenario of analysis being used as a means of social and political control, with opposing political opinions being treated as pathological. To a certain extent this probably happens already when politics is discussed in analysis. And the ongoing computerization of health and police records, together with the right of courts to access 'confidential' patient notes, adds another dimension to such fears. Perhaps the reluctance of many analysts to get further mixed up in politics could be understood in this light.

I expect Samuels would argue, however, that he is not supporting the sort of analytic practices I am describing above. In fact he would probably regard his proposals to selfconsciously politicize analysis as aiming to counteract such malpractice. But if this is the case, he fails to show how those proposals might actually help that aim be achieved.

He advocates the introduction of 'political discussion' into ordinary analytic work for instance without identifying what he means by this. Is he talking about 'discussion' in its ordinary sense – an exchange of personal political views between client and therapist? If he is, it is hard to see how this type of discussion could ever be therapeutic – for the reasons outlined above. Or does he have some specialized type of discussion in mind? He might for instance envisage the specific use of political discussion to facilitate dialogue between different parts of the client's psyche. This looks more therapeutically promising, and it does seem to tally with the one relevant piece of clinical material he presents.

That material, it will be recalled, involved an Italian man who dreamed of a beautiful, isolated, deep, clear lake. He associated the lake to himself and contrasted it with the Adriatic coast and its tourism and pollution. Samuels used this material to facilitate a dialogue between a part of the client that wished to withdraw from the emotional pollution of the world, and another that wished to engage with it in political activity. This material seems at first sight fairly innocuous. It also seems similar to the sort of work many of us are doing or trying to do already. But, as we have seen, Samuels treats the client's political potential as possessing a special innate or constitutional factor. So at this point he would have to be very careful not to allow a theory-driven privileging of political action to lead him to underestimate the importance of the call for withdrawal from the world in his client's dream material.

Of course there are practitioners of holistic medicine – Engel (1977), Pietroni (1996), Broom (1997) etc. – who rely on a 'bio-psycho-social' model of health. They do link mind, body and social concerns in their work, and their practices may be informed by analytic understanding. But they would not claim to be practising analysis when they work in this way. Analysts who wish to continue practising analysis tend to refer their clients to colleagues for medical treatment rather than risk falling prey to therapeutic omnipotence by consulting with them themselves – even if they are medically qualified. I believe that analysts who engage politically with their client's material risk falling prey to a similar therapeutic omnipotence.

At this point a further question arises: 'Why stop at politics?' Why is political discussion any more therapeutically central, important or innately determined than discussion about physical health, the desire to retreat from the world, or any number of other subjects?

Hillman revisited

But if political discussion in therapy is no longer sanctioned by appealing to the special status of 'political potential' in individuation, then how can analysis be protected from Hillman's attacks on it? Furthermore could the above account of my two analyses not be regarded as lending further ammunition to those attacks?

It is true that my first analysis was indirectly ended via the intrusion of politics. Hillman would presumably regard this as symptomatic of individual therapy's healthy wish to put an end to itself. It seems to me, however, to be more symptomatic of the difficulty my analyst and I had in working with the unconscious processes underlying our shared political material and was the result of a *departure* from standard analytic practice. If I am highlighting the failures in both my analyses, it is in the hope that something useful can be learned from them – not in order to attack analysis. In fact I benefited in different ways from both analyses, despite their difficulties.[3]

Hillman it will be recalled objected to analysis on the grounds that it reinforces a Cartesian world-view of ourselves as isolated masters of a soulless world. And this may well be true of a kind of psychotherapy that emphasizes ego strength at

3 At this point I would like to thank both my analysts' heirs for kindly granting permission to publish this sensitive material – and also Andrew Samuels whose 'response' to this paper alerted me to the wisdom of seeking that permission.

the expense of the unconscious. But analytic psychotherapy, it seems to me, asserts the precise opposite of this. It posits the otherness of the unconscious at the heart of the self and thereby subverts the sovereignty of the ego. This is profoundly undermining of the kind of isolated individualism Hillman opposes, especially when that unconscious includes a collective (Jung) or linguistic (Lacan) element. In addition, of course, the relational aspect of much contemporary analytic practice further undermines individualism. For all these reasons I would argue that Hillman is mistaken when he regards the apparent analytic exclusion of politics as a symptom of its resistance to the overthrow of the Cartesian world-view. That view has been subverted already. Hillman, however, is presumably quite aware of these arguments. It seems likely therefore that his opposition to analysis springs from personal frustration with its rigours rather than from high-minded philosophical principles. But whatever Hillman's motivation, Samuels' 'defence of analysis' on the grounds of an appeal to innate political potential now begins to look unnecessary.

I will move on next to consider how political material is treated in the course of an ordinary contemporary analysis. Is it possible to adequately address the client's legitimate political concerns without revisioning analytic theory and practice along the lines suggested by Samuels?

An ordinary analytic case

Peter was a young man in his late twenties with a socialist/feminist political orientation in five-times-a-week analysis. He lived in shared, cooperatively managed accommodation with a number of other like-minded men and women. He reported that a housemate had been expelled after some 'girlie magazines' had been found in his room. Peter was terrified that if he betrayed feelings of sexual attraction towards any of the women they would experience this too as oppressive, and he himself would be expelled. Consequently he spent a lot of time alone in his room and avoided emotionally meaningful interactions with his housemates wherever possible. When these did occur he felt painfully oversensitive to their nuances and became terrified by the violence and intensity of the feelings and fantasies they aroused in him. This led him to withdraw further, worsening his problems.

One day Peter shamefully reported that in a general election in his teens he had nearly voted for an extreme right-wing political party. He desperately wanted to understand this action that was so contrary to his current political beliefs. The thing that disturbed him most was the party's racist agenda, which led it to advocate the forced expulsion of immigrants.

When he thought back to his life at the time, he recalled the following incident. His father (an alcoholic) had hit him, his mother and his numerous siblings throughout his life. One day after dinner when his father went to attack his mother in a drunken state, Peter intervened physically and forced him off. His father reacted by attacking a different brother and furiously declaring that if Peter ever interfered in such a way again he would kick him out of the house. From then on he lived in constant fear of his father's threat.

With very little help from me, he was able to see that by nearly voting for the far right political party he was unconsciously identifying with his father. In other words he was hoping 'his party' would expel foreigners in the way he himself had feared being expelled. He went on to make some links with his present living situation: his fear of being thrown out again, his guilt about his relief that it was his housemate not him who had been expelled and so on.

He then remarked that he had attempted to cope with his mother's depression and lack of availability by becoming extremely self-sufficient from a very early age. This could be regarded, as a forced expulsion of his own dependency needs from his conscious psyche. The denial (expulsion) of his own needs in both his current living situation and his previous political belief system clearly reflected his continued use of this defensive strategy. He was greatly relieved to begin to understand the significance of his previously incomprehensible political flirtation in this light, and went on to address other therapeutic issues.

I suspect this clinical vignette illustrates how many analysts might currently work with similar political material presented in a session, and I trust that Samuels too would probably find little to disagree with in the handling of this case so far. As we have seen he does not specify what type of 'political discussion' he wishes to encourage in therapy so it is hard to be sure of this. But it seems unlikely he intends the analyst to get drawn into a discussion of the relative merits of hard right as opposed to hard left politics in a situation such as this. Since his teens Peter has simply replaced one harsh set of political beliefs with another, leaving the under-lying splits in his psyche unaltered. Discussing politics in this way would therefore not be therapeutic and could easily reinforce those splits.

There are those who believe all meaningful analytic work must take place within the here and now of the transference relationship (see, for example, the contributions of Proner and Hinshelwood to the present volume). Such analysts would no doubt attempt to relate Peter's political dilemmas to that relationship, hoping to resolve the underlying splits in his psyche there. And in fact Peter and I did go on to address the way his conflicts manifested themselves in the therapeutic relationship. But many therapists besides Samuels would reject the reductive formulaic use of transference interpretations (see Kast in the present volume; Peters, 1991) without espousing any 'radical revisioning' of analysis. How might Samuels' views differ from theirs?

At times I became identified in the countertransference with Peter's split-off libidinal desires. This happened, for instance, when he first mentioned his housemate's expulsion. I found myself then wanting to argue the case in favour of pornography and against the version of feminism prevalent in the group of people with whom he lived. Perhaps Samuels would advocate actually getting involved in a political discussion at this point. He might justify this as an exploration of Peter's feelings about the oppressive nature of the politically correct regime within which he lived, and/or an attempt to improve the relationship between different parts of himself.

If I had got involved like that at this point, however, I believe there would have been a danger of simply returning Peter's projected feelings to him undigested. In fact he was strongly identified with the socialist/feminist regime within which he lived initially. So, if I had argued in favour of pornography at this point, I could well have entrenched his identification with a harsh superego. He might have believed then, with some justification, that I was filled with dangerous sexual desires, not him; and the reintegration of those desires would have got blocked.

But Samuels might agree that under these circumstances it is better to wait until the client shows more awareness of the needy/sexual part of his psyche. Only then might he feel able to embark on a fruitful discussion of the conflict between that side *of the client* and the other more moralistic one. Such a 'political discussion' might conceivably have taken the form of a consideration of Peter's conflicting attitudes to pornography. But if this is all Samuels is suggesting then it is hard to see how his position differs from that of many other ordinary therapists. In fact, slightly later, when Peter had talked about his (fear of betraying) feelings of sexual attraction to his housemates, we were able to address this split together. But the groundwork for this had already been laid by then through his recognition that the immigrants he had wished to expel in his teens also represented needy parts of himself.

This piece of clinical material appears to illustrate that it is possible to work with a client's political material without either denying its importance or radically revisioning therapeutic practice.

CITIZEN AS THERAPIST TO THE WORLD

Although most of the above considerations seem to militate against Samuels' project to politicize analysis, there is another factor that appears to operate in its favour. Quite often in an analysis, material arises which has clear political connections. My dream of Freud, the garden, the tree and the Israeli air force quoted above is a case in point.

It will be recalled that in that dream the Israeli air force was about to bomb the desolate garden, and my feeling was that this was in order to make way for a commercial building development. The garden was effectively going to be concreted over. Firstly, then, the dream could be regarded as referring to the end of nature at the hands of the military industrial complex (see, for example, Giddens, 1991).

But it could also be interpreted as a reaction to the Arab–Israeli conflict. From this perspective the garden could represent a ruined Eden, with the plum tree corresponding to the tree of knowledge: I am then identified with the Palestinians who are about to be driven from the devastated Holy Land by the Israeli air force.

A third political interpretation concerns the Freud–Jung split. It will be recalled that at the time of the dream I had just moved from a Freudian to a Jungian analyst. The Israeli air force from this perspective is in the position of Jung in his conflict with Freud. I am then in danger of being caught in a conflict of loyalties between my new Jungian analysis and my original psychoanalytically dominated training, which I feel I will have to leave.

A fourth political interpretation concerns the demise of communism, which was in the process of succumbing to the cost of the arms race at the time of the dream. Freud would then stand for my Marxist Freudian analyst, who was being threatened by the capitalist-backed Israeli air force.

The dream could thus be regarded as a countertransference in Samuels' sense to all these political situations. This observation seems to support Samuels' conception of 'citizen as therapist to the world'. I cannot see though that acceptance of the notion of 'citizen as therapist to the world' would actually require any change in analytic practice. What could my analyst have done about these political interpretations of the dream apart from acknowledge my feelings about them, and help me address any unconscious elements in them? After that surely it would be up to me to decide what, if anything, to do in terms of political action *outside analysis*. In addition feminism has long acquainted us with the notion that the personal is political (see Orbach, 1998). So even here there is little new in what Samuels is suggesting.

Other interpretations

Partly for completeness' sake, it seems important to acknowledge that other interpretations of this dream are also possible and could prove therapeutically more fruitful than those above. The tree could stand for mother with the air force in the place of the oedipal father. Both could stand for parts of the self. A transference interpretation involving my two analysts (represented by Freud and the Israeli air force) is also clearly possible. And the plum (bum) tree could even allude to the first stage of the alchemical work. An archetypal interpretation is also possible with the disembodied voice representing God expelling Adam and Eve from the Garden of Eden. And the purple skin of the ripe plums could refer back to the purple clothes in the dream I shared with my first analyst. . . .

It is small wonder perhaps given such a plethora of possible interpretations that many therapists turn to the security of a formulaic method of working with dreams, systematically prioritizing one type of interpretation over another. If the therapist resists this defensive manoeuvre, however, then the interesting question of how the analytic couple (see Carvalho, present volume) decide which interpretation to actually pursue does arise – given that only one at a time can actually be worked with. Preferably of course this is the one most likely be therapeutic and open up unconscious material. Ideally that interpretation probably comes out of a mixture of the client's feelings and associations and the analyst's ability to sense the presence of the unconscious. All too often, however, the couple's defences or preconceptions seem to be the determining factors.

My own analyst actually emphasized the purposive nature of the dream. The old was being cleared to make way for the new. In effect she was telling me to put the past with my mad analyst behind me. Although kindly meant, this interpretation tended to block the work both of mourning and of understanding what had happened in my first analysis. This contributed to leaving us partially stuck in a paranoid-schizoid way of relating. From my analyst's side it is conceivable that her difficulties coming to terms with the emotional effects of the Holocaust played a part. I can only speculate that perhaps she had had to concrete over important aspects of her own past and that she was advising me to do likewise. In this sense, perhaps, her own unresolved traumas interfered with her ability to listen to my comments on the Arab–Israeli conflict in a way that would help me to resolve my related ones.

CONCLUSION

If there is one conclusion to be drawn from the above experiences and reflections, it is that it is extremely difficult to be there for another person without imposing our own conscious or unconscious agenda upon them. And yet as analysts this is precisely what we aspire to do. Of course at times we all fall short of that ideal. But it is hard to see how we could either directly discuss politics with our clients, or systematically ignore their political concerns, without straying further from it.

SUMMARY

In the course of this chapter I have argued that it is analysts' specific theoretical preoccupations, not something intrinsic to the analytic process itself, that has led them to sometimes neglect their client's legitimate concerns about the outside world. On this view the radical revisioning of analysis proposed by Samuels is unnecessary. In fact it could be harmful if it simply replaces one privileged piece of theory with another. I have gone on to use case material (both my own and that of a client) to illustrate what I consider to be some of the dangers of political discussion in analysis. In particular I have suggested that political discussion is by its nature likely to encourage the intrusion of the analyst's own views and judgements into the analytic process. This could tend to reinforce splitting processes in the client and distract from the analyst's task of listening therapeutically to the client's material. I have gone on to question Samuels' simplistic suggestion that the existence of the analytic frame automatically confers protection from those dangers.

I have also pointed out that Samuels is very unclear about exactly what he means by 'political discussion' in therapy. I have tried to identify a type of discussion that uses political issues to encourage dialogue between different parts of the client's self and suggested that this could in fact be therapeutic. I have argued, though, that this is possible in normal analytic practice, and in this sense we already have the tools to deal with political material, and therefore do not need to radically revision therapy.

I have also suggested that it is possible to treat certain aspects of Samuels' proposal to politicize analysis as a defence against James Hillman's damning criticisms of contemporary analysis. I have gone on to show why I believe those criticisms are themselves ill-founded, and Samuels' defence against them therefore unnecessary.

Finally I have addressed Samuels' notion of citizen as therapist to the world. I have tried to show that there are strong grounds for believing that material on both the client's and the therapist's side may reflect the impact of political events. I have also implied that it is as therapeutically important to try to understand unconscious elements in that as in any other analytic material. In addition it may well be therapeutic for the analyst to acknowledge the client's emerging feelings about such events. But the notion of citizen as therapist is already implied in the well-known feminist equation of the personal and the political.

It should go without saying that some of the psychological concepts discussed in this paper could be usefully applied in the world of politics. I am thinking in particular of the mechanism of identification with the aggressor, and of the use of endless conflict as a defence against mourning and fears of engulfment. Despite years of analytic endeavour, however – Gross (1913), Freud (1931), Reich (1933), Orbach (1978, 1998) etc. – the world has yet to show up for its first therapy session, as Samuels would put it. So I shall have to leave it to those with greater therapeutic ambitions than myself to devise a way of getting it there. Meanwhile I hope I may be forgiven if I stick to the more modest task of listening to my clients' concerns and attempting to attend to the unconscious processes at work in both them and myself: that task is arduous enough.

REFERENCES

Bion, Wilfred (1967) *Second Thoughts*. London: Heinemann.

Broom, Brian (1997) *Somatic Illness and the Patient's Other Story*. London: Free Association Books.

Engel, George (1977) 'The need for a new medical model: A challenge for biomedicine'. *Science*, Vol. 196, 29–36.

Fordham, Michael (1993) 'On not knowing beforehand'. *JAPA*, Vol. 38, no. 2: 127–136.

Freud, Sigmund (1912) *Recommendations to Physicians Practising Psychoanalysis*. Standard Edition, Vol. 12. London: Hogarth Press.

Freud, Sigmund (1931) *Civilisation and Its Discontents*. Standard Edition, Vol. 21. London: Hogarth Press.

Giddens, Anthony (1991) *Modernity and Self Identity*, Cambridge: Polity Press.

Gross, Otto (1913) 'Zur Uberwindung der kulturellen Krise'. *Die Aktion*, Nr. 14, III Jg., 2 April 1913, col. 385.

Grosskurth, Phyllis (1985) *Melanie Klein, her Work and her World*. London: Hodder & Stoughton.

Hauke, Christopher (2000) *Jung and the Postmodern*. London: Routledge.

Hillman, James (1994) 'Man is by nature a political animal, or: patient as citizen', in S. Shamdasani and M. Munchow (Eds), *Speculations after Freud*. London: Routledge.

Klein, Melanie (1961) *Narrative of a Child Analysis*. London: Hogarth Press.

Meltzer, Donald (1978) *Richard Week by Week*, The Roland Harris Educational Trust; and in *The Kleinian Development*, London: Karnac, 1998.

McLeod, John (1997) *Narrative and Psychotherapy*, London: Sage Publications.

Orbach, Susie (1978) *Fat is a Feminist Issue*. London: Hamlyn.

Orbach, Susie (1998) 'It's official: The personal will be political', *Guardian*, 12th August, p. 7.

Peters, Roderick (1991) *The Therapist's Expectations of the Transference. JAPA*, Vol. 36, no. 77–92.

Pietroni, Patrick (1996) *Innovations in Community Care and Primary Health*. London: Churchill-Livingstone.

Reich, Wilhelm (1933) *The Mass Psychology of Fascism*. Harmondsworth, UK: Penguin.

Reik, Theodore (1949) *The Inner Experience of a Psychoanalyst*. London: Allen & Unwin.

Samuels, Andrew (2001) *Politics on the Couch*. London: Profile Books.

Searles, Harold (1959) 'The effort to drive the other person crazy', in *Collected Papers on Schizophrenia and Related Subjects*, London: Maresfield Press.

(c) Response

Andrew Samuels

It is ironic, though a little sad, that, in a piece extolling the virtues of conventional analytical thinking about practice, Bob Withers manages utterly to bust the confidentiality and right to privacy of both of his analysts. Each of these practitioners was instantly recognizable to me and, I would imagine, to many of the people who will read this book. Purely from the point of view of debate, I am glad that Withers, while making his position clear, has slipped up in this way, because it makes it so much easier for me to counter any implicit or explicit propaganda claims in his comment on my chapter that I am in some way an incompetent or one-sided clinician with a tendency to return people's feelings to them 'undigested'.

It is not clear to me that Withers realizes that he has in fact got a 'position'. This is part of the trouble when proposing innovations in practice and technique – the people who stick up for the old ways do not realize that theirs is as partial and polemical a view as that of the person who critiques it. Withers' point of view should not be regarded as self-evidently correct, as above debate or as reflecting some sort of natural law about therapy.

Returning to the quite harrowing accounts of his analysts' work with him, I have a few observations to make. The analyst who became psychotic was, we are told, a Marxist. It is not at all clear from Withers' account what he is trying to tell us. Her psychosis and her Marxism seem, for him, to be connected. Surely this is primarily a case of an analyst not being well enough to practise and the only sensible response on Withers' part would have been to report her to the relevant authorities?

The analyst who supported Israel seems to have been completely unable to deal with the political material with which she was faced. This can only strengthen my case that, without making all of analysis revolve around the political dimension of experience, the profession had better start to think of responsible ways of working with this relatively new type of material with which we now are faced every day.

En passant, I would point out how 'political' Withers' personal analytical material was in both analyses. His political selfhood was crying out for recognition. He needed an informed and sensitive analysis of this material that, without neglecting its manifold symbolic meanings, apprehended (and respected) it just as it presented itself, on its own level and in its own terms.

Similarly, the client called Peter was in urgent need of what I have called 'discussion' in order to help him find his way through the vicissitudes of living in the kind of communal house described. What happens is that, when political discussion goes on within therapy or analysis, both participants are deeply affected by the process. But the analyst knows of the risks of over-influencing the client (we know that *some* influence is inevitable). The therapeutic vessel is crucial for this to take place and it is the decisive factor that makes such discussion different from political discussion in everyday life. By discussion, I mean a verbal interchange with the political material as its focus and with the psychological (emotional and fantasy) side of things very much to the foreground. If this definition does not satisfy, then all I mean is ordinary relational interaction in analysis but with reference to the political.

Withers is well aware that the current state of the field leads to manifold understandings of the same phenomenon. I think that what we need is some kind of new approach to interpretation, that I have called 'plural interpretation'. It would not be a case of presenting the client with a multiple-choice task, more of highlighting the tension between different points of view when making an interpretation so that the client can share in the task of evolving and constructing an understanding of what is going on. (In this way, a contribution is made to the politics of the therapeutic relationship, rendering it more transparent and democratic – though without denying difference.)

These new thoughts about clinical practice also make a contribution to the politics of the profession and this is a good note on which to end because, whilst writing against what he calls the 'politicization' of therapy, Withers is making a highly politicized intervention of his own into a faction-ridden and highly disputatious field. He is no more reliable a guide to good-enough practice than I am!

Analysis and implicit homophobia

Introduction

The debate within analytical psychology and psychoanalysis has thankfully moved on (in most quarters) from the question of whether homosexuality per se is perverse or pathological. But this movement itself brings a dilemma in its wake. The analytic theories once used to justify the characterization of homosexuality as pathological are revealed as having been applied in the service of prejudice – once homosexuality is accepted as a healthy sexual variant. Is it possible that other currently accepted analytic theories are being similarly, if less obviously, applied?

One analytic theory places what Jung called the 'conjunctio', Freud the 'parental intercourse' and Bion the relationship between the 'container and the contained', at the centre of the healthy psyche. In her paper Chess Denman argues that the heterosexual framing of this theory betrays a deeply held prejudice against homosexuality. Analysts who espouse it, she claims, can never fully accept their homosexual clients. In reality the theory is the product of a cultural valorizing of heterosexual sex, not of analytic neutrality or scientific observation.

Richard Carvalho accepts that homosexuality can be a healthy form of sexual expression and heterosexuality at times deeply pathological. But he argues in favour of maintaining a model of the heterosexual conjunctio, at least in an abstract form, as a useful way of representing psychic life. In particular he regards the otherness of the heterosexual couple to each other as a helpful way of symbolizing the otherness of the conscious to the unconscious, and the ego to the self. He sees no reason in principle why the abstract template of the conjunctio could not be fulfilled by a homosexual intercourse. But he argues that we will not be in a position to know if this does in fact occur until we have tracked the effect of contemporary changes in patterns of parenting on the unconscious over several generations.

Denman's impatience with this position can be understood in the light of her conviction that meanwhile analysts are damaging their homosexual clients, by using an inappropriate model to gauge their psychological health. In making her case Denman covers wide range of issues. She refutes the idea that the psyche has a particular centre at all. She argues that the appeal to ethological and biological paradigms by supporters of the theory masks a cultural bias. She goes on to question the usefulness of the notions of perversion, of pathology and even of unconscious phantasy in analysis. All these, she believes, can and have been used to attempt to force the client to conform to the analyst's belief of what constitutes psychic health or psychic reality. She concludes by arguing in favour of some sort of public acknowledgement of, and atonement for, the damage this has caused.

These are deeply contentious issues, and Carvalho concedes that these concepts and related theories have in fact at times been used in the way Denman describes. He argues, however, that this is not a consequence of the theories and concepts themselves but more of their insensitive application by individual analysts. He goes on to emphasize the importance of interpretation as a collaborative enterprise. He also attempts to establish a less value-laden conceptualization of perversion. In addition he tries to ground theories about the conjunctio in the discourses of ethology and biology without denying their cultural components. In all these ways he seeks to ensure that the concept of the conjunctio can be uncoupled from the oppressive practices Denman rightly condemns. If this can be done, atonement for the theory becomes unnecessary.

(a) Analytical psychology and homosexual orientation

Chess Denman

INTRODUCTION

This chapter discusses aspects of the attitude of analytical psychology to homosexual orientation largely from a critical standpoint. It is divided into three parts. In the first part some key statements about homosexuality are discussed, next a clinical case is discussed and finally a number of clinical and political questions are addressed.

SOME KEY STATEMENTS

Homosexual orientation is not pathological – it is a normal variant

Nothing that is inherent in homosexual orientation makes it a priori a pathology. Those who have wished to pathologize it have generally proceeded in two ways. The first involves appeal to a 'natural' state of heterosexuality from which homosexuality deviates. The value of this appeal turns on the sense of the word natural that is being used. Natural might be being used to mean usual or common but, being unusual cannot be equated with pathological or else, for example, being called Yolanda would be pathological. Natural can mean without man-made or cultural intervention, brought about entirely by nature but such a use of the term cannot equate with lack of pathology since it is natural to have appendicitis, die, get cancer etc. – all pathological states of affairs. Finally invoking the world 'natural' may involve an appeal to the proper or moral way to do things but to do so is to enter a moral domain not a medical one and confusing pathology and morality can lead to abuses such as the soviet tendency to label dissidents as schizophrenics who were suffering with a desire to rebel against the state.

The second way in which people have tried to pathologize homosexual orientation is to argue that it is associated with (co-morbid with) some other pathology (often a character pathology like fickleness, seductiveness, lying, etc.) and that the co-morbidity can be ascribed to common psychic causation. For example, homosexual orientation in men is due to having a close, binding mother and a distant, hostile father which also results in superego weakness and consequently fickleness etc. However, studies of non-clinical homosexual populations show no evidence of increased character pathology. Furthermore there are competing theories of the origins of sexual object choice with differing consequences for presumptive pathological co-morbidity. A plausible theory of the origin of sexual object choice may well turn out to be that sexual object choice is to some extent biological in origin, to some extent culturally determined and to some extent conditioned by developmental sexual experience. In different individuals the balance between these elements probably differs. Some people's sexual object choice seems evident very early and, in consequence (although not entirely logically) gets labelled genetic. In others there is considerable plasticity of object choice and sexual fantasy life responds to different experiences. However, in none of these pathways, when they lead to homosexual object choice, is there any necessary associated pathology. Thus homosexual orientation is not itself a pathology; nor is it necessarily co-morbidly associated with any other pathology.

So, is homosexuality ever pathological? It is sometimes suggested that there may be some homosexualities which are pathological and others which are not and, on first reading, it seems inherently unreasonable to resist this idea. One such seemingly sensible position in the field is that both heterosexual and homosexual organizations can be either pathological or normal. However, taking up this position generally involves judging sexual behaviour by some standard. Generally this standard involves suggesting that some or all of the following activities are pathological: sex for money, casual sex, sex in groups, sex involving pain and humiliation, and, oddly, abstaining from sex. A second look at this list reveals it as the negative of heterosexual Christian marriage that is: free, committed, dyadic, egalitarian, and procreative. So, the standard of judgement for sexual pathology turns out to be a heterosexual one even when the gender of the participants involved is ignored.

Heterosexual orientation needs as much explanation as homosexual orientation

Special attempts to explain homosexual orientation generally tend to assume it is problematic, whereas heterosexual orientation is not thought problematic and consequently rarely 'explained'. In consequence theoretical attempts to explain homosexual orientation in particular carry within them risk of pathologizing bias exactly because heterosexuality is not subjected to a similar analysis. This is not to say that such explanations should not be attempted, but rather that they should be attempted with care. The commonest example of such a situation is a case report. If the patient is gay or lesbian, homosexual orientation may be reported as a feature of the case. Were the patient heterosexual this fact would not be reported but assumed and then discovered by the reader if/when a sexual partner was mentioned. Here homosexuality shares its 'marked' status with non-white skin colour, female

sex and the number 99. A marked term is one that is unusual or needs special mention. The unmarked term is the one which deserves no comment.
Consider:

> 99 is nearly as much as 100
> 100 is nearly as much as 99

Both are true but the second seems odd because 100 is the unmarked term.
Now look at:

> boys deserve as good an education as girls.
> whites are just as intelligent as blacks
> heterosexuals should have as many rights to equal employment as homosexuals

It is homosexuality's status as a marked term which makes it seem in need of special explanation next to a presumptive heterosexual norm. With these initial civil rights points in mind we can move on to consider psychological aspects of sexual orientation.

Homosexual object choice does not imply psychic contrasexuality

Freud and Jung, in common with many other psychological commentators and indeed popular lay opinion, subscribe to the idea that homosexual orientation is a consequence of exaggerated psychic contrasexuality. Hence the characterization of homosexual men as effeminate and lesbians as mannish. However homosexual object choice is not necessarily the consequence of a psychic identification with the opposite sex to one's own. That is lesbians are not all mannish and gays not all effeminate (and not all mannishness in lesbians or effeminacy in gays is a consequence of contrasexual identification). Indeed, a moment's thought reveals that locking same-sex object choice onto contrasexual gender identification is necessarily incoherent. Consider a lesbian who identifies as a man, acts mannishly and desires a woman. Who shall her partner be? Theory allows only for another butch lesbian or for a straight woman settling for second best. While such a theory might have fitted the world of Radclyffe Hall in *The Well of Loneliness*, it does not reflect the lives of today's lesbians.

This formulation which ties object choice to gender identity also serves to erase the possibility of any real homosexual attraction. In this view all homosexuality is, in truth, psychic heterosexuality, contrasexual identification and denial of the reality one's own gender. So it is not surprising that the idea, that homosexuals try to repudiate or deny their true (biological) gender is a charge often made against homosexuals in pathologizing accounts. In fact homosexuals know their gender identity for what it is and establish a secure gender identity at the same age as heterosexuals establish it. Gender identity (knowing what sex one is), however, needs separation from gender role which is behaving in ways culturally associated with that sex. Homosexuals' security in their gender identity can be combined with elements of boundary crossing in their gender role (creating, as a result, identities based on camp, not effeminacy, in gay men; in women producing not mannish lesbians but dykes). Such role-stretching may lead to nicely judged parodic plays on the way our culture does gender – for example, daddy dykes, and drag queens. But these plays only work because the established gender identity of the 'actor' is being juxtaposed against their gender role.

Some analysts, particularly Jungians who appeal to the concepts of animus and anima, are attracted by the notion that bisexuality allows some conceptual freedom from rigidly dimorphic nature of the sexual and gender-based stereotypes in our culture. However, it is important to realize that for Jung and Freud bisexuality meant plasticity of gender identification and not plasticity of object choice. Neither, even at their most liberated was able to question the linkage between gender identity and object choice, choosing to preserve at least psychic heterosexuality at any price.

Homosexual sex acts are not pathological but are psychically specific

Currently in psychoanalytic circles homosexuals appear to have gained a degree of acceptance. However, sadly, this is based on an avoidance of acknowledging the sort of sex they are having. When it is discussed, homosexual sex is often more or less subtly denigrated. Anal sex is seen as degraded or degrading. Lesbian sex is either caricatured as consisting in intimate sensual exchanges reminiscent of mother–baby interaction, with its in-built connotations of regression, or it is caricatured as a poor reflection of heterosexual sex (for example, involving the use of dildos) inviting suggestions that the 'real thing' might prove more satisfying. So, on the rare occasions it is discussed, homosexual sex is often pathologized relative to a heterosexual norm. In an attempt to respond, some gay and some straight commentators have tended to argue that homosexual sex is just like heterosexual sex. This is an argument which has often involved failing to investigate or dwell on the details of homosexual sexuality, preferring rather to announce that homosexual sexuality is at least potentially 'whole object related' in the same way as heterosexual sexuality, without enquiring what contribution the specifically homosexual aspects of an erotic exchange make to its object-relational quality.

However, the kind of sex people have, its details, who comes when and as a result of what act, is important psychically and homosexuals have sexual experiences which cannot be interpreted from a heterosexual template or reduced to a common (heterosexual) core. Sadly this is exactly what happens in much of the psychoanalytic literature on homosexual sex, which readily reveals both heterosexist and misogynist assumptions. Consider a man who is being anally penetrated. He is often described as being in a passive feminine position, directly analogizing him with a straight woman. What is wrong with this? Well, for a start we might notice that a woman who is being vaginally penetrated might take very great exception to being described as passive. Second, to be anally penetrated by a man as a man is not the same as to be vaginally penetrated by a man as a woman. The experience is sui generis and an understanding of its erotic nature and the ways in which that erotic nature act on psychic experience is not furthered by its reduction to a heterosexual prototype.

Homosexual experience also involves, probably to a greater degree than heterosexual experience, some sex acts which seem beyond the pale. Fisting, the insertion of a hand into the vagina or anus, is often taken as such an act, as well as sadomasochistic acts involving pain, or dominance and submission. Commentators have either been content to point to these acts as further evidence that homosexuality is perverse or have tried to 'rescue' homosexuality by dividing it into normal and perverse types. The difficulties of that project have already been discussed. However, it is also important to point out that, on closer inspection, people who indulge in acts like fisting or SM talk about them as having the same kind of individuating and erotic properties which are ascribed to straight sex. Therefore a strong but entirely tenable view is that that no sexual act is, as such, perverse, although some are illegal (rightly or wrongly) and, in our culture, others are immoral.

Heterosexual (and analytic) assumptions about what constitutes good (healthy, object-related) loving relationships are culturally, not psychologically, determined and homosexual culture may be different from heterosexual culture

Cultural forces shape the expression of sexuality and this is important because psychoanalytic theory's blindness to the structuring role of culture in its own constitution has made its theories of homosexuality and heterosexuality culpably inadequate. It is therefore worth thinking about the current cultural forces which may shape homosexual sexual expression. One powerful set of cultural forces acting on gays and lesbians is to do with being in a minority, often oppressed or misunderstood, and imparts an acute sense of difference. Even in childhood, before claiming a gay or lesbian identity, some homosexuals report having felt different from other family members. So there is often a considerable psychic stress on finding others who are similar, or on breaking out from confining restrictions. As a result sex, for some, is a group event (rather than a dyadic one), fulfilling needs for group bonding. In others there are elements of ecstatic experience–self-shattering which may serve needs to do with breaking out of conformist concealment. It is a reasonable consequence of this kind of argument that, for some, it may be individuated if not 'object-related' to have repeated anonymous sexual encounters. Here Jungians do have a decisive advantage over analysts in the Freudian tradition. Jung's concept of individuation can offer the capacity to overcome the culturally limited hegemony of the notion of object relations.

It can be hard at first to see that anything could be wrong with the term 'object relations' – arguing against it, like arguing against motherhood and apple pie, seems to involve standing up for paedophilia, perversion, chaos and the abuse of children.

However, arguably the heterosexual ideal of Western culture, a faithful loving union for the purposes of child-rearing, contains perverse elements. It represents an idealization and romanticization of a culturally necessary move by men in early medieval times as culture moved away from a tribal to a feudal system. Increased actual and social mobility made it necessary for the men to lock up their wives for fear of their impregnation by roving males. In doing so they were protecting their sexual assets, but even more importantly ensuring the paternity of their children. Such a situation is not 'natural', 'innate' or 'right'; it is, rather, expedient. As society has changed and women's choices have expanded, the ideal of romantic love has come to replace the chastity belt as enforcer of this strategy. The perversion then lies in the binding of all parties to the male imperative and the blinding of all parties to the expediency involved.

Heterosexual unconscious phantasy (the internal parental couple) is not at the foundation of psychic life – healthy or otherwise

The romantic ideal of philoprogenitive heterosexual union has been exalted in one strand of psychoanalytic theorizing based on the work of Klein and Meltzer. It argues that there exists in the psyche an unconscious phantasy of the parents and their sexual and baby-making activities. The nature of this phantasy and the reactions of the individual to it are held to be centrally important in structuring unconscious and conscious mental life. There are Jungian versions of this theory, and Jung's theory of the conjunctio seems ready-made to fit. This theory, if it is right, puts heterosexuality at the centre of the psyche and in relation to it we might ask two relevant questions. First, is it a true description of human psychology? And second, if it is, is it a logical consequence that homosexual sexuality is always in some way at odds with psychic nature? Commentators who accept that it is a valid description differ on this point, but it is becoming fashionable to argue that (in the language of this story) it is possible for a homosexual to have a satisfactory internal object relation with the parental couple and in consequence be healthy.

The idea of the internal parental couple as a central structuring feature of the mind is, however, not a true or a useful way of characterizing or judging psychic life. Indeed it is worse than false. It is a pernicious way of describing psychic life for lots of reasons but, pertinently to the current debate, because a logical consequence of centring theories of psychic functioning around a heterosexual sex act is necessarily to pathologize homosexuality, however much its proponents argue that this is not a logical consequence of the theory. Closer inspection of theoretical writings on homosexual orientation which derive from this tradition always reveals the carving out of, at best, a second or an eccentric place in the psychoanalytic pantheon of adjustment for homosexuals; and this is indeed a logical necessity in terms of the theory.

There are advantages to homosexual orientation as well as disadvantages – just as for heterosexual orientation

Homosexual orientation is not, as Freud put it, 'assuredly no advantage', because some psychic and individuation experiences are more readily available to homosexuals than they are to heterosexuals. For example, some homosexuals, knowing, from an early age, that they are 'different', find the task of recognizing their essential separateness from their parents, and thereby accepting the inevitability of death and the necessity of facing this experience alone, easier than do heterosexuals. The AIDS crisis drew out this strength in homosexual men who, in ways which I think would not have been seen so readily in a heterosexual community, were able to mobilize a rich, flexible and caring network around the many affected members of the gay community. Another area of potential advantage concerns the lived experience of oppressed status. While, in large part, this experience is psychically damaging, it does confer a lively awareness of the operation of unconsciously wielded power. Lesbians, for example, have been consistently able to keep drawing issues around oppressed minorities to the attention of the larger feminist movement. By the same token, just as homosexuals are able to individuate in some areas more readily than heterosexuals, so also homosexual therapists will be able to add to the largely heterosexual world of therapy a better and more rounded perspective in areas (and this is the important point) which will extend beyond issues solely to do with sexual orientation.

FORDHAM'S PAPER 'THE ANDROGYNE'. HOW DO THE VARIOUS FALLACIES AND DIFFICULTIES DISCUSSED SO FAR AFFECT CLINICAL WORK?

Before considering Fordham's paper it is important to note that many analysts argue that in relation to all aspects of their patient's life they take a morally neutral stance, neither condemning nor condoning but analysing. Frequently a moment's inspection of their case material reveals that this is, at best, a self-delusion and that an attitude of approval or disapproval, at the very least, conditions what to interpret as pathological and what to interpret as beneficial. It is important to make this point because the adoption of a morally driven stance is particularly evident in writings on patients who are homosexual. These texts, including the one which follows, are littered with asides which denigrate the homosexuality of the patient and downplay any adaptive functions it performs.

To look at this and other issues in a more detailed way I want to analyse the case of James in Fordham's paper 'The Androgyne: some inconclusive reflections on sexual perversions' (Fordham, 1988). In this paper Fordham sets out to explore the psychology of Jung's concept of the androgyne in relation to sexual perversion. He disscuses two cases, one of a homosexual man and one of a heterosexual man who has some homosexual phantasies.

Fordham certainly holds a pathologizing view of homosexuality. The first thing to note is that he moves straight to homosexuality as the paradigm perversion:

> we seem not to have gone much further than the notion, initiated by Freud, that any sexual activity that prevents genital heterosexual intercourse or replaces it, must be counted a perversion. That could be somewhat bettered by adding that, in perverse sexual activities, infantile sexual phantasies and practices are exploited . . .

Next it is clear that Fordham adheres to the idea that homosexuals are not experiencing a genuine homosexual desire but are identified with the opposite sex. He says:

> Thinking of the functioning of the archetypes in this way helps us to recognise some of the roots of the process of identification with the opposite sex in both men and women and how, if excessive it can lead to lesbianism and homosexuality.

In the main body of the paper Fordham discusses James, introducing him as someone who

> had a male lover, and the couple were stable, which made their relationship 'respectable'. They had lived together for several years, and it was, on the whole, mutually satisfactory.

Fordham's text shows us ample evidence of the tendency to judge homosexual relationships by heterosexual standards of fidelity, but the ironic use of the term respectable in quotation marks denigrates the relationship and underlines the way that its homosexual nature disqualifies it forever from real acceptability.

Next Fordham tells us that in relation to sex acts

> They seemed to be based mainly on part object relationships, by which I mean they were activities to produce comfort when skin contacts were important, whilst genital, anal, or oral acts produced excitement.

Fordham clearly intends to signal by the use of the term 'part object relationship' the unsatisfactory nature of the sexuality expressed. However, it is difficult to see from the text what about the sexuality described is psychically any different from heterosexual sex in which cuddling (presumably what Fordham means by skin contacts) is certainly described as comforting and in which genital, anal or oral acts are thought disappointing if they are not exciting. Fordham therefore pathologizes James' sex life on what he presents as objective grounds. However, closer inspection reveals that Fordham gives us no independent grounds for judging it pathological other than that it is homosexual.

Later Fordham comments, 'At no time did James explore his life with the aim of curing himself of his homosexual practices.' The term 'practices' is especially revealing here: by characterizing James' sex life as 'practices' Fordham manages to represent it as a part object affair by disarticulating it from the relationship in which it was embedded, a relationship he has previously characterized, albeit cynically, as stable and mutual. Finally, Fordham reveals his underlying theory of James' psychic structure, arguing that, owing to certain difficulties, James had sexually become his mother's penis and suffered from bisexual homosexuality.

Fordham goes on to describe a more worrying sexual act on the part of the patient.

> He practised one other perversion, apart from genital masturbation he found great satisfaction in anal activities, passing big stools and letting them squeeze down his legs. As an alternative, he would go into a wood and defecate there or find a place where there was as much liquid mud as possible, undress and roll about in it. He also liked his bed to be dirty as well as the room in which he worked.

Now, analytically this is important material which needs understanding. James' interest in shit (one he shares with Jung) may be a vital clue to the location of as yet undiscovered valuable aspects in his psychic life. Fordham, however, does not in any way analyse this set of observations, merely adding them after he comments on his failure to elucidate the reasons why James does not have enduring sexual relations with women. So the material, fascinating though it is, serves no central purpose in the text and is put to no further use. Baldly put, then, at this point in the text, a text written by someone who wants his patient to be heterosexual, the addition of this 'other perversion' serves no purpose other than to attack the patient – as though Fordham is saying, 'look at this dirty boy', describing the material in a way that wreathes him in cleanly scientific distance while allowing him to debase and degrade his patient.

It is worth asking if it is not Fordham who is 'part object related' here? Fordham's case description ill-treats James gratuitously, attacking and vilifying him, denying and ignoring his stable union with another person by calling it 'homosexual prac-tices'. Fordham identifies his patient with a part object (mother's penis) and he treats his patient, and particularly his patient's partner, like a part object. Yet, despite this view, he continues in an analytic relationship with his patient, never for a moment considering what these attitudes might mean for their relationship.

How might all this have played out clinically? Fordham hopes towards the end of the paper that James will become heterosexual, although he comments that this is rare in homosexuals in analysis. It is hard, reading the paper, to imagine that some of Fordham's countertransferential wish for this change in his patient and, worse, some of his contemptuous attitude towards James did not permeate the analytic situation. Fordham tells us that, as the transference developed, he got bored with his patient. He investigated this phenomenon and discovers that his patient was 'conducting his analysis on the basis of a conception of how an analysis should proceed'. In relation to this description of the transference/countertransference situation, the analysis of Fordham's attitude might make it possible to go a little further in thinking about the boredom.

One possibility is that Fordham is bored because his patient wishes to comply with Fordham and please him as much as he can, although he knows that Fordham, probably like his father, will never wholly approve of his individual nature and of the flowering of his self. Another possibility is that Fordham, not his patient, is conducting the analysis on the basis of his (pre)conception of how an analysis should proceed, and, knowing as he does all about how part object related his patient is, has left no room for anything new. But a final possibility, and perhaps the most likely, is that Fordham is bored because he cannot bear to be near his patient, whom he hates and despises for being a shitty gay wanker, but, since he is wedded to a notion of analysis, neither can he part. It will be a miracle if Fordham's analysis helped his patient and I am left worried for the man.

Presented with evidence of homophobia by senior or founding figures in the analytic community, many people make one of two moves. One is to argue that views have moved on since the paper was written, the other that it is unrepresentative of the author's work. However neither of these will work in Fordham's case since this paper is amongst the later ones he produced. Nor is it convincingly possible to argue that views have moved on very far. Certainly it is the case that such easily expressed and unguarded hatred is more rarely expressed these days, but sadly it is not hard to give references to recent work by respected theorists (see, for example, Bollas, 1996; Covington, 1999) which continue to reveal ample latent or overt homophobia.

Another move, when defending homophobic theorists, is to argue that it is possible to separate the wheat of theory from the chaff of personal prejudice. On closer inspection Freudian, Jungian and Kleinian thought all rely on presumptive heterosexuality as a founding moment in all psychic development using various notions about the Oedipus complex, the primal scene, the conjunctio or the egg and sperm race! It is hard to see how this privileging of heterosexuality which, ironically for psychologists, rests on a prejudiced conceptualization of the part biology plays in psychology can ever allow for a proper or successful threshing.

PRACTICAL AND CLINICAL CONSIDERATIONS

What are the implications of differing attitudes to homosexuality for issues of analytic politics and therapeutic practice? Traditionally discussion of these issues has crystallized around a number of key questions.

Should homosexual candidates be allowed to train as analysts?

Some analysts and organizations have felt that analysis should be reserved for heterosexual and preferably married individuals. Such individuals, they feel, have demonstrated a suitable quality of object relations. Other more homophile trainers think that gay and lesbian candidates should be encouraged to train as analysts. A range of more or less tolerant positions exists about the kind of gay lifestyles which will be acceptable in applicants, with a general preference for lifestyle choices which resemble the 'standard' of heterosexual marriage. At the more radical end some have argued that, insofar as sex life is relevant to the process of assessing an application to train, homosexual candidate's sex lives should be assessed from the basis of an understanding of the erotic and relational wellsprings of homosexuality. To do otherwise would both unfairly exclude suitable candidates and deprive the training organization of the advantages they could bring.

Certainly the main advantage in training gay men and lesbians as analysts will be to the organizations which train them. For the candidates themselves the resultant exposure to sustained but secretive (even unconscious) hostility and rejection can be personally destructive, leading to concealment or downplaying of a homosexual identity which may have been a hard-fought victory. The irony is that, as things are currently organized in some trainings, the desire to train may have pathological elements and the process of training may be pathogenic. Analytically, for these candidates, the task must be to question the internalized homophobia which may be stimulated by the experience and may even drive the urge to train.

Is it all right for gay men and lesbians to have children?

Some analysts have argued that the children of homosexuals are more likely to be homosexual or to be psychologically damaged because of the confusion they will have about gender, parenting or reproduction; and this is a common lay view. In fact there is no evidence that the children of homosexual couples are more likely to be maladjusted than the children of heterosexual couples. The possible homosexual orientation of these children would not be an argument against the arrangement, since there is nothing wrong with it. But there is no evidence of an increased incidence of homosexuality in these children.

In relation to the issue of possible 'confusion' in the children of gay men and lesbians there is often appeal to various biological theories of psychic development – what we might term internal couple arguments. Presumably the underlying argument here lies in the presumptive pathological consequences of the contrast the child notices (unconsciously) between its innate internal phantasy of parental intercourse and the actual parents it observes. This paper has argued that the concept of internal unconscious phantasies of heterosexual intercourse is incorrect and pernicious but, even if it were correct, there would still be no simple step from the

existence of such an unconscious phantasy to necessary pathology if this unconscious phantasy is not realized in actual life. Research studies show that the most
important mediator of the health of children brought up in homosexual relationships
is the degree to which the couple are open with the child and others about their
relationship.

How should homosexuals who wish to become heterosexual be treated?

Traditionally two views have been taken of ego-dystonic homosexuality. Some
interpret it as evidence of a deformation of nature by social pressure and aim
to reverse the ego-dystonic quality of a sexual orientation taken as given. Others
interpret the request as a recognition of the limited nature of the patient's current
sexuality and encourage the exploration of heterosexuality. One way to gain some
purchase on the question is to consider a putative case of ego-dystonic heterosexuality. In such a case, efforts to assist the individual in changing to a homosexual
lifestyle are unlikely to be undertaken in the absence of good evidence of a strong
homosexual fantasy life which might indicate that the heterosexual orientation was
more social sham than true preference. Such a thought experiment should reveal
that, only when a homosexual reveals a strong, persistent, sexually arousing fantasy
life of a heterosexual nature, preferably masturbatory and ideally with covert forays
into the heterosexual world, should an analyst start to consider the possibility of
exploring a change of orientation.

Fortunately there is no evidence that psychodynamic or any other kind of psychotherapy is capable of altering sexual preferences to any great extent. So little damage
can be done to a basic sexual preference either way. Sadly, however, analysts
have managed to convince gay men to marry with horrible and life-destroying
consequences some years down the line when the underlying orientation reasserts
itself.

How should an analyst respond to questions about their sexual orientation?

Gay patients, many aware of analytic prejudice about homosexuality, ask questions
about the sexual orientation of and attitudes towards homosexuality of their analysts.
Should these questions be explored, addressed and responded to, or should the
analyst confine themselves to an analysis of the fears behind them? This is not
a question which allows of a simple answer. However, it is important to notice that
many straight analysts reveal their sexual orientation, for example by wearing a
wedding ring, and, like all normative statuses, heterosexuality is generally assumed
to be the analyst's orientation. Evidence that the analyst is not usual in this respect
may come from a public position, books in the consulting room or wearing a gay
symbol. Such evidences may seem more provocative than the kinds of evidences
of heterosexuality which heterosexual analysts give off, but it is controversial

to suggest in consequence that a homosexual analyst should be especially discreet.

In relation to discussing theoretical attitudes to sexuality it is arguable that the history of analytic oppression of homosexuals needs to be acknowledged. The theoretical and technical issues here seem similar to those which might be raised by a Jewish patient who learned of Jung's support for national socialism, or a black patient who took issue with his patronizing view of primitive cultures. These patients, and gays and lesbians, are right to enquire if a central aspect of their psyche will be regarded as pathological and invalid. Many of them may be aware of the ways in which friends and others were damaged by being pathologized. In such circumstances, enquiry about the analyst's attitude may represent not only fearful transferences but also sensible self-interest. Failure openly to discuss the issue, as one analyst suggests (Limentani, 1991), may amount to deception and, at worst, to obtaining money by false pretences.

CONCLUSION: SHOULD THE WORLD OF ANALYTICAL PSYCHOLOGY TAKE ANY SPECIAL ACTION IN RELATION TO ITS OWN HISTORY?

Homophobia has damaged lives and continues to do so. Jungians have been complicit in this by active hatred and, as is often the Jungian way, by silence in the face of the homophobic prejudice of others. Most importantly, homophobic practice is prejudicial to the successful treatment of certain patients. Sadly, it seems self-evident that the Society of Analytical Psychology, because of its close links to Freudian and Kleinian ideas and to the Institute of Psycho-analysis, has been more homophobic than other Jungian organisations. This is not a legacy to be proud of; nor is it a legacy to be silent about. Particularly now, at a time when we are potentially facing a moral backlash fuelled by a hatred arguably more perverse than the objects of its rage, Jungians could help by speaking up loudly against moralizing witch-hunts, and pointing out the dangers of objectifying and dehumanizing any individual. They could acknowledge the homophobic views of the founder of their society and of some contemporary members of the organization. Then, having acknowledged them, they could treat these views in the same way and with the same seriousness that, it is to be hoped, they would treat racist views.

In such a way they might atone publicly for their own history and free themselves to start the fascinating work of elaborating the way that all different kinds of sexuality condition existence for good or ill.

REFERENCES

Bollas, C. (1993) 'Cruising in the homosexual arena', in C. Bollas, *On Being a Character*. London: Routledge.

Covington, C. (1999) Talk given to the Brighton Psychotherapy Group.

Fordham, M. (1988) 'The Androgyne: Some inconclusive reflections on sexual perversions'. *Journal of Analytical Psychology*, Vol. 33, 3.

Hall, R. (1982) *The Well of Loneliness*. London: Virago.

Limentani, A. (1991) 'Neglected fathers in the aetiology and treatment of sexual deviations'. *International Journal of Psycho-Analysis*, Vol. 66, 573–584.

(b) A comment on Denman

Richard Carvalho

Denman has written a deeply felt chapter in which she takes to task various societal and analytical assumptions which define homosexuality as pathological a priori. She is right to emphasize that heterosexuality can on occasion be deeply perverse and may need careful scrutiny to demonstrate this. How much any individual's sexuality may be pathological or not, or any attendant phenomenology be defined as 'co-morbid', must depend upon scrupulous and rigorous analysis of the individual concerned and not on a-priori assumption. We must as ever approach the individual on all occasions without knowledge, memory or desire and always remember that interpretation should never fail to be, as its etymology suggests, a consensual negotiation rather than the delivery of a higher truth. In addition, we need to remember how deeply ignorant we are about minds, psyches and brains and that such ignorance puts us all in great difficulty at the point at which we wish to define what is 'pathological' against any bench-mark of 'normality'.

I broadly agree, therefore, with the main thrust of Denman's first section, and can only concur that the language that she cites from Fordham's 'Androgyne' (in her third section) is indeed deprecatory, while his attitude emerges as prejudiced and contemptuous. I do, however, have a different understanding of the issue of the unconscious phantasy of the parental couple, and this in turn informs my thinking as to whether or not the sexual behaviours that she mentions might be seen as individuated. It also informs my thinking about the more political points that she raises in her final section.

The central issues in the paragraph on the unconscious phantasy of the parental couple are: (1) whether or not there is an unconscious phantasy of the parents and their sexual and baby-making activities; (2) whether this is a romantic ideal, one in which the heterosexual union has been exalted; (3) whether this phantasy is central to the structuring of unconscious and conscious life; and (4), if it is true, whether or not it puts heterosexuality at the centre of the psyche.

I think that it is probably fair to say that Denman leaves no doubt as to her answer to these questions, and you might say 'fair enough' given the airing that the equally firm opposite view has had. Despite my grounding in the view with which she disagrees, I found it very difficult to answer these questions with certainty.

I will assume in what follows that a reader of controversies is as thoroughly conversant with the literature to which Denman refers as she assumes they are.

Turning to issue (4), various analytic schools have developed the theory that the process whereby the infant's innate or archetypal competence is embodied is through the metaphor of a parental copulation. The abstraction may be most familiar in the form that Bion bequeathed: preconception (signed as the astrological sign for Mars or the biological symbol for masculine) + realization (Venus or feminine) → conception, as well as in Fordham's earlier version, deintegrate + realisation → conception. Interestingly, Jung's 1921 version, which may be found in the definition of the primordial image in *Psychological Types*, is by far the earliest: something in the infant finds something else in the environment to produce a mental content at some level of awareness, the primordial image. This is a 'concretization' which may either be stuck as such or be thought about and graduate to an 'idea', something more abstract and more flexible in the service of thought.

Those who propound this kind of model assume that these processes, which in themselves are completely abstract and gender/sexuality-free, can only be grasped metaphorically in the embodied form of the objects around us. Jung says 'the self is felt empirically not as a subject but as an object' (*CW*, 9i, para. 315). In his 'Psychological approach to the Trinity', Jung suggests that the trinity is a metaphor for the unfolding of the unconscious self, which is here symbolized as God, to yield the individuating self, symbolized as the Son, through the mediation of the Holy Ghost. Though the latter may sometimes appear as a mother this seems a largely sexuality-free formulation, unless possibly homosexual, while of course thoroughly male-bound. ('The psychological aspects of the Kore' offer us some sort of trinity with Demeter, Kore and Hecate, but I'm not sure that it addresses the area we are looking at.)

Several questions arise: is there an archetypal (i.e. abstract, unsaturated drive) to individuate? Is there any way of embodying such a drive that is not trinitarian? (I am leaving out the fourth, diabolical, element so as not to complicate what is already difficult enough.) And then, given that the first dyad we are likely to meet is a parental couple, do we and they form that trinity? And is the idea of such a trinity innate, as its being archetypal would imply? Jung is sometimes inconsistent about the innateness of the archetype, which he usually ascribes to the commu-nalities of central nervous structure and function, and sometimes attributes them to societal influences. Were they to turn out to be innate, however, would this imply that we are ready-wired for competition (envy and jealousy)? Or do we come as blanks who discover competition and their attendant emotions when we arrive in the world and as we develop?

I am less inclined to dismiss the 'sperm race' than Denman. There does seem to be some evidence that simple organisms compete and that, in an Aristotelian sense, that is a part of their 'psyche', i.e. a function of their make-up, much as metabolism is a large part of the 'psyche' or function of the liver (Wilkes, 1988). If the liver had a (conscious) mind, it would 'know' what it was doing, just as a spermatozoon might know about killing off its potential siblings in the female genital tract if it were wired up to a brain. Similarly, it is in neither the sperm's nor the egg's interest (or rather that of their DNAs) to help each other replicate, and there is evidence to suggest that they each try to disable the other. Things have evolved so that, while female DNA knocks out the male's capacity to make an emotional brain, the male eliminates the female's to construct a cortex, and between them they do the job, like Jack Spratt and his wife (Vines, 1997). But the point is that 'competition' and 'envious' behaviour are wired in in a way we might, after Jung, call 'psychoid' from the preconception of the organism. This does not require awareness, but it does imply a 'knowledge' of the existence of competition – another couple, just as the chick's freeze response to a predator silhouette implies 'knowledge' of predators. Psyche without mind.

To the Kleinians and Jungians who say that they have an overwhelming mass of clinical evidence to support the idea that there is an innate knowlege of objects in the infant and that their expectation of preconception meeting realization is personified by some shadowy apprehension of a parental couple, I suspect that Denman would say that this is simply because such analysts find what they expect to find. I am not sure that at the moment there is an answer to that, so that the answer to the question, 'Is it true?', must come when we are less ignorant. Nor can ethology, anthropology or the neurosciences help us much, despite the astonishing strides in the latter over the last 30 years or so. The questions that the neurosciences can address are at present much simpler, but they do support a view that the neurological processes underlying sexuality in general and homosexuality in particular can be independent of the external environment and its objects, and so, by inference, of any pathology of thinking (Panksepp, 1998).

So, however strong our views of the matter either way or in any direction, we cannot say with scientific exactitude that (1) there is or is not an unconscious phantasy of the parents and their creativity and procreativity, nor can we say that there is or is not an abstraction that is embodied in them. If there were, would it necessarily be idealized in the way that Denman seems to suggest it necessarily is in her point (2)? I suppose that if the existence of such a phantasy could be demonstrated to be true beyond any reasonable doubt, it is also true that it would be as likely to be subject to any abusive or defensive manoeuvre such as idealization that any other truth may be, rather as 'good enough mothering' has been idealized in certain quarters.

What if we could say with certainty that there is an unconscious phantasy of the parental couple? Does it put heterosexuality at the centre of the psyche? This is Denman's point number (4). One of the problems for the epistemological child is 'the facts of life' which, as I see it, should not be a problem for the homosexual any more than they should be for a single male or female, for someone who has chosen a life of celibacy, or indeed for someone who is for any reason unable to conceive, of either sex. The facts of life are common to us all and, as I see them, are these: that we are all to some extent dependent (Fairbairn's mature dependency), and as infants, utterly so; that we all appreciate that the failure of this dependency is potentially death; that dependability has its limits and failures; and that these limitations include obligation to other dependants (rivals) and partners, as well as the needs of the object.

So far, it has not been necessary to specify any gender to the rivals for the sake of the argument. What is important here, however, is that Bion and Money-Kyrle have refined an argument as to the development of thinking, which, if it is true, puts the facts of life squarely at the centre of the individual's capacity to function. For the sake of brevity, the argument suggests that, if the infant has a satisfactory experience of his or her object and is not overwhelmed by unbearable emotion that is not metabolized by the present mother or left too long by one who is absent, the absence can be filled with a thought, the memory perhaps of the nipple or teat in the mouth and the expectation of return. If, however, for whatever reason, conditions are too adverse and the infant is overwhelmed, then the 'object' that seems to have occasioned the catastrophe is evacuated and a spurious substitute is installed in the mind in an attempt to negate the absence, and with it, the facts of life.

Those who argue for this theory of thinking would argue that it explains those individuals who, when they present for analysis, find the facts of life intolerable: they are enraged by their dependency and/or deny it or the value of what can be offered them as contemptible; they are incensed at the limitations of the analytical setting and relationship which are seen as arbitary and cruel; our failures in the slightest regard are seen as intolerable and cynical spite, as is any evidence, such as the existence of other patients, let alone of family life, that anyone else exists in the analyst's life. And it is a commonplace that strenuous attempts, to the point of delusion, may be instituted to deny these facts of life: it will be known as a fact that we have no other patients and that we do not move from our consulting rooms between sessions, even and especially at weekends, while our absences are dealt with by not having had a mind for us, the analysis or what has transpired over its course. The thought has been evacuated, and such individuals often reproach us with the feeling, therefore, that 'they are back at square one'. There may also be evidence of the spurious substitute. A common experience, for instance, is that when an interpretation is made, the patient already knows it, or that it is defective and/or that it does not go quite far enough. Usually when these are the case and we are with patients who are motivated to negotiate an interpretation as interpretation always needs to be, the patient can give us evidence of the area of disagreement, even if it cannot be clearly articulated. The individual for whom separation is a disaster cannot do this, and is likely to have great difficulty in permitting any thought at all.

The theory that I am describing would suggest that the patient has constructed alternative facts of life in which he or she already has the equivalent of our thought and that which 'generates' them in their mind. Furthermore, since babies do not have such abstractions as 'thought' available, this is likely to be a version of the expedient whereby the infant mobilizes the idea that a nipple in the mouth can be equated to a tongue in the mouth or a turd in the bottom, with the advantage in the latter case that a turd in the bottom may seem satisfyingly like father's penis and/or a baby inside mummy.

This brings us to the final facts of life which I have not yet mentioned. These are that there are certain ways in which we may not compete. It is a fact of life that I am not as good an analyst as X, am not as talented as Y, do not have the same understanding as Z etc., etc., etc. Men cannot bear children or lactate. Nor can babies, of course. And the final fact of life: that the only way that babies can be made is by the meeting of male and female gametes from adult genitals. If the baby for whom separation, along with any rivalry which implies it, is intolerable succumbs to the need to remedy the intolerable by insisting that tongues are nipples and produce milk, that turds are penises that are babies and that the not-thought is generative thought, and therefore creativity are, according to this theory, seriously impaired.

Notice that I am not arguing for the truth of this formulation on the same grounds that I demurred earlier. What I wish to address here is Denman's idea that were (1) and (3) to be true, i.e., that the couple and the abstraction it represents could be validated and that they were important for the structuring of psychic life, this would, as she says, (4) put heterosexuality at the centre of psychic life. It would seem to me rather *that it put facts at the centre of reality* and would be no more prejudicial to homosexuals than the fact that swallows migrate to Africa is prejudicial to humans. Babies cannot procreate, whatever their delusions; humans cannot fly, whatever theirs. To suggest that this is about sexuality rather than evidence seems to me pejoratively to confuse the homosexual with the child, as if to be homosexual were also to be as unable to deal with the facts as a child might be.

There is a final question that Denman poses, which is that if it were true that the phantasy of the parental intercourse is central to psychic organization, this necessarily implies that homosexuals are at odds with nature. As I see it, the same argument obtains as in the last paragraph. Perhaps any *pathological* sexuality, whether asexuality, hetero- or homosexuality, *might* turn out to be at odds with nature, though I would think it more clinically helpful to connote it as wanting to defy reality and its evidence, because this implies something that at least in principle implies the possibility of arriving at a different, negotiated consensus, whereas 'being at odds' suggests unnegotiable defect. But, if Panksepp's (1998) account is right, then homosexuality is a part of nature as a function of neural organization and chemistry, and need be at odds neither with it nor with reality and evidence, any more than celibacy, single status, asexuality, heterosexuality or being a swallow need be.

If, then, we were to eschew a facile definition of homosexuality as 'against nature' or perverse, how might we regard 'perversion' or 'deviancy' conceptually? (It's difficult to avoid the language of 'generation'.) I would like to suggest an analogy with 'perverting the course of justice', and put forward the idea that Bion's theory of thinking would indicate that our clinical enquiry should be aimed at understanding the ways in which those who come to us for help may be 'perverting' the facts of life and therefore perverting the course of thought. Does the celibate perhaps harbour the illusion that he or she is one of their parents who is withholding conception from their other parent? Is the man who insists on regular, monotonous sex with his wife in the missionary position sustaining the illusion that he is his father in relation to his mother? Is the Don Juan of fleeting, casual sexual encounters someone who, by insisting on the interchangeability of his partners, is able to deny separation while sadistically subjecting them-as-his-mother to devastation? Are there instances where the fister of either sex is insisting on their possession of a very big, grown-up penis which can hurt? Or where the fisted may be identifying with the parent to be hurt? Would all of these be examples of denying separation, dependency or the threat of rivalry?

On the other hand, we need to be in a position to recognize, as Denman rightly suggests we need to be able to when it is true, that there is something importantly healthy in what our patients are describing which has nothing to do with perverting the course of reality and thought. As Denman suggests, we need to develop new 'standards of judgement for sexual aesthetic, etiquette and . . . pathology'. As I understand the theory of thinking that I have outlined, it would enable practitioners and patients of 'sexualities other than heterosexuality' to evaluate dispassionately whether the practices and relationships under scrutiny had to do with the *use of objects*, in Winnicott's meaning where the object is perceived as an entity independent of the subject, or more to do with *object-relating*, as he idiosyncratically uses this term, that is to denote a relationship where the object is not perceived at all as having any existence independent of the subject's projective identificatory omnipotence, but is entirely disposable by that subject. We have seen that 'object-relating' in the more usual sense is central to the formation of the 'primordial image' (though Jung did not use the term) and therefore the beginning of individuation, and I would not therefore see object-relating and individuation as alternatives or antithetical, as Denman seems to, although the concretization needs to be surrendered to yield the individuated 'idea'. What, however, is a crucial consideration is the extent that the projective identificatory processes are in the service of binding the object into inseparability, and the extent to which their motivation is claustral, i.e. anti-thought, anti-reality, anti-function, anti-mind. To the extent that any practice is any of these things, anti-reality/function/mind, however ostensibly 'normal', it might be thought of as 'perverse'. It might be understood as an attempt to 'turn' truth around to suit the subject. Etymology helps.

The advantage of a theory of mental organization of the sort that Jung, Fordham, Bion and Money-Kyrle have elaborated might seem to be that, far from implicitly glorifying heterosexuality and implicitly denigrating 'deviation' from it, it offers us a pragmatic means of assessing 'perversion' and its absence at a much more profound level than arbitrary assertions on the basis of what a majority or substantial minority are up to (on which basis, a majority insistence on genocide would be acceptable), or on a doctrinal decision as to what was moral or not (so that, presumably, the hard line at the Vatican, in the shadow of SS. Paul and Augustine, would be that any sex not explicitly aimed at procreation was perverse, deviant and immoral). The fact that practitioners who have used a theory may have not used it in a dispassionate or unprejudiced way does not imply that the theory itself is gender/sexuality biased, any more than Marxism necessarily implies oppressive totalitarianism or Christianity the slaughter of unbelievers.

What is important is that the individual be in touch with reality and evidence, so as to be able to function both in an internally creative world and in the external world with a sense of well-being. Being at odds with the evidence usually makes most of these difficult for the people who consult us, whatever their sexuality, especially where specious versions of reality are used to protect the individual from reality. It is much easier to confront these if we understand that the reality from which they are having to protect themselves, whatever their sexuality, has usually been unbearable, often with very considerable deprivation that makes separation and the idea of the exclusive, generative couple seem like an intolerable insult. It follows that it is only in analysing the meaning of an individual's behaviour including their sexual activities, rather than by insisting on their phenomenology as pathological by definition, that we can judge whether or not they are ways of substituting spurious reality for one that is intolerable, or ways of achieving object-relating that in other language Jung thinks is necessary for individuating ('individua*ted*' almost certainly *is* an exalted ideal!) Presumably it is on the same criteria that we should assess any candidate for training, homosexual or otherwise: are they individuating, or is individuation blocked by an insistence on a plausible, claustral concretization which precludes the facts of life in whatever form?

As for the question as to whether homosexual couples should have/adopt children the fact is that they are already doing so, and perhaps a more interesting question is as to whether Segal's or Denman's views will be born out by the natural experiment in whose midsts we find ourselves, just as we find ourselves in the midst of a neuroscientific revolution which will, one hopes, dispel the need to split into camps of defensive certainty. If the apprehension of the 'trinity' as an abstraction is innate, does it matter how it is incarnated? If it is an innate expectation, how close a fit does there need to be between expectation and realization? And what will happen as the external lineaments of the facts of life that incarnate the putative archetype change with homosexual parental couples, with IVF, with cloning . . . ? Again, some think that there is evidence we may derive from the 'experiment' of single motherhood about the importance of the father as a real, external figure; but these observations largely derive from the theories of which Denman is suspicious. We need the cooperation of other disciplines that are innocent of our prejudices.

In the meantime, we creep, forward, we hope, rather than back, in ignorance that we should always repent, and hope that we learn from our experience and from the harms that our culture-bound assumptions and prejudices, including political correctness, inflict on individuals and society. I fear that public penitence and atonement could be a full-time activity and may be better replaced by careful revision in the light of the facts of life as they become available to us. That requires of us all a real tolerance and readiness to revise our views from whatever initial cherished viewpoint we start off.

Just a final point on language: I realize that the word 'homophobic' is with us to stay with its present lexical meaning, but it troubles me as a coinage because etymologically it means 'fear of the same', rather than 'fear or hatred of homosexuals' which is what it has been coined to mean. This seems to me to rob us of the capacity to refer to the possibility that some compulsive or defensive heterosexuality might derive from 'fear of the same' ('homophobia'), a repudiation of the attraction perhaps to the parent or other members of the same sex, rather than from the 'natural' sources to which Panksepp refers, this being presumably normal 'heterophilia'; or perhaps from thinking that some homosexuality might derive defensively from 'heterophobia', fear, possibly of the attraction to the parent or to members of the opposite sex, rather from Pankseppian normal 'homophilia'. There is another important issue latent in these etymologies, aside from that of sexual object choice: we might notice that most prejudice is based on fear and hatred of otherness – heterophobia: fear of those who are of other countries, other tribes, other race, other gender, other sexuality, other schools of thought, other schools of analysis even. All these are examples of 'heterophobia' in the etymological sense – all with stupid, tragic consequences.

REFERENCES

Jung, C. G. (1921) 'Psychological Types'. *Collected Works*, Vol. 6. London: Routledge and Kegan Paul.

Panksepp, J. (1998) *Affective Neuroscience*. Oxford: Clarendon Press.

Vines, G. (1997) 'Where did you get your brains?' *New Scientist*, 2nd May, pp. 34–39.

Wilkes, K. (1988) *Real People*. Oxford: Clarendon Press..

(c) Response to Carvalho

Chess Denman

Carvalho's chapter packs a very large number of ideas into a small space making a comprehensive response difficult. In consequence I shall confine myself to a few selected areas. Carvalho is careful to avoid any suggestion of prejudice against homosexuality and, I am sure that he does not, consciously, hold prejudiced views. However, as is very common in current discourse around this topic his chapter does reveal a bias against homosexual orientation or, rather, a bias towards heterosexual orientation. A core notion at the centre of all the arguments around this topic is that of perversion and Carvalho's chapter can be read as an attempt to produce a definition of perversion that is free of any direct judgement about the acts being performed but is rather a description of a certain state of mind. However, I argue that the whole concept of perversion (along with a whole host of pathologizing terms in psychoanalysis, such as manipulation, or defence) is unhelpful and is, in practice, most often used to attack patients rather than to help them.

For this reason it is important to correct Carvalho's representation of me right at the start of his chapter as 'emphasiz[ing] that heterosexuality can on occasion be deeply perverse'. This is incorrect and rests on a misreading of my chapter. The term perversion at once judges and forecloses. Take Carvalho's description of some acts of fisting as possibly involving fantasies about big painful penises. He might be right, but his line of speculation reveals that he has not talked to many fisters about what the activity means to them. If he did he would discover a set of discourses about trust, another about skill and yet a third about ecstatic experience. He would also discover a wide range of ideas about penises and about penetration (along the lines of not every penis penetrates and not everything that penetrates is a penis) and ideas about how fisting relates to penile penetration. Talking in detail to people about their sexuality involves finding mutual terms of discussion and negotiating a space of mutual debate. This is instantly made difficult by the use of terms like unconscious phantasy, which assign privileged knowledge to the analyst leaving the patient's direct experience only second place.

It is worth being clear that I am suggesting that the whole theoretical and analytic edifice built around the concept of unconscious phantasy inherently involves an imposition on the patient of a preconceived metapsychology the truth of which is, from the analyst's point of view, non-negotiable. The ill-effects of this position are in proportion to the distance between the analyst's and the patient's experience. Where both share the same – or largely the same – world-view little (or at least less) distortion is imposed by the metapsychology used. As world-views diverge the difficulties multiply so that, for example, Carvalho's use of fisting as a potentially perverse act is the most worrying precisely because Carvalho is speculating about the unconscious meaning of an act with which he is apparently unfamiliar.

But, if the analyst cannot bring to bear his or her metapsychology on the patient's material, what is he or she to do? To my mind there are two potential routes out of the dilemma of how to take a truly non-judgemental view of the patient. The first is to be aware of and to acknowledge the inherent biases in one's metapsychology by discussing these with patients and perhaps by suggesting to some patients that a different kind of therapy or analyst would be more appropriate. This route is blocked if, as I think Carvalho does, one argues that there are no biases inherent in the metapsychology being used. A second route involves a wholly different paradigm for the analytic enterprise, which eschews the notion of depth entirely in favour of an existential or intersubjective position. In my view some American Jungians, including some variants of Hillman's archetypal psychology, approach this position

It will come as no surprise therefore that I reject the notion that it is in any way helpful to talk about infants as 'mobiliz[ing] the idea that a nipple in the mouth can be equated to a tongue in the mouth or a turd in the bottom' and Carvalho is right to suppose that I believe that suggestion and biased observation account for the data on which these theories are built. Carvalho, discussing these theories, suggests that the evidence is not all in yet and that we should on this account suspend judgement. However, I think that the notions behind the theories espoused by Bion, Meltzer and Fordham are both logically and philosophically incoherent. In Wittgenstein's terms they are non-sense and for this reason no amount of evidence gathering is capable of validating them

Carvalho argues that the theories of Bion, Meltzer and Fordham offer a 'profound and pragmatic means of assessing "perversion" and its absence at a much more profound level than arbitrary assertions on the basis of what a majority or substantial minority are up to'. The notion of a deeper viewpoint than that of the common mass is to my eye somewhat chilling. It sets the analyst up above all others in his or her capacity to spy out such things as anti-reality.

I think most analysts would object at this point. There is a huge analytic literature on the way in which analysts should suspend judgement and maintain a neutral stance, and it is indeed ironic that this same analytic perspective that can make profound and pragmatic judgements avows dispassionate open neutrality while at the same time holding on to a rigid and moralizing metapsychology. Bion's injunction that we should be free from memory and desire, cited approvingly by Carvalho, is held up as an example of analytic openness and neutrality. On closer inspection though, Bion's injunction enjoins us to something at once impossible, and inhuman – for memory and desire are the greater parts of our humanity. When we purge ourselves of them we lose any of the recall on which humility might be based and any of the tangle of desire on which kinship with our patient could be established. Surely therefore this was not what Bion meant. He must have meant some memories only: some desires only should be absent from the room. If so, which memories, which desires to exclude? And who shall arbitrate their exclusion? Giving up rigidity, certainty and preconception, if you like, involves accepting, however sad it may be, that there is no site of profundity or pragmatics that is apart from the majority or the substantial minority.

Of a part with the general theme of wished-for purification by clear separations between truth and anti-truth, reality and anti-reality is the idea that theories can be separated neatly from the uses to which they are put. Carvalho attempts to wash clean the Bion–Meltzer–Fordham fusion from its homophobic past by arguing that the uses of a theory do not contaminate the theory itself. So, for Carvalho, Marxism does not necessarily imply totalitarianism nor Christianity the slaughter of unbelievers. However, for me when a theory has been put to terrible use we simply must bring ourselves to distrust the theory or at least to treat it with extreme suspiciousness. Theories do not exist in another plane from the world we live in but only in our minds. That their presence in some minds has motivated acts of clear immorality makes them risky objects at best.

I want now to turn to biology which figures largely in Carvalho's chapter. Passages in it imply, I think, that homosexuality may have a biological substrate. I think also that there is an implication that this means homosexuality is in some way 'natural'. What worries me here is the idea, which I would tend to resist strongly, that if homosexuality were chosen by someone for entirely social reasons it would in some way be less legitimate. But Carvalho uses biology to bring up another notion, which is, at base I think, the idea that the structure of the natural world patterns the structure of the psychic world and, to an extent, that the structure of the natural world sets norms for the structure of the psychic world.

For example, Carvalho tells us that something called female DNA 'knocks out the male's capacity to make an emotional brain, the male eliminates the female's to construct a cortex', having previously speculated on what a sperm would know if wired up to a cortex. Behind these ideas, which I find a bit far-fetched, lies the notion that the natural world structures the way our mind works. Later in the chapter, Carvalho lists 'facts of life': 'Men cannot bear children or lactate . . . and the final fact of life: the only way that babies are made is by the meeting of male and female gametes from adult genitals'. Carvalho's use of these facts is obscurely put but he does seem to mean that these special facts are at 'the centre of reality'. That is to say that the natural order patterns the psychic one. Or rather, that if it does not pattern the psychic one then a denial of reality is occurring which distorts the mind and that we call this denial 'perversion'.

The core of this argument seems ultimately to be no more than 'it's natural' which after a lot of complicated working comes to be 'it's natural we should think this way'. In this way nature is somehow taken to have a voice, to structure the core of our thoughts. However, this is wrong. Nature has no voice, no meaning of its own. It only takes on the many meanings we read into it. If a sperm were wired up to a brain and the brain to a mouth, nothing intelligible would be said; nor, indeed, can livers think. To me this means that we cannot turn to nature to judge behaviour.

To put it another way Carvalho expresses some of the Bion–Meltzer–Fordham view in this area in terms of the fantasy of a 'best truth'. What he does not tell us is why the centre of reality or truth is composed of the union of sperm and egg rather than of any other selected fact but it is clear that he thinks this is the case. However, there is no 'centre' to 'reality'. For reality stretches out as far as anyone can see without intrinsic meaning or reason and, while what we make of it may be dominated in our minds by one or two chief ideas, this is at best a fleeting and local matter even within a single psyche. What we make of reality is always a social matter, always something done in communication with another. This means that there can be no profound or pragmatic means of judgement free of the social struggles and the behaviour of other majority or minority groups.

Last, I want to discuss atonement. Carvalho worries that saying sorry publicly will become a full-time activity, although the total absence of such activities so far rather militates against this fear. Instead of atonement Carvalho favours further, more dispassionate, even stately, revision of views as evidence becomes available and implies that this will require tolerance on all sides. It might seem churlish or strident or 'deeply felt' to disagree with the call for measured theoretical agnosticism which permeates Carvalho's chapter. But it is worth reflecting on what this seemingly even-handed tolerance might mean for gay men and lesbians, or people with other alternative sexualities? I argue that, Carvalho's arguments notwithstanding, the core of the Bion–Meltzer–Fordham position is a celebration and elevation of heterosexual coitus, and the metapsychology it spawns is inevitably one which sets 'at the centre of reality' a heterosexual ideal. This ideal tends to treat as odd, curious, abnormal or perverse other kinds of sexuality, either in the mind or in the body. From the starting point of this metapsychology with its essentialist roots tolerance will always fail.

But should we analysts not atone, even if it be time-consuming? Do we not owe it to our patients and to the patients of our predecessors? The main value of atoning would lie in the healing value of saying sorry publicly to the many gay men and lesbians who, like Fordham's patient, were subjected to analytic abuse and anti-therapeutic treatment, to the candidates refused admission to training, to the analysts hiding (even as I write) in the closet. For me the first part of atonement is acknowledging the past. As professionals we need to acknowledge that we are members of a group that has damaged people by following the homophobic views of analysts of the stature of Klein, Meltzer, Guntrip, Balint, Casement, Jung, Bollas and Fordham. Saying sorry would do those we have hurt a lot of good and that is reason enough to do it, whatever length of time we might need to take

(d) Reply to Denman's response

Richard Carvalho

Not forgetting the substantial areas of agreement to which I alluded in my original response, I would like to address what I feel to be a misunderstanding about the concept most familiar in the form of container/contained. This is an abstraction, which seems usually to be personified by the Oedipal situation

Bion's model of container/contained arose as an attempt to account for disordered thinking. Something completely inchoate from an un-realized psyche meets a coherent response, probably at a psychosomatic level, often in a suitably attuned mother who is likely to be in a state that Winnicott characterized as primary maternal preoccupation. The coherent response may well be provided by a foster-carer or adoptive parent and, as society changes and as homosexual couples begin to adopt, 'mothering' and 'fathering' will presumably increasingly be provided by men and women respectively. Up until now, however, it has seemed that this process whereby something *metaphorically* characterized as 'male' is contained in the comprehension and sense of something conveyed *metaphorically* as 'female' has found its isomorph in an adult heterosexual intercourse. Not a lot has been written about what form its personification takes when other versions of adult intercourse (sexual and other) are available as metaphorical templates. Of and as itself, there is nothing idealized about this. Indeed, most of the literature, including Bion and Money-Kyrle, concerns the failure of the maternal environment and the causative and consequent attacks on linking.

I think that a much more potent source of idealization is likely to be the fact that what has to be tolerably embodied is archetypal, unconscious material which remains of its essence unknowable and unattainable to conscious processes. As a result, as consciousness emerges out of unconsciousness, two mutually uncomprehending and exclusive realms emerge: these are the realms of conscious process, and unconscious process. It is the latter (unbounded, omnipotent and omniscient, and therefore idealized) that is projected onto the carers, their bodies and their relatings, presumably whatever genders may be involved, though we perhaps do not yet know the outcome of this experiment. The result is a 'supremely good object' and a 'supremely creative intercourse' in Money-Kyrle's language. These would correspond to the mother archetype and the conjunctio between conscious and unconscious in Jung's terminology. These personify the creative capacities of the individual, which are both them and not them: as processes to a large extent beyond their conscious awareness and control, they are not theirs to conjure at will, so that they have to be waited for. In this respect, therefore, they can be likened to a parental intercourse. Whatever genders this may turn out to involve, it will inevitably be experienced as exclusive. It is evident that sexuality is not the issue here – homo- or hetero-sexuality, but the idealized contents of a self beyond omnipotent control of the ego. As such, they will also be the objects of envy, as will be, therefore, the phantasized couple in the intercourse which personifies them, whatever their genders.

This, to repeat, as I understand it, is an abstraction: something (archetypal of the unknown self) meets something else (in the environment) which defines the something in the subject self. This something else is probably a carer, and the meeting is a bit like what is phantasied to go on between the something else and a rival (intercourse or whatever that is dimly taken to mean beyond rivalry for what we are not getting ourselves so that we fear someone else might be). My excursus into biology is explained by the fact that, in my view, to the extent that organisms are adapted to the environments in which they live, their adaptation appears as if it involves innate 'knowledge': the baby 'knows' that the nipple is there; baby chicks 'know' that hawks are predators; all life 'knows' that rivals are likely to survive at each others' expense. All this is 'psyche' in Aristotle's sense of the word, signs of being 'animate', perhaps even 'psychoid', to use Jung's term. It IS nature, and when nature develops a central nervous system with cortical function which is complex enough to have a mind, nature does indeed evolve a voice. By dwelling on the biological, incidentally, I do not in anyway wish to minimize the importance of the social or cultural environment which is both the creation and the context of our biology.

The model I have been suggesting is that creative process is personified by heterosexual parental intercourse. Were this to be vindicated by experience (and we are of course, lamentably ignorant) then it is the abstraction I have stressed that the model would put at the heart of psychic functioning, not the objects that embody it in whatever gender combinations. As I have already suggested, we will increasingly be in a position to evaluate how flexible the archetypal process is with respect to the ethological complement it requires to personify it: will the deintegrative process which has hitherto been 'male' in relation to a 'female', 'containing' realization be as easily personified as rex and rex, or regina and regina as they have hitherto as rex and regina? Will it turn out that what has been archetypally 'mother' up till now can as easily be embodied by men, and what has been 'father' be represented by women? Presumably it will be three or four generations before we have the answers to this sort of question. But, in the meantime, what matters adaptively is the resulting functioning of the individual, and I regret that I was not apparently clear enough in my expression of the notion that, as an abstract idea, 'perversion' seems entirely unhelpful. What matters in any individual on any given occasion is not the formal attributes of an activity, whether analysing, interpreting, intercourse in any position involving whatever organ, doing the washing up or walking in the park. What matters is whether it constitutes facilitation, obstruction or evasion of adaptation or ongoing individuation. Certainly, interpretation as Denman presents it, as a non-consensual activity where one person's view is forced upon another, would not be in the service of individuation. In fact interpretation, as its etymology suggests, should be a consensual negotiation – inter = between, pretium = price, i.e., barter as to the value or meaning of a statement or communication. The activity that Denman describes sounds to me more like violation of the trust put in the analytic intercourse, executed without love or skill. It is certainly not in the service of individuation and is emphatically technically crass.

There are many other interesting issues to take up in Denman's original chapter and her response to my reply. I shall take up just one of them. This is that theories that may be thought to have been propagated in a climate averse to homosexuality might not be purged but should rather be expunged. The abstraction that I am suggesting is that the core of this theory of thinking may turn out in the light of experience to be wrong. But to put such a theory on the Index because it may have been misapplied, or invoked by individuals in the service of their prejudice, would seem to me to be descending to the inquisitorial level that Denman so rightly deplores. It would be equivalent to expunging Russell's theory of sets which is, I gather, thought to be inconsistent in certain quarters, on the basis of his having been a misogynist womanizer, rather than modifying or even rejecting it on the basis of what could be proved or disproved of his mathematics.

Approaching religion

Introduction

This chapter explores contrasting approaches to Jung's view of religion. A particular emphasis is placed on academic attitudes to religious aspects of his work.

Roderick Main argues that suspicion of Jung's views on religion have contributed in the past to his exclusion from a largely rational, secular academy. He goes on, however, to assert that the proliferation of the scientifically dominated world-view promoted by that academy is felt by many to pose a threat to the spiritual dimension of their existence. This may have contributed to a compensatory rise in the popularity of 'irrational' phenomena such as New Age religion and religious fundamentalism.

The time is therefore right, Main claims, for academia to reconsider Jung. There has always been a strong scientific strand to his thinking. But the religious element, which in the past worked against him, may now actually operate in his favour. Academics and others are urgently searching for ways of understanding the current upsurge of the irrational without denigrating it. And Jungian thought may be in a position to act as a bridge between these two previously disparate worlds.

Melanie Withers is a welcome but late contributor to the book. The timing of her contribution has in some ways been fortuitous, however – Jungians might even say synchronous. It has given her the chance to offer a different view to Main's thesis in the light of the terrible events of September 11th, 2001 and the potency of religious fundamentalism. Withers contends that Jung's approach to the irrational is in danger of replicating some of the problems it attempts to resolve. In particular, if analytic theories assume the status of literal or scientific truth, rather than narrative analysis, figures such as Jung and Freud can themselves come to stand as icons against the terrifying realities of life and death they seek to explain. She further argues that transformation can only occur at the level of the social imaginary with an acknowledgement that doctrinal certainty is at best illusory and at worst oppressive.

(a) Analytical psychology, religion and the academy

Roderick Main

INTRODUCTION

In recent years, analytical psychology has had some notable success in becoming integrated within the academy (see, for example, Kirsch, 2000: 55–56, 121–23). One major factor contributing to this is the appearance of an increasingly rigorous level of scholarly work on Jung by sympathetic academics (e.g., Ellenberger, 1970; Homans, 1979; Shamdasani, 1995; Bishop, 1995, 2000). Another is the increasing willingness and ability of some post-Jungian thinkers to engage with prevalent academic discourses on their own terms – for instance, in philosophy (e.g., Papadopoulos and Saayaman, 1991; R. Brooke, 1991), politics (e.g., Samuels, 1993, 2001), literature (e.g., Rowland, 1999), or social and cultural theory (e.g., Adams, 1996; Hauke, 2000). However, even in the midst of this success, one can frequently notice considerable caginess, not to say embarrassment, when academics encounter the religious component within analytical psychology. Often, this religious component is alone sufficient grounds for academics to disregard Jungian contributions to their fields. Such embarrassment, though possibly less frequent and acute, is not absent even within religious studies, where Jungian theory provides more often the object than the method of study and where more rationalistic theoretical or methodological frameworks usually keep the religious attitude within Jungian thought safely pinioned. It is true that many commendable studies of the relationship between analytical psychology and religion have continued to appear – some with a more academic, others with a more clinical emphasis (see, for example, Heisig, 1979; Stein, 1985; Ryce-Menuhin, 1994; Lammers, 1994; Corbett, 1996; Palmer, 1997). However, this on its own does not seem to affect the overall academic disquiet about the religiosity embedded in Jungian theory.

The problem was highlighted a few years ago, when there was a discussion in the *Journal of Analytical Psychology* on 'Analytical psychology and academic studies' in which the contributors shared their reflections on the problems and potentialities of teaching Jungian ideas in the academy (see Tacey, 1997a, 1997b; Brooke, 1997; Papadopoulos, 1997; Ulanov, 1997). David Tacey, the primary contributor, concluded his 'Reply to responses' by arguing that the powerful 'academic resistance to Jung' that he and others experience 'must be viewed as a "religious" problem'. In Tacey's view, 'Jung's response to the world and psychic reality is fundamentally religious':

> No amount of fancy post-modern footwork by the cleverest Jungian intellectual will manage to take this religious attitude away from Jung. And that is, I think, what ultimately sticks in the throat of the secular academy, and why it so fiercely opposes Jung, no matter how spruced up or reconstructed he is made to be. (Tacey, 1997b: 315–316)

I have no difficulty agreeing with Tacey's characterization of Jung's outlook as 'fundamentally religious'. As articulated by Jung, such core concepts as the collective unconscious, archetypes, individuation, and the self presuppose a dimension of reality that is intelligent, purposeful, and irreducible to material, social, or cultural terms (see Jung, 1928–54: passim). Jung frequently equated his psychological concepts with traditional religious ones (see, for example, his analyses of the doctrine of the Trinity, 1942/1948; the symbolism of the Mass, 1942/1954; and the problem of evil, 1952a). He even designated experience of numinosity as the most important factor in therapy (Jung, 1973: 376–377). However, the religious aspect of Jung's outlook is only half the story, for his outlook is also, and no less 'fundamentally', secular, by which I here mean concerned with natural, specifically scientific, and human-centred principles and methods of explanation rather than supernatural ones (see, for example, Jung, 1947/1954, 1952b). Jung's claim to be an empiricist and a phenomenologist (1938/1940: para. 2), his concern for the actualities of lived human experience (1938/1940: para. 88), and his refusal to engage in theological speculation (1938/1940: para. 2) are all part of this. It is mainly this secular aspect within Jung's theory that recent post-Jungians have so ably appealed to and drawn on in their attempts to integrate analytical psychology into the academy.

This doubleness, at once religious and secular, is, I think, a tremendous potential both in Jung's own thought and in subsequent analytical psychology. It emerged, historically and biographically, out of Jung's lifelong struggle to resolve the tension he experienced between the claims of traditional religion and secular modernity, as he himself and many later commentators have related (e.g., Jung, 1961; Homans, 1979; Charet, 1993; Main, 2000). As an outlook that attempts to remain true to both the religious and the secular attitudes, Jung's psychology arguably embeds insights from both, as well as about how the two sides can productively co-exist (Main, 2000: 92–97). In the following, I shall suggest a few reasons why this double nature of analytical psychology may be valuable, both for analytical psychology's engagement with the academy and for the academy's engagement with religion. First, I should explain why I think there may currently be an opportunity for these improved engagements.

RELIGION AND THE ACADEMY

Granted the basic problem voiced by Tacey that the academy is primarily oriented towards secular modes of thought, while analytical psychology embeds an inalienable religious aspect, nevertheless, the antipathy of the academy towards analytical psychology has often been exacerbated by at least two conditions. One is the academy's largely negative image of religion and the other is analytical psychology's frequently unsophisticated representation of itself. However, both of these conditions have considerably changed in recent years.

At the end of the nineteenth and beginning of the twentieth century, there was a widespread view among intellectuals (e.g., Marx, Nietzsche, Freud) that religion no longer had any positive relevance as a force in the world and might, with luck, eventually disappear. This post-Enlightenment view has informed thinking through-out much of the academy, tacitly as well as explicitly. However, at the beginning of the twentieth-first century, religion remains a major player on the world stage; it is neither disappearing nor, looked at from a global perspective, declining. It is true that some manifestations of religion, such as church-going in Britain, may have waned, but others, such as the numerous forms of fundamentalism and alternative spirituality appearing throughout the world, are currently burgeoning (Beckerlegge, 1998: 8–11). Quite apart from these explicit manifestations of religion, there is also a growing awareness of 'implicit religion' where a religious-style commitment informs secular activities (e.g., in politics, sport, or consumerism) (Hinnells, 1995: 234–235). Both explicitly and implicitly, religion remains inextricably bound up with politics, economics, ethics, health, life-styles, and culture generally. In the face of this unexpected persistence of religion, those working in the academy can scarcely afford to dismiss religious issues from serious consideration. Any theoretical approach, such as analytical psychology, that has a record of engaging seriously with religious phenomena may find it an opportune time to try to gain the academy's ear.

Underlying much of the antipathy of the secular academy for religion (and of religion for the secular academy) is the assumption that there is a fundamental and clear-cut conflict between their core values. If both try to explain the same phenomena (e.g., the natural world, society, human beings), but do so in incom-patible ways (e.g., one appeals to natural, the other to supernatural principles), then, it would seem, one outlook must be right and the other wrong. However, contemporary work on the relationship between religion and science (science being the prime exemplar of and influence on the secular approach) tends to recognize conflict as only one mode of engagement among other equally important modes such as independence, dialogue, and integration (see Barbour, 1998: 77–105). If religion and science do not necessarily conflict, then the ascendancy of science – and of the secularity that science supports – need not negate the potential value of religious approaches to understanding. The double nature of analytical psychology, then, may be a sign not of inner contradictions but of a theoretical complexity that better approximates to the experiential complexity of human life.

Furthermore, work in the history of science has demonstrated in detail the profound historical interdependence between religion and the very science that is so often set against religion by champions of secular modernity (see J. Brooke, 1991; Brooke and Cantor, 1998). With the increasing recognition that the modes of thought, the institutions, and the canonical figures of secular modernity have roots in religious soil, it becomes less easy to separate off and dismiss the dimension of religion even from the most hardcore secular fields. In the light of these developments in the history of science, the value of theoretical models, such as analytical psychology, that are conscious of and articulate about their past and present participation in the religious dimension, may increasingly come to be appreciated.

Another important factor is the postmodern challenge to the hegemony of the post-Enlightenment rationalism that has dominated the academy. As the limits of this rationalism have become apparent, so other kinds of rationality as well as avowedly non-rational approaches to understanding have begun to receive more attention. Thus, there has been a burgeoning of interest in and respect for the thought-worlds of pre-modern, non-Western, and other formerly marginalized cultures (see, for example, Tambiah, 1990). In such a climate, there is clearly space for the respectful reconsideration of religious attitudes and outlooks. Indeed, Tacey, when discussing the 'religious problem' of Jung and the academy, noted with a measure of optimism the 'spiritual possibilities in postmodernism itself', particularly in philosophical discourses of the 'Other' (Tacey, 1997b: 316). His suggestion that Jungians might vigorously and creatively contribute to this debate has recently been taken up by Christopher Hauke (see Hauke, 2000: especially pp. 205–215).

ANALYTICAL PSYCHOLOGY AND RELIGION

At the same time, recent years have seen some aspects of work on analytical psychology become considerably more sophisticated, so that those involved with the discipline, should they wish to do so, are now equipped to present a much more acceptable case for its religious aspect. The rigorous scholarship mentioned earlier has played a large part in this. Perhaps more formerly than now, there has been a tendency among adherents of analytical psychology to idealize Jung and to treat his insights and formulations, especially on religious topics, as having the status almost of revealed doctrines. Some have even written of his psychological model as a new religious dispensation (e.g., Edinger, 1984). Not surprisingly, these kinds of attitudes have prompted some equally uninhibited attacks on Jung (e.g., Noll, 1994, 1997). One value of some of the recent scholarship has been to introduce a moderating voice into these debates, presenting historical data or theoretical perspectives that make it harder to sustain either inflated or wildly denigrating religious images of Jung and analytical psychology (see, for example, Storr, 1999; Segal, 1999a, 1999b; Shamdasani, 1999). As more historical sources become available and are responsibly examined, a more realistic picture of the origin and development of Jung's thought has begun to emerge (e.g., Shamdasani, 1995, 1998). In particular, the kind of contextual work initiated by Ellenberger (1970) has helped more accurately to locate Jung and analytical psychology within the history of ideas, revealing numerous affinities and continuities between Jung's work and the work of others within the same historical milieu. If Jung sometimes emerges as less original than formerly supposed, he also appears as less eccentric. For instance, his interests in spiritualism, occultism, Gnosticism, and oriental religions, which have often provided the grounds for his being summarily dismissed as a mystic, were by no means idiosyncratic in late nineteenth- and early twentieth-century Europe (see, for example, Webb, 1976; Charet, 1993; Shamdasani, 1994; Hanegraaff, 1996).

The prospect of gaining a better hearing for the religious side of analytical psychology may also have improved as a result of the recent successes in integrating its secular side. The more analytical psychology proves itself to the academy on the academy's own terms, the harder it becomes to dismiss analytical psychology, even when it brings its religious aspect to the fore. Particularly valuable in this respect is the increasing sophistication with which exponents of analytical psychology can engage in debates about epistemology (e.g., Papadopoulos, 1984, 1997; Nagy, 1991; R. Brooke, 1991, 2000a; Kugler, 1997). Jung himself stands out among the early depth psychologists for the extent to which he was aware of and willing to engage with epistemological issues. While his own presentation of his epistemological position can be criticized for some dubious logical moves and historical misrepresentations (see, for example, Heisig, 1979: 103–145; Voogd, 1984; Bishop, 2000), various modified versions of it, as well as other positions inspired by it, can surely take a respectable place within the field of philosophical debate. At any rate, the vigour and intelligence with which contemporary post-Jungians are taking up and pursuing epistemological questions can only gain respect for the discipline that can prompt such deep and lively discussions. Moreover, whatever their secular starting point, once the specifically Jungian contribution enters the picture, such discussions tend towards a position where secular and religious assumptions are on an equal footing. For one of Jung's repeated arguments in this area is that the assumptions underlying the prevalent materialistic outlook are subject to precisely the same kinds of epistemological criticism as those underlying the religious outlook (Jung, 1939/1954: paras. 762–765; see also Main, 2000: 96). Indeed, for Jung, any thoroughgoing epistemological discussion cannot avoid addressing religious and theological issues.

ANALYTICAL PSYCHOLOGY AND THE ACADEMIC STUDY OF RELIGION

I have argued that analytical psychology has a double nature, inalienably involved in the spheres of both religion and secularity but fully identified with neither. However, it is the secular aspect of analytical psychology that has received most attention when integration of the discipline within the academy is attempted. Nevertheless, I have suggested that because of changes both in the academy's perception of religion and in analytical psychology's representation of itself, a climate may now exist in which the religious aspect of analytical psychology can be brought more effectively into the intellectual mainstream. I shall now briefly suggest some ways in which an acknowledgement of the religious attitude within analytical psychology might be turned to account in the study of two of the most prominent contemporary manifestations of religion: New Age spirituality and religious fundamentalism. These two areas have been singled out as especially problematic by both Tacey (1997b: 315) and Samuels (1998: 31–32). Part of their special interest for analytical psychology, I think, is that, like analytical psychology itself, they can be understood largely as responses to secular modernity (see Marty and Appleby, 1991; Heelas, 1996).

New Age spirituality

Tacey describes the New Age as 'simply the re-emergence of the religious impulse in a predominantly secular time' (Tacey, 1997b: 315), a view which, if we replace 'simply' with 'among other things', finds ample support in recent scholarship on the New Age (e.g., York, 1995; Heelas, 1996; Hanegraaff, 1996). In addition, the New Age is a response to secularity that has many significant points of similarity with the response of analytical psychology. For instance, both have an ambivalent but largely oppositional relationship to secular modernity. Both tend to react against the reductive tendencies of modern science while at the same time selectively appropriating ideas from modern science. Both place considerable importance on notions of psycho-spiritual transformation. Both engage eclectically with non-Western, pre-modern, and esoteric traditions. Both frequently frame contemporary experience in terms of myth. Both prioritize personal experience over institutionalized beliefs. Above all, both locate authority in the individual self (see Main, 2002; also York, 1995; Heelas, 1996).

These affinities may be the result partly of Jung's direct influence on the New Age, partly of shared heritage, and partly of shared contemporary concerns (see Main, 2002). However, the very presence of the affinities means that those oriented within analytical psychology potentially have access to the inner thought-world of the New Age. For example, when New Agers evince interest in holistic science, creative visualization, spiritually oriented therapies, paranormal phenomena, alchemy, astrology, the *I Ching*, Indian and Chinese religions, indigenous African and North American religions, myths from across the world, myth-centred reinterpretations of Christianity, or UFOs, the underlying principles and aspirations in these interests should not be too unintelligible to Jungians. Indeed, the literature of analytical psychology, especially its more classically oriented literature, is replete with these topics. Whether or not a particular exponent of analytical psychology shares or approves of such interests, the fact remains that they are woven into the history and theory of the discipline in a manner that could prevent summary dismissal and facilitate understanding when they are encountered in their New Age forms.

More specifically, Paul Heelas, in an extensive study of the New Age Movement, identifies 'self-spirituality' as its defining characteristic (1996: 18–19). The precise extent to which the understanding of 'self' and 'spirituality' in this formulation equates with the way the terms are understood in analytical psychology is less important than that the two terms are conjoined. Very rarely in any contemporary academic discourse would the self be designated spiritual. In analytical psychology, however, such designation is usual. Arguably, then, the religious dimension of analytical psychology, as embedded in the notion of a spiritual self, provides an insider appreciation, less accessible to secular perspectives, of what is possibly the central tenet and motivation of the New Age.

Of course, there are also important differences between analytical psychology and New Age spirituality. Tacey, for instance, has recently argued that the New Age differs from Jungian psychology especially in its one-sided celebration of the feminine (an overcompensation for the former one-sided commitment to patriarchal values) and in its naive elevation of bliss over suffering (Tacey, 1999: 36–42). It could be replied that the New Age is an expansive movement in which people participate in varying ways and at varying levels of sophistication (just as they do in analytical psychology and in religions), and it is certainly possible to point to some New Agers who do not exhibit the attitudes mentioned by Tacey (Main, 2002). Nevertheless, the differences Tacey identifies, as well as others, undoubtedly do exist in many cases and are important to bear in mind. Indeed, detailed awareness and discussion of such differences might be helpful in forestalling a tendency discernible in some analytical psychological writing of too readily denigrating the New Age for its superficiality and commercialism (for recent examples see Young-Eisendrath and Miller, 2000: 2, 4, 147, 176). Such criticism, itself often superficial, may serve to push the New Age out of consideration before it has been sufficiently understood. This would be unfortunate, since the New Age, if nothing else, is a very real social movement and as such a fit area for investigation by a culturally engaged analytical psychology (see Tacey, 2001). Clearer appreciation of the religious aspect of analytical psychology and its relation to secular modernity can serve here by providing the basis for a fairer assessment of the real similarities and differences between analytical psychology and the New Age.

Religious fundamentalism

The recent rise of fundamentalism within almost all the world's major religions stands in an often-noted relationship to the rise of secular modernity (Marty and Appleby, 1991; Beckerlegge, 1998: 16–22). Put simply, with the increasing dominance of secular values, traditional religious identities come under threat and respond by entrenching themselves. Moreover, they often do this in a way that leaves a seemingly unbridgeable gulf between religion and secularism. This presents a difficulty for those who wish to understand or engage with fundamentalism from an academic perspective. For the academy is, or fundamentalists often perceive it to be, a pre-eminent representative of the very secularity which fundamentalists oppose. Conversely, academics aligned with the values of secular modernity are unlikely to be able lightly to put aside their own deep opposition to the fundamentalist attitudes.

Analytical psychology has avoided any radical split between the religious and the secular domains. Indeed, it arguably has its origins largely in Jung's attempt to hold these two domains together. This may give exponents of analytical psychology certain potentialities for understanding phenomena such as religious fundamentalism – an area into which, with few exceptions (e.g., Brooke, 2000b), they have not yet ventured.

First, exponents of analytical psychology can empathize with religious fundamentalism in a way that secular academics usually cannot. However, in this case the capacity for empathy stems from a mediated rather than direct affinity. Few if any exponents of analytical psychology would share such extreme values and attitudes of religious fundamentalism as commitment to scriptural literalism, non-tolerance of religious diversity, and anti-individualism (Hinnells, 1995: 177–178; Marty and Appleby, 1991: vii). However, fundamentalists are also likely to hold, less distinctively but just as essentially, that there is a transcendent reality, that knowledge can be divinely revealed, and that emotional commitment to revealed knowledge can justifiably override rational criticisms of it. Here, in this terrain that fundamentalism holds in common with much mainstream religion, there is some affinity with analytical psychology. For analytical psychology also recognizes and attends to a transcendent reality, accepts the possibility of revealed knowledge, and acknowledges the validity of non-rational modes of apprehending and evaluating truth. To be sure, major differences remain. In analytical psychology, there is less dogmatism and certainty in the characterization of the transcendent; the revelations (e.g., in the form of dreams) are individual and relevant primarily to very specific circumstances; and the valuation of emotional awareness is a help-ful complement rather than a defensive alternative to reason. However, that analytical psychology respects these principles (in a way that the secular academy mostly does not) provides some participatory access to the world of thought of fundamentalism. That it nevertheless does not one-sidedly identify with them ensures that sufficient critical distance is maintained to generate academic understanding.

Second, because analytical psychology incorporates both secular and religious attitudes, it can help contain the impulse to pursue one or other attitude to extremity. A sensibility influenced by analytical psychology would find it difficult either to forget the sphere of religion when moving in secular contexts or to forget the need for intellectual openness when moving in religious contexts. It could dialogue with both sides and even facilitate dialogue between the two sides. Above all, it could exemplify the possibility of a non-polarized position. This resource is present in relation to any manifestation of religion but is especially relevant in the case of fundamentalism where the tendency to polarization is so strong.

Third, because Jung and subsequent exponents of analytical psychology have themselves often had to struggle with the tension between the religious and the secular and have had to resolve in themselves tendencies towards the polarization and splitting of these domains, they may be in a position to appreciate some of the psychological dynamics that can be involved. Particularly helpful might be an understanding of the role of projection and projective identification in creating and sustaining the split. Simply put, the religious attitudes of the fundamentalists may be extreme partly because they are affected by not only their own religious needs but also the unconscious – and hence undifferentiated, split off, and projected – religious needs of the secularists. (Conversely, of course, the critical rationalism of the secularists may be extreme partly because they are affected by the unconscious critical rationality of the fundamentalists.) Awareness of such unconscious dynamics operating in this context may be sharper in analytical psychology than in other depth-psychological approaches for at least two reasons. One is because in analytical psychology there is an assumption that the unconscious of each person contains 'an authentic religious function' (Jung, 1938/1940: para. 3). The possibility that secularists may be projecting their unconscious religiousness onto and into fundamentalists would be less likely to occur to adherents of theories which have usually considered religious needs to be inessential, pathological, and, in favourable cases, eradicable. The other reason is that Jungians may have experienced being caught in the same dynamic as the fundamentalists. For as Tacey observes, many academics may 'project their own largely unconscious devotional, religious, or belief life upon the Jungians and condemn them' (Tacey, 1997a: 281). As well as being condemned, Jungians may sometimes have been pushed by this into more extreme and obdurate expressions of religiosity than their theoretical inheritance requires.

CONCLUSION

Contrary to many confident predictions at the beginning of the twentieth century, religious phenomena are neither disappearing nor, looked at from a global perspective, declining. They continue to exist as a major force on the world stage and need to be engaged with intelligently. Analytical psychology has a long tradition of such serious engagement. In particular, analytical psychology, because it partly emerged out of tensions between traditional religion and secular modernity, embeds some potentially useful strategies and wisdom for responding to the complex and sometimes dangerously conflicting interactions between these domains. Because of changing academic perceptions of the relation of religion to modernity and changing self-presentations of analytical psychology, there may currently be an opportunity for analytical psychology within the academy to be more forthright about its religious component. I have offered a few brief indications of how a forthright acknowledgement of this religious component could be useful for the academic understanding of New Age spirituality and religious fundamentalism. However, to conclude on a qualifying note, it needs to be borne in mind that the kind of religious sensibility embedded in analytical psychology by no means accounts for the entire phenomenon of religion. Religion is a multidimensional phenomenon (Smart, 1997), and Jung and subsequent exponents of analytical psychology have tended to focus on only some of its dimensions (in particular the experiential and mythic), while paying less attention to others (such as the social, economic, and political). What analytical psychology can offer, modestly but importantly, is a helpful additional perspective in the academic engagement with contemporary religion.

REFERENCES

Adams, M. V. (1996) *The Multicultural Imagination: 'Race', Colour and the Unconscious.* London: Routledge.

Barbour, I. (1998) *Religion and Science: Historical and Contemporary Issues.* London: SCM Press.

Beckerlegge, G. (1998) *Religion at the End of the Twentieth Century*, Milton Keynes, UK: Open University Press.

Bishop, P. (1995) *The Dionysian Self: C. G. Jung's Reception of Nietzsche.* Berlin: Walter de Gruyter.

Bishop, P. (2000) *Synchronicity and Intellectual Intuition in Kant, Swedenborg, and Jung.* Lampeter, UK: The Edwin Mellen Press.

Brooke, J. (1991) *Science and Religion: Some Historical Perspectives*, Cambridge, UK: Cambridge University Press.

Brooke, J. and Cantor, G. (1998) *Reconstructing Nature: The Engagement of Science and Religion.* Edinburgh: T. & T. Clark.

Brooke, R. (1991) *Jung and Phenomenology.* London: Routledge.

Brooke, R. (1997) 'Jung in the academy: a response to David Tacey'. *Journal of Analytical Psychology*, Vol. 42, no. 2, 285–296.

Brooke, R. (Ed.) (2000a) *Pathways into the Jungian World: Phenomenology and Analytical Psychology.* London: Routledge.

Brooke, R. (2000b) 'Emissaries from the underworld: Psychotherapy's challenge to Christian fundamentalism', in P. Young-Eisendrath and M. E. Miller (Eds), *The Psychology of Mature Spirituality: Integrity, Wisdom, Transcendence.* London: Routledge.

Charet, F. X. (1993) *Spiritualism and the Foundations of C. G. Jung's Psychology.* Albany, NY: State University of New York Press.

Corbett, L. (1996) *The Religious Function of the Psyche.* London: Routledge.

Edinger, E. (1984) *The Creation of Consciousness: Jung's Myth for Modern Man.* Toronto: Inner City Books.

Ellenberger, H. (1970) *The Discovery of the Unconscious: The History and Evolution of Dynamic Psychiatry.* London: Allen Lane.

Hanegraaff, W. (1996) *New Age Religion and Western Culture: Esotericism in the Mirror of Secular Thought.* Leiden: Brill.

Hauke, C. (2000) *Jung and the Postmodern: The Interpretation of Realities.* London: Routledge.

Heelas, P. (1996) *The New Age Movement: The Celebration of the Self and the Sacralization of Modernity.* Oxford: Blackwell.

Heisig, J. (1979) *Imago Dei: A Study of Jung's Psychology of Religion*. Lewisburg, PA: Bucknell University Press.

Hinnells, J. (Ed.) (1995) *The Penguin Dictionary of Religions*. London: Penguin.

Homans, P. (1979) *Jung in Context: Modernity and the Making of a Psychology*. Chicago, IL: The University of Chicago Press.

Jung, C. G. (1928–54) *Psychology and Religion: West and East, Collected Works of C. G. Jung*, 20 vols, edited by Sir Herbert Read, Michael Fordham, and Gerhard Adler, executive editor William McGuire, trans. R. F. C. Hull, Vol. [hereafter *CW*] 11. London: Routledge & Kegan Paul, 1986.

Jung, C. G. (1938/1940) 'Psychology and Religion', *CW* 11: 3–105. London: Routledge & Kegan Paul, 1986.

Jung, C. G. (1939/1954) 'Psychological Commentary on "The Tibetan Book of the Great Liberation"', *CW* 11: 475–508. London: Routledge & Kegan Paul, 1986.

Jung, C. G. (1942/1948) 'A Psychological Approach to the Dogma of the Trinity', *CW* 11: 107–200. London: Routledge & Kegan Paul, 1986.

Jung, C. G. (1942/1954) 'Transformation Symbolism in the Mass', *CW* 11: 201–96. London: Routledge & Kegan Paul, 1986.

Jung, C. G. (1947/1954) 'On the Nature of the Psyche' *CW* 8: 159–234. London: Routledge, 1991.

Jung, C. G. (1951) *Aion: Researches into the Phenomenology of the Self. CW* 9ii, London: Routledge, 1991.

Jung, C. G. (1952a) 'Answer to Job', *CW* 11: 355–470. London: Routledge & Kegan Paul, 1986.

Jung, C. G. (1952b) 'Synchronicity: An Acausal Connecting Principle', *CW* 8: 417–519. London: Routledge, 1991.

Jung, C. G. (1961) *Memories, Dreams, Reflections*, recorded and edited by Aniela Jaffé, translated by Richard and Clara Winston. London: Fontana, 1995.

Jung, C. G. (1973) *Letters 1: 1906–50*, selected and edited by Gerhard Adler in collaboration with Aniela Jaffé, translated by R. F. C. Hull. London: Routledge & Kegan Paul.

Kirsch, T. (2000) *The Jungians: A Comparative and Historical Perspective*. London: Routledge.

Kugler, P. (1997) 'Psychic imaging: a bridge between subject and object', in P. Young-Eisendrath and T. Dawson (Eds), *The Cambridge Companion to Jung*. Cambridge, UK: Cambridge University Press, pp. 71–85.

Lammers, A. (1994) *In God's Shadow: The Collaboration between Victor White and C. G. Jung*, New York: Paulist Press.

Main, R. (2000) 'Religion, science, and synchronicity'. *Harvest: Journal for Jungian Studies*, Vol. 46, no. 2, 89–107.

Main R. (2002) 'Religion, science, and the New Age', in J. Pearson (Ed.), *Belief Beyond Boundaries*, Aldershot, UK: Ashgate; Milton Keynes, UK: Open University Press, pp. 173–222.

Marty, M. and Appleby, R. (1991) *Fundamentalisms Observed*. Chicago, IL: University of Chicago Press.

Nagy, M. (1991) *Philosophical Issues in the Psychology of C. G. Jung*. Albany, NY: State University of New York Press.

Noll, R. (1994) *The Jung Cult: The Origins of a Charismatic Movement*. Princeton, NJ: Princeton University Press.

Noll, R. (1997) *The Aryan Christ: The Secret Life of Carl Jung*. New York: Random House.

Palmer, M. (1997) *Freud and Jung on Religion*. London: Routledge.

Papadopoulos, R. (1984) 'Jung and the concept of the Other', in R. Papadopoulos and G. Saayaman (Eds), *Jung in Modern Perspective: The Master and His Legacy*. Bridport, UK: Prism Press, 1991 (1984), pp. 54–88.

Papadopoulos, R. (1997) 'Is teaching Jung within the university possible?: a response to David Tacey'. *Journal of Analytical Psychology*, Vol. 42, no. 2, 297–301.

Papadopoulos, R. and Saayaman, G. (Eds) (1991 [1984]) *Jung in Modern Perspective: The Master and His Legacy*. Bridport, UK: Prism Press.

Rowland, S. (1999) *C. G. Jung and Literary Theory*. London: Macmillan.

Ryce-Menuhin, J. (Ed.) (1994) *Jung and the Monotheisms: Judaism, Christianity and Islam*. London: Routledge.

Samuels, A. (1993) *The Political Psyche*. London: Routledge.

Samuels, A. (1998) 'Will the post-Jungians survive?', in A. Casement (Ed.), *Post-Jungians Today: Key Papers in Contemporary Analytical Psychology*. London: Routledge.

Samuels, A. (2001) *Politics on the Couch: Citizenship and the Internal Life*. London: Profile Books.

Segal, R. (1999a) 'Comments on Storr's and Shamdasani's articles'. *Journal of Analytical Psychology*, Vol. 44, no. 4, 561–62.

Segal, R. (1999b) 'Rationalist and romantic approaches to religion and modernity'. *Journal of Analytical Psychology*, Vol. 44, no. 4, 547–60.

Shamdasani, S. (1994) 'Encountering Hélène: Théodore Flournoy and the genesis of subliminal psychology', Introduction to T. Flournoy, *From India to the Planet Mars: A Case of Multiple Personality with Imaginary Languages* (1899), edited by S. Shamdasani, with foreword by C. G. Jung and commentary by Mireille Cifali, tr. D. Vermilye. Princeton, NJ: Princeton University Press.

Shamdasani, S. (1995) 'Memories, Dreams, Omissions'. *Spring: Journal of Archetype and Culture*, Vol. 57, 115–137.

Shamdasani, S. (1998) *Cult Fictions: C. G. Jung and the Founding of Analytical Psychology*. London: Routledge.

Shamdasani, S. (1999) '*In statu nascendi*'. *Journal of Analytical Psychology*, Vol. 44, no. 4, 539–546.

Smart, R. N. (1997) *Dimensions of the Sacred*. London: Fontana.

Stein, M. (1985) *Jung's Treatment of Christianity: The Psychology of a Religious Tradition*. Wilmette, IL: Chiron.

Storr, A. (1999) 'Jung's search for a substitute for a lost faith'. *Journal of Analytical Psychology*, Vol. 44, no. 4, 531–538.

Tacey, D. (1997a) 'Jung in the academy: devotions and resistances'. *Journal of Analytical Psychology*, Vol. 42, no. 2, 269–283.

Tacey, D. (1997b) 'Reply to responses', *Journal of Analytical Psychology*, Vol. 42, no. 2, 313–316.

Tacey, D. (1999) 'Why Jung would doubt the New Age', in S. Greenberg (Ed.), *Therapy on the Couch: A Shrinking Future*. London: Camden Press.

Tacey, D. (2001) *Jung and the New Age*. London: Brunner-Routledge.

Tambiah, S. (1990) *Magic, Science, Religion, and the Scope of Rationality*. Cambridge, UK: Cambridge University Press.

Ulanov, A. (1997) 'Teaching Jung in a theological seminary and a graduate school of religion: a response to David Tacey'. *Journal of Analytical Psychology*, Vol. 42, no. 2, 303–311.

Voogd, S. de (1984) 'Fantasy versus fiction: Jung's Kantianism appraised', in R. Papadopoulos and G. Saayaman (Eds), *Jung in Modern Perspective: The Master and His Legacy*. Bridport, UK: Prism Press, 1991.

Webb, J. (1976) *The Occult Establishment*. La Salle, IL: Open Court.

York, M. (1995) *The Emerging Network: A Sociology of the New Age and Neo-pagan Movements*. Lanham, MD: Rowman & Littlefield.

Young-Eisendrath, P. and Miller, M. (2000) *The Psychology of Mature Spirituality: Integrity, Wisdom, Transcendence*. London: Routledge.

(b) Religion and the terrified

Melanie Withers

Events of 11 September 2001 above the skies of New York reminded the world of the enormous potency of religious belief. To appalled eyes, two planes crashed into the World Trade Centre, a third into the Pentagon and a fourth into a field somewhere in Pennsylvania. Casualties were great. What is more, none of this was accidental. Muslim fundamentalist suicide pilots, believing in guaranteed instant entry to paradise as a result of their actions, allegedly carried out these acts and were acclaimed as heroes among their sympathizers. Others condemned them as murderers and as madmen.

To the affluent West, secure in global domination, and complacently willing to believe that its secular ideology and cultural values were universally desirable, it was a shocking reminder of 'otherness'. Yet to those excluded, whether for reasons of poverty or politics, it was to religion, rather than consumerism or science that groups and individuals now returned in an attempt to counter perceived impoverishment: framing it in terms of the spirit.

INTRODUCTION

Dr Main's chapter eloquently proposes that Jung might have something to offer to a world so schismatically divorced from itself. Taking up Jung's interest and commitment to both science and mysticism he attempts to rehabilitate a thinker who was often derided for his religious attitude, but who nevertheless, according to Main, retained a commitment to empirical and phenomenological exploration. In so doing he positions Jungian thinking as a dynamic to understand and potentially integrate what is disavowed and denigrated about religious belief by secular academic thinking within psychoanalysis and other disciplines. Project Jung is born.

In this response I want to suggest that this approach is both helpful, and Main's chapter speaks for itself on that account, and trapped – caught additionally in its own ideology and in the person of its creator. Furthermore, I want to consider that both academic, here epitomized by psychoanalysis, and religious thinking fail to address something of the human condition which remains caught up in the dynamics of terrifying uncertainty.

SCIENCE AND RELIGION

It can be argued that both Freud and Jung explored their theories in scientific terms and attempted to account for them according to scientific criteria. Psychoanalysis as a scientific discipline was charged with the resolution of problems. In attempting to uphold the status of analytic 'truth', and in maintaining a belief that madness could somehow be treated as understandable, psychoanalysis promoted a vision that it could make the irrational known. Freud, in particular, wished to unite the romantic and rational (see 'A Case of Hysteria', 1901: 15). His approach in *Totem and Taboo* (1913) was to make use of the powerful biological, anthropological or psychological theories to secularize what had been the domain of religion. In offering a new vision of the self as able to be internally aware and ultimately in control, he mirrored the cultural desire for autonomy and mastery of the laws of science. To acknowledge a limitation of these ideas could be not only seen as heretical but also at times denied altogether.

That Jung's notions are entangled oppositionally with Freud's is nothing revelatory, but it is in the nature of psychoanalytic understanding to hold in tension what is split off and projected. Both Freud and Jung encourage a belief that meaning can be symbolized and contained, though in different ways. Ehrenwald (1991) and Parker (1997) maintain Freud's aversion to religion is as much to do with his split from Jung and his hostility to the use of mysticism, countering as it did his adherence to a materialist view, than anything to do with individual belief. Jung however, was a determined mystic, who continued to believe 'there has not been one whose problem in that last resort was not that of finding a religious outlook on life' (Masson, 1988). In attempting to account for the ubiquity of religious belief, he posited the collective unconscious and a notion of archetypes as potentialities, free from any culture or historical process – something latter-day Jungians have struggled to account for, for example by reference to DNA (Samuels, 1985; Stevens, Controversy Eight in the present volume). Despite Jung's apparently 'transcendent' approach, his theoretical stance may be as amenable to scientific justification as Freud's, not least in his belief that acceptance of religion was a necessary part of the analytic 'cure' (Parker, 1997). It is my view that he remains as much as Freud trapped into a modernist narrative.

RELATIONSHIP AND THE CONSTRUCTION OF KNOWING

The decline of religion, at least in the West, has left us with few beliefs about what is ethically appropriate in therapeutic or pastoral relationships. The problem is that there is no moral certainty as we now live in a predominantly secular age and can offer only relativist certainty as to beliefs about moral activity.

> In philosophy, ethics means the study of moral conduct for living a good life.
> . . . It is only in our own time that ethics has more or less become reduced to a

set of rules for living without treading on other people's toes. (Jostein Gaarder, *Sophie's World*, 1995)

Post-Freudian and post-Jungian developments[1] look at the psychic relationships *between* people rather than the internal world of the individual alone. It might be argued that Jung extends this notion to include the relationship or otherwise to God. Disturbance is no longer a matter of sexual repression and unrestrained desire; rather it is the impoverishment of human relationships, which creates psychic pain. If people are said to be constructed through the other (Gergen and McNamee, 1993; Hauke, 2000) then individual experience can be formed only through relationships – or the lack of them. Otherness, however, is increasingly conceived of as that which is disavowed or unconscious within the self. Postmodern theory collapses the space in between. If certain beliefs have to have the status of 'other', whether to the cleric or the academic, they can be subject to interpretation. What is repudiated, however, is that they are one and the same, held in dialectic tension. Thanks to the influence of psychoanalytic thinking we can no longer dissociate from those secret desires which repel us – our unconscious contains that which we consciously disown – to our continuing horror. As Eliot and Frosh (1995: 3) point out:

> what is starting to become terrifying about postmodernity is not so much the gaps and absences in people's lives but the way everything is wrapped up together into a space that denies distance.

We live with a fundamental terror at the heart of the analytic enterprise in that madness and sanity live entangled with one another and are inextricably related. To return once again to the secular and to religion it becomes clear that in this reading, each is the mirror of the other, and as such we are left compelled to inhabit a landscape of secular-religiosity at once uncomfortable and mutually corrupting.

The above is couched in the familiar language of identification and projection and is dependent on a notion of individual autonomy somehow being able to control anxiety through knowledge. But, as has been repeatedly recognized, there remains something unending about the unconscious dynamic. One could always go on tinkering with the mechanism. Additionally the problem with the analyst's credibility resting on the mastery of internalization and identifications made in the past is that one is exposed to more madness as time goes on.[2] For the analyst to take up positions of expertise is to reinforce a religiosity about psychoanalysis and run the risk of foreclosing on madness. For if psychoanalysis is enabled to work with

---

1   Fordham's (1985) notion of deintegration and reintegration requires a real 'other' for the contents of the collective unconscious to be deintegrated into (see Urban, Controversy One in the present volume).
2   Witness the alarming accounts of acting out by senior members of the profession (Bartell and Rubin, 1990; Godley, 2001).

neurotic anxieties and what is repressed, this leaves those disavowed psychotic fears threatening to engulf us under extreme circumstances (Fordham, 1985).

Postmodernism argues for something beyond: in that within the failure of symbolization and science, that which cannot be interpreted or known, we come face to face with the Real – an overflow of what must be repudiated or 'abject' (Kristeva, 1987) and which cannot be spoken of in our culture. By suggesting that the nature of psychoanalytic knowing is something of a false consciousness (Lacan, 1977) anyone who claims to know is rendered obsolete. Far from reassuring us about the potency of unconscious understanding, we become further exposed to apocalyptic vistas of inherent helplessness from which there is only imaginary escape. We cannot recruit Freud for reassuring visions of accessible autonomy or ultimate mastery. Is it any wonder then that some turn to Jung's mystical and transcendent ideas in order to escape the disappointing entrapment of the earthly?

EXISTENTIAL ANXIETY AND THE DYNAMICS OF POWER

Whilst writing an earlier version of this chapter my computer was struck by lightning. Just such an unpredictable event raises the spectre of existential uncertainty to which we are all subject and which is deeply disturbing to our illusion of mastery (Lipman-Blumen, 1994). Furthermore, the ultimate capacity to foresee future events is catastrophically undermined by the evening news every night. (Would anyone working in the World Trade Centre have got out of bed on 11 September 2001 for example?) Human frailty is brought into sharp relief by such events, and the usual foreclosure on awareness of our one-day death becomes impossible to avoid.

Existentialist thinking, according to Lipman-Blumen maintains that always percolating below the surface of our existence is a terror of death. It can be argued that attempts to overcome the potential paralysing effects of such anxiety are seen in a variety of powerful narratives circulating around belief. Religious ideas and mystical gurus no less than academic thought and psychoanalytic practice, can be considered as a defensive features in a search for the kind of 'truth', which will prolong the illusion of control. As Elliot and Frosh (1995) remind us, however, ideas need not be only in our own heads – as postmodernism no longer offers us the security of a 'centred self' (Kennedy, 1998), but rather must be constituted through society, and made manifest in the kinds of power dynamics Lipman-Blumen holds as reducing existential chaos. Power in this formulation is not to do with individual autonomy like an acquired commodity, nor does it reside within individuals whether organized into groups or not. Rather it is constructed through relationships and comes to characterize the processes, which exist amongst these. These relationships offer the promise of security, which we need, both to protect ourselves against existential anxiety operating at an *un*conscious level and to maintain our capacity for action. Even if we cannot control the unpredictability of life, power relationships as sanctioned and legitimized by society sustain the delusion that someone or something can. Lipman-Blumen lists five strategies for reducing existential anxiety, which will be considered in terms of religious and psychoanalytic thinking.

Submission to a sacred force or being

For vast numbers of the world's population, adherence to a sacred deity provides the major focus of daily life. Islamic thinking continues to rise, whilst evangelical Christianity and the New Age belief as noted by Main continue to attract devotees. Paradoxically, by forgoing individualistic thinking, by surrendering personal independence and by acknowledging powerlessness, believers are given the tools to live by and structures to survive all eventualities. The benefits are threefold. The faithful can expect relief from the burden of responsibility and security from life's anxieties by continuing to hand over such concerns to an omnipotent being. Moreover, that most annihilating of visions – the endless void of death – can be avoided by the security of an afterlife. It is understandably seductive.

What is less obvious is how apparently secular figures can fulfil such a role too. There is a tendency for some within psychoanalysis to revere figures such as Freud in particular, by investing him with the status of the all-powerful, all-seeing deity who invented psychoanalysis. Followers draw strength from the evidence that others share their point of view, so to question Freud, for example, assumes the status of virtual heresy. This may not be because his thinking is necessarily 'right' or 'wrong', but because without it all that is left is to elect some other figure into the gap – hence the interesting splinter groups, which forever spring up in the analytic world. Nevertheless, Freud's shortcomings, and his resolute opposition to matters spiritual, leave obvious openings for subsequent recruitment. In attempting to rehabilitate Jung, despite some unfortunate difficulties around his anti-Semitic views (Samuels, 1992), and his behaviour with Spielrein (Ehrenwald, 1991), the desire is to find a figure within psychoanalysis who can be substituted for Freud on the subject of religion. Jung, as the founding father of analytic psychology with clear mystical and scientific strands to his work, is a strong candidate, and his followers remain dedicated to his ideas with a religious fervour greater even than devotees of Freud (Tacey, 1997). So the transference to a superior deity is replicated – and Jung is elevated to the status of yet another cult figure (Noll, 1994).[3]

Allegiance to a religious or secular ideology

This is somewhat similar to the previous category but with less obvious deification. It can most easily be understood as the 'truth' of religion or a psychoanalytic theory, for example, to which adherents commit and invest their own belief system. In

---

3 'According to Bowlby, Anna Freud worshipped at the shrine of St Sigmund, and Klein at the shrine of St Melanie' (Grosskurth, 1986).

return, ideology, whether sacred or secular, offers explanations, meaning and structures within which to work and to understand life's events. It also offers illusory control – for if the explanations are correct, outcomes can be predicted. Believers therefore contend that the ideology will prevail and will lead to a better tomorrow. As such the text can be given sacred status to which followers return in moments of stress or indecision. (The original 'words' of Freud and Jung are revered at times in ways reminiscent of the Bible or the Koran.) A psychoanalytic theory as much as a religious one contains within it its own protective structure to shield believers from any evidence disproving its findings, via defensive mechanisms such as denial or disavowal.

Secular ideologies, just like religious ideologies, have a community of believers. This not only reinforces confidence in the theory, but also ensures conformity to norms and values. As the membership of the community grows, and as individuals join in defence against isolation and exclusion, the success of the ideological approach is confirmed. Moreover rebel elements are quickly expelled. The psycho-analytic movement, no less than the religious, is bedevilled by schisms which, though painful, ensure the purity of the original thought within the organization concerned. So the dominant discourse is resurrected. Foucault (1980) demonstrates how regimes of truth are inextricably bound up with forms of sovereignty and domination. Such ideas assume proprietary hold on knowledge and the power relationships with which they are imbued. Nevertheless ideas located more directly in economic, political and situational features are more vulnerable to being replaced, whereas spiritual theories – claiming as they do to be above such earthly concerns – are capable of withstanding direct assaults on their integrity. In this way religious ideas are more easily able to claim universal 'truth'.

Subordination to a religious or secular institution

Church, temple and mosque, government, school and workplace provide the setting for our daily lives. In providing the illusion of existential order through highly structured arrangements regulating behaviour, thoughts and actions, institutional hierarchies clarify the ambiguities around our status and place on the world stage. Regulatory bodies fulfil this function by embodying values and, via a system of agreed norms, rewards and sanctions, ensure members adhere to the values inscribed (Menzies-Lyth, 1988). By submitting to the regulatory practices, whether within Church or via a professional psychoanalytic organization, members facing ethical dilemmas or uncertainty around how best to proceed are offered the security of guidelines and codes of conduct – whilst unruly or subversive elements can be expelled.

In addition such institutions provide meaning for our very existence. If we can continue to subscribe to a particular belief – that we are 'here' in order to glorify the word of God, to help others via analytic insight, or advance academic thinking by writing papers, to name a few – we can be protected from alternative ideas that our lives are futile, irrelevant and pointless. In such ways can our beliefs become located within political and powerful institutional frameworks, which we challenge at our peril for in such ways can we be protected from despair.

Those who have devoted themselves to promoting Christian or Islamic, Freudian or Jungian ideas via the political and institutional structures of our culture are therefore trapped existentially amidst forces which may be too terrifying to address – for that way, potentially, lies psychosis.

Subjugation to a human ruler benign or otherwise

In most societies individuals and groups subject themselves to a human ruler perceived as being wise, compassionate and benevolent. In seeking the protection of leaders thought to be more intelligent, skilful and powerful than themselves, people aim to have individual burdens and responsibilities lifted from their shoulders, though at the same time they long to be free.

Freud, of course, would interpret this as a desire to replicate the parent–child relationship with which we are all so familiar and which we have all used to deal with underlying aspects of existential anxiety, albeit with varying degrees of success. It remains the case that from childhood we become conditioned to follow our parents' dictums. Exchanging safety and security, if not love and care, for obedience and subordination is difficult over time, however; Jung's notion of individuation versus subordination here represents something of this struggle. As adults we may well attempt to renegotiate the power balance. Sometimes we simply replicate our difficulties with our own children – or 'swap' leaders for a more benign one better able to represent our needs. Tacey (1997: 274) comments on how those who reject hard-line knowledge epitomized by Freudian and Lacanian patriarchal authority turn to Jung as representative of maternal 'womb of gnosis' where understanding is contained in 'last night's dreams'.

That we may have little choice over who leads us also replicates aspects of parent and child relating. We do not ask to be born to those particular parents, for example; and again it could be argued we are supremely conditioned to make limited fuss about leaders who oppress us and whom we have little opportunity to challenge. The person of the priest, as representative of a particular ideology to which we are committed, matters less than his or her message – it is the leadership function to which we cleave. In psychoanalysis, analytic notions of blank screen relating similarly ensure that the particular character or personality of the analyst is less important than his or her function as companion in our journey into the unconscious. It is clear that troubled and vulnerable people entering treatment do not make a distinction between analysis as ethically principled and their analyst as morally sound. So the analyst, of whatever persuasion, is given the status of priest, confessor and absolver and anxiety can be suspended for another day.

Assumption of control over other people, situations, resources and institutions

The final strategy for subduing existential anxiety comes in our capacity and desire to take control over other peoples' lives. To assume responsibility when another is unable to do so has the double advantage of convincing both parties that everything is under control. That this is omnipotent and ultimately a delusion passes almost unnoticed, such is the need to limit existential anxiety. However, such a position is dependent on a sense of internal mastery, the 'knowing of the self' usually gained through reflection, whether via spiritual meditation or personal analysis – included here are optional and additional features such as the internalizations of doctrinal study, or psychoanalytic training.

Socialization practices too contribute to the way in which some accede to positions of power. It can be argued that young males are frequently socialized to repress displays of feeling and to exert self-control more rigorously than females. Subsequently men are channelled into positions where they exercise control over weaker males and most women. It is notable that women constitute the majority of religious believers; and most psychoanalytic practitioners, of whatever persuasion, are female. However, almost all religious leaders are male, and men too are to be found in senior roles within psychoanalytic and similar organizations. Such social conditions create the complex apparatus whereby men are able to access decision-making power in resource-rich institutions.

Religious leaders and those at the forefront of leadership (including those within academia or psychoanalysis) are then highly vulnerable, at a gendered and political level, to attempts to hang on to their power. By controlling resources they are able to reward and attract loyal followers and oppose those who challenge their hegemony. Such power, as manifest in a capacity to put grand designs into action, may convince even those beset by their own existential anxiety that they are powerful enough to withstand it. But, as always, the danger of this strategy is in subscribing to one's own press release: the potential for megalomania arises through believing in one's own omnipotence, or being seduced into that position by the needs of others.

Existential conceptions of power relationships as dualistic permeate this account. Transfers of power can occur according to definitional or situational features, but participants are either subordinate or dominant within the relationship. It is my contention that both religion and psychoanalysis attempt to deny both neurotic and psychotic anxieties inherent in an understanding of the human condition. By putting forward powerful arguments and figures to support their individual cases, they attempt to circumvent the kind of existential anxiety outlined above.

Additionally they attempt to produce conflicting views – often denigrating what the other has to say. Such rivalry too seems important. Although it might be comforting to believe perhaps in Jung as the universal healer able to contain and work with all splits and schisms in the understanding of oppositional attitudes, there is something revitalizing about the struggle to engage with difference. Maybe it is better to endlessly 'resurrect the image of the rival' (Borch-Jacobsen, 1991: 94) than face the 'abyss of desire'. When one ceases to care then perhaps that ultimately represents the death we so much fear.

NARRATIVE AND THE IMAGINATION

It seems unlikely that the unpredictability of human existence is about to change, and recent events can only intensify the uncertainty; but at least confronting the fact of existential anxiety weakens our predisposition to choose unconscious remedies. Although there will always be the undeniability of fact which brings into focus the realities of our lives,[4] there are fewer certainties as to what we can reliably believe in. At its most simplistic, are we not creating necessary narratives by which to live? I am suggesting that such narratives whether religious or secular are mechanisms used over centuries to make meaning, secure protection and satisfy desire in an existence where we have limited control (McLeod, 1997). But what Foucault (1979) reminds us of is the multiplicity of positions it is possible to take rather than the dominant one. As such, any narrative may approximate only to an understanding of the complexities of the world *as we currently see it*. That these may not be enduring gives uneasy security, in that we can dream up subsequent more meaningful ones as the situational features of our lives move forward. Although we may be trapped individually within a limited cultural imagination, the capacity to think beyond has always been a feature of collective human existence. The words spoken in analysis set off a chain reaction in the other, outstripping their original speaker. Contemporary psychoanalytic thinking continues to focus on the imaginative and innovative in the psyche (Castoriades, 1995). In everyday life he argues that we use imaginative perceptions of each other to escape the framework of organizations that have been imposed upon us. Eliot and Frosh (1995: 6) put it thus:

> Whether at the level of individual fantasy or global social transformations, self and society interlock through this structuration of imaginary representations. Although self-generated, however, these same imaginary creations necessarily escape the memory, control and conduct of human subjects. From this angle social organisation always outstrips the self-referential representational activity of human subjects; or to put the matter slightly differently, the social imaginary always exceeds the domain of unconscious fantasy.

They maintain that the self-referential nature of psychoanalysis *is* appropriate to the postmodern cultural context where meaning is constantly shifting and cast adrift. It is possible then to conceive reflexivity as the imaginative capacity to think beyond

---

4   Witness how terminal illness focuses the priorities of life's desires – much too could be illustrated with reference to those condemned to death or determined on a suicide mission.

the cultural, political, social or religious distortions imposed upon us by the necessity of intersubjective identity. Jung's work, possibly more than Freud's as Main suggests, is well placed to consider what lies at the margins of our current understanding – but only at the level of speculative and hallucinatory narrative. The danger, which remains, is to give any plausible commentary on the human condition the status of 'truth', for this is to close down any manoeuvre for creativity and future thinking. By all means let us return to our masters – but let us not be seduced by their writings as universal.

CONCLUSION

It is increasingly clear that those who, for whatever reason, are disqualified from Western affluence, which they have little hope of attaining, turn instead to religious and spiritual values for a unifying comfort, relegating Western practices to the corrupt and morally redundant. As Foucault (1979) illustrates, where there is dominance within any discourse of power there too will be found resistance. Similarly, psychoanalytic understanding, existing largely speaking in an a-spiritual world, has repeatedly championed individual insight and exploration of the unconscious as the road to integration, and, at times, has dismissed religious fervour as either neurotic anxiety or the lunatic ravings of a culture bent on the subjugation of a largely ill-educated population. Jung may be one of the few to attempt a bridge, as Main suggests, and his work offers some explanation of how each projects the shadow onto the other. Nevertheless, his ideology is always in danger of becoming positioned by his followers (and maybe himself) in those discourses of power outlined above when a particular kind of knowledge around spiritual belief becomes privileged. Although empathic, this continues to sidestep some more pressing anxieties around existence and subsistence in deprived areas.

These are to be found most obviously in Third World countries, where it is easier to trace the rise of religious fundamentalism to a concept such as envy, as the majority of the population are excluded from access to the world's riches. Additionally, in facing imminent exposure to death, whether through famine, poverty or dispossession, the embracing of an 'afterlife' is an attempt to deny the daily horror of annihilation. Yet this too fails and is liable to return in the face of the great Satan, as embodied by the West, threatening traditional existence.

In the West itself, hermetically sealed from too much proximity to death, it is easier to deny that we all suffer from a terminal illness (although there is perhaps a guilty identification with those living in poverty-stricken regions). Increasingly however, as Main points out, the rise of interest in New Age philosophies reminds us of a different kind of spiritual deprivation closer to home. Although less obvious to track, it might be argued that what is at stake is not just a reawakening of attitudes to the spiritual, but a commentary from those who feel unable to find values of the soul in the consumerist, patriarchal culture of the West (Tacey, 1997). What differentiates one group from the other is the no small matter of choice.

Religion and psychoanalysis operate against a background of real suffering, and in their mutual spiritual, reflexive aspects attempt to transcend and reformulate something of human oppression. Both address the transformation of self-awareness as well as representing those powerful relationships into which we sink to manage our anxiety. Each offers the promise of a brave new tomorrow, but as Parker (1997: 79) mentions:

> It is not individual transformation, which accomplishes the destruction of religious neurosis, as Freud thought, but social transformation, which accomplishes the spiritual transcendence of our need for neurosis.

That this seems likely, is as far away as ever.

REFERENCES

Astor, J. (1995) *Michael Fordham. Innovations in Analytical Psychology*. London: Routledge.

Bartel, P. A. and Rubin, L. J. (1990) 'Dangerous liaisons: sexual intimacies in supervision'. *Professional Psychology: Research and Practice*, Vol. 21, no. 6, 442–50.

Borch-Jacobsen, M. (1991) *Lacan: The Absolute Master*. Stanford, CA: Stanford University Press.

Castoriades, C. (1995) 'Logic, imagination and reflection', in A. Eliot and S. Frosh *Psychoanalysis in Contexts*. London: Routledge.

Ehrenwald (1991) *The History of Psychoanalysis*. New Jersey: Jason Aronson.

Eliot, A. and Frosh, S. (1995) *Psychoanalysis in Contexts*. London: Routledge.

Fordham, M. (1985) *Explorations into the Self*. London: Academic Press.

Foucault, M. (1979) *The History of Sexuality*, Vol. 1. Harmondsworth, UK: Penguin.

Foucault, M. (1980) *Power/Knowledge: Selected Interviews and Writings, 1972–1977*, (edited by Colin Gordon). New York: Pantheon Books.

Freud, S. (1901) *A Case of Hysteria*. Standard Edition, Vol. 7. London: Hogarth Press, 1981.

Freud, S. (1913) *Totem and Taboo*, quoted in A. Richards *The Origins of Religion*, Pelican Freud Library, Vol. 13. Harmondsworth, UK: Penguin.

Gaarder, J. (1995) *Sophie's World*. London: Phoenix House.

Gergen, K. and McNamee, S. (Eds) (1993) *Therapy as Social Construction*. London: Sage.

Godley, W. (2001) 'Saving Masud Khan'. *London Review of Books*, 22 February, 3–7.

Grosskurth, P. (1985) *Melanie Klein, her Work and her World*. London: Hodder & Stoughton.

Hauke, C. (2000) *Jung and the Postmodern*. London: Routledge.

Kennedy, R. (1998) *The Elusive Human Subject*. London: Free Association Books.

Kristeva, J. (1987) *In the Beginning was Love: Psychoanalysis and Faith*. New York: Columbia University Press.

Lacan, J. (1977) *Ecrits: A Selection*, trans. A. Sheridan. London: Tavistock.

Lipman-Blumen, J. (1994) 'The Existential Bases of Power Relationships: the Gender Role Case', in H. L. Radtke and H. J. Stam (Eds), *Power/Gender Social Relations in Theory and Practice*. London: Sage.

Masson, J. (1988) *Against Therapy*. London: Fontana.

McLeod, J. (1997) *Narrative and Psychotherapy*. London: Sage.

Menzies-Lyth, I. (1988) *Containing Anxiety in Institutions*, Vol. 1. London: Free Association Books.

Noll, R. (1994) *The Jung Cult: The Origins of a Charismatic Movement*. Princeton, NJ: Princeton University Press.

Parker, I. (1997) *Psychoanalytic Culture*. London: Sage.

Samuels, A. (1985) *Jung and the Post-Jungians*. London: Routledge.

Samuels, A. (1992) 'National psychology, national socialism, and analytical psychology: Reflections on Jung and anti-semitism, Part 1', *Journal of Analytical Psychology*, Vol. 37, no. 1, 3–28.

Tacey, D. (1997) 'Jung in the academy: devotions and resistances'. *Journal of Analytical Psychology*, Vol. 42, no. 2, 269–283.

The body, analysis and homeopathic medicine

Introduction

History will regard Edward Whitmont as a pioneer in the integration of analytical psychology and complementary medicine. On a theoretical level for instance, he was the first person to apply Jungian insights to the study of homeopathic remedies (see, for example, Whitmont, 1947, 1950). In the present paper – first published just before his death in 1998 – Whitmont argues for a closer integration of analysis with homeopathy.[1] In particular he claims that homeopathy can sometimes assist the individuation process when an insufficient separation of ego from self has impaired the patient's capacity to symbolize. This is a particular issue with borderline and psychosomatic patients, where important material may remain unavailable for conventional analytic work as a result. He illustrates his contentions with reference to related case material.

As well as these practical proposals, Whitmont argues that alchemy can be regarded as the common ancestor of both homeopathy and Jungian analysis. In this way he attempts to establish it as a theoretical bridge between the latter two disciplines. He rejects Jung's notion that alchemy worked via the projection of the contents of the alchemist's unconscious into their materials, however. Instead he opts for a more concrete explanation of its workings involving the 'subtle body'. He believes the same model can be applied to homeopathy. On an analytic level he links this subtle body to Jung's notion of 'psychoid substance'.

Withers acknowledges the importance of Whitmont's groundbreaking application of analytic ideas to homeopathy. But he argues against this 'concrete' element in his thinking. Instead he contends that Jung's psychological approach to alchemy can be fruitfully applied to understanding homeopathy. He uses notions from the developmental school of analytical psychology to illustrate this in relation to Whitmont's own case material. In this sense, he claims, Whitmont underestimates the explanatory power of analytic theory. On a practical level too he argues that Whitmont may be too quick to dismiss the therapeutic potential of the analytic method in borderline and psychosomatic cases.

---

1 British and American spellings of the word 'homeopathy' have recently been standardized, but this leaves an inconsistency with earlier British spellings.

REFERENCES

Whitmont, Edward (1947) 'Lycopodium: a psychosomatic study'. *Homoeopathic Recorder*, March.

Whitmont, Edward (1950) 'Sepia analysis of a dynamic totality'. *British Homoeopathic Journal*, July, Vol. XL, no. 3.

(a) Alchemy, homeopathy and the treatment of borderline cases

Edward Whitmont

Fundamental to alchemy is a true and genuine mystery which since the seventeenth century has been understood unequivocally as psychic.

> But I do not imagine for a moment that the psychological interpretation of a mystery must necessarily be the last word. If it is a mystery it must have still other aspects. (Jung, 1955–6: para. 213)

In this chapter I shall present a method that, over approximately one hundred and fifty years of clinical experience, has proven itself highly effective, not only in the treatment of physical malady, but also for what we now call borderline and psychotic conditions. For reasons of space I am offering just two case examples from many in my personal experience to illustrate the therapeutic potential of homeopathy for the practising psychotherapist.

Homeopathy, hitherto overlooked by analytical psychologists, may be considered an extension or modern technique of alchemy and of the spagyric arts. Unlike psychotropic medication, the homeopathic approach seemingly does not operate on the level of material chemistry. It seems to work through the 'subtle' or 'vital energy' body, which Paracelsus called the Archaeus. Consequently, it does not limit itself to or interfere with neurotransmitter or hormonal activity but affects the psychosomatic totality in a direct, holistic normalization of psychoid dynamics. The indications for homeopathic medicines are always based on the psychophysical totality of the patient. Even in the treatment of organic disorders, primary emphasis is placed upon personality type and psychological make-up. Classical homeopathy tends to support the individuation process by overcoming the blocking effects of psychoid engrams. It is therefore highly syntonic with psychoanalytic work.

PSYCHOTHERAPY AND THE BORDERLINE PROBLEM

The goal of psychotherapy is self-awareness (Jung, 1955–6: para. 674), realization of one's essential nature. This rests on the premise that psychopathology, as well as frequently also organic suffering, could be alleviated through self-awareness and maturational development. Such a development requires a capacity, sooner or later, for self-observation based upon an adequately functioning ego capable of confronting one's shadow. As Jung sees it, such ego development rests upon a separation between one's 'natural', that is, biologically, instinctually and emotionally determined motivations and affects on the one side, and one's capacities for consciousness, that is, a sense of personal identity and an ability to think rationally and exert willed control over one's actions. Even though he does not explicitly speak of borderline pathology (a term not yet in use at that time), Jung emphasizes that the quest for self-awareness necessitates this dissociative experience as a 'requirement of any psychotherapy that goes at all deep' (Jung, 1955–6).

This first separation stage makes possible, and is eventually to be followed by, the second step: an eventual conscious differentiation and reconciliation of hitherto primitive and potentially pathological affect dynamic into an ethically self-fulfilling personality that can perceive spiritual, ethical and transcendental meaning.

In the borderline pathology the embodiment or incarnation through deintegration of the transpersonal Self, into a complex of identity able to tolerate the stress of polar opposites is inadequate. In consequence of severe early environmental or prenatal traumatization or retardation of psychobiological development, an initially adequate centre of conscious identity failed to solidify out of the psychoid, semi-animalic that is, affect-determined state of unconsciousness (Jung, 1955–6: para. 695). Since affectivity operates to a large extent in terms of biologic-somatic functioning (autonomous nervous and hormonal activity), it possesses itself of a certain fixity and 'imprints' itself in reflex, hormonal, neurotransmitter, organ and peripheral muscular structuring and spasticity. Since the initial ego nucleus is of the nature of a body-ego, this organic fixation may interfere with or even prevent further ego–affect separation and shadow confrontation which, even under the best of circumstances feel like mortification and figurative death (Jung, 1955–6: para. 674). In these states the attempt to bring about such a self-witnessing and mortifying separation carries the threat of a fragmentation of the personality and feels intolerable and impossible to approach. The extremest form of this non-incarnation we encounter in the so-called hospitalism. Infants raised under strict biologically adequate conditions, proper nutrition, and hygiene, but without hugging, cuddling and loving physical touch, fail to develop and frequently even die. Lacking bodily experience of loving acceptance, the Self withdraws from the intended full incarnation. In less extreme cases, a slowed or inadequate ego development fails to establish full cortical control over the limbic and reptilian brain functions. An insufficient scope of the magical-mythological psychoid stratum becomes psychologized. Emotionality remains 'characterized by marked physical innervation . . .' and a 'peculiar disturbance of the ideational process' (Jung's definition of affect: Jung, 1921: para. 681). Emotion is not sufficiently transformed into feeling, nor obsession into thought, drive into willing, and paranoic fears into perception, attention and reflection. Instead of developing into 'voluntarily disposable functions' (Jung, 1921), affects and drives remain largely bound up in what Jung called the body psychoid. The elementary motivational force fields continue to behave and to be experienced like extraneous, quasi-macrocosmic rather than microcosmic, psychological factors. The weak ego remains merged with and feels threatened by the 'demons' of obsessive complexes and, when the rigid defence system is threatened or tampered with, lives in fear of being carried away or swamped by these 'demons'.

In this state of affairs psychotherapy is limited at best to supplying to the adult a regression experience for the sake of an encounter with the unmetabolized and largely unconscious affects in an environment of safety and 'holding' support. The ego/non-ego confrontation, which Jung considered the first step necessary for individuation and ethical choice and responsibility, cannot be attained at this stage. Moreover, the adult or adolescent no longer has the child's plasticity. The distortions and deficiencies have become not only conditioned reflex activities but are encoded in the substance and functioning of musculature, posture and the innervation of organs and neurotransmitter systems. The activities of organs and of the hormonal and autonomic nervous system are altered, first, on the level of the 'subtle body' (which corresponds to the body-psychoid), shown to be 'real' by Kirlian photography. Later, indeed, a persistence of these engrams may change what at first was only functional into gross organic pathology.

This dynamic is only to a limited extent accessible to cognitional approaches. In order to modify the pathology of the psychoid, psychotherapy is in need of complementary modalities of precognitional nature. To varying extents, bioenergetics, art therapy, hypnosis and therapeutic regression, and (for the treatment of addictions) acupuncture have endeavoured to fill this gap. Psychotropic medication also addresses itself to the organic level, even though by means of material, chemical interference, always fraught with the risks of side effects and functional if not organic damage.

Yet the centuries-old spiritual tradition and experience of the spagyric arts not only considered our problem of soul–body evolution of primal concern, but also claimed to have discovered effective ways of dealing with it. Some part of what they shrouded in esoteric language, accessible only to intuition or personal initiation has in our time been developed into an experimentally and clinically verifiable highly effective modality. Paradoxically, however, homeopathy has until now not been given attention by Jung and the Jungian school, even though it was anticipated and, in principle, spelled out by alchemy.

THE *MEDICAMENTUM SPAGYRICUM*

In the alchemist's view, the creation of the *lapis*, which we consider equivalent to the individuation process, required first the separation of the mind from the *unio naturalis* and subsequently as a second step the reintegration of the soul-substance into a *unio mentalis*; and the alchemists considered that the first part of this process, the separation, could be aided by a medicine, a *medicamentum spagyricum*.

The alchemists held the *prima materia* of the human state to be the *unio naturalis*, called chaos, *nigredo*, *massa confusa*, and 'hard to dissolve convolution of body and soul'. From this 'original semi-animalic state of unconsciousness', the mind was to be extracted and separated by dividing this *unio naturalis* into a pair of opposites consisting of 'instinctuality and rational mind'. That division would bring into existence a soul capable of opposing and resisting the influence and compulsions of the body and its instincts (Jung, 1955–6: para. 695).

Remarkably, the medicine, an *arcanum* or *medicamentum spagyricum*, which was to bring about this separation, was to work by dint of 'similarity, not oppositeness' (Jung 1955–6: para. 677). Since this medicine was considered the physical equivalent of the *lapis* and the heavens it was called '*caelum*' and *pharmakon athanasias* (Jung, 1955–6: para. 770) and was to set free a *substantia coelestis* in man. As *caelum* it was held to represent the pure non-corrupt archetypal substance (*Ursubstanz*) of the world (Jung, 1955–6: para. 429) which could make ill as well as heal (Jung, 1955–6: paras. 607, 640) all fragmentations of body and soul (Jung, 1955–6: para. 429).

This 'heavenly' *medicamentum spagyricum* was produced by extracting a *quintessence* from various substances, but the specific nature or contents of the *arcanum* were not indicated. However, it was affirmed to be of physical nature (Jung, 1955–6: paras. 678, 773), yet also called a 'substance and yet not a substance' (Jung, 1955–6: para. 715). Moreover, while great stress was put upon the fact that the *arcanum* is of physical nature, yet, paradoxically, it was emphasized that it is alive, that it possesses an anima and a spiritus, and even a human-like nature (Jung, 1955–6: para. 773).

Thus, in a chapter called 'The operations of nature in the aqua philosophica, as in a seed' the *Tractatus aureus* ascribed to Hermes Trismegistus states:

> Now the Bodies of the Metals, are the Domiciles of their Spirits; which when they are received by the Bodies, their terrestrial substance is by little and little made thein [sic], extended and Purified and by their Vivifying Power the Life and Fire, hitherto lying-Dormant, is excited and stirred up. For the life which dwells in the Metals, is laid as it were asleep, nor can it exert its Power, or shew it self, unless the Bodies be first Dissolved, Exalted, and turned into Spirit, (for that the Spirit does only Vivifie;) being brought to this Degree of purity and spirituality, and at length to perfection, by their abundant Virtue, they communicate their tinging property to the other imperfect Bodies, and Transmute them into a fixed and permanent substance. This is the property of our Medicine, into which the Bodies are reduced; that at first, one part thereof will tinge ten parts of an imperfect body; then an hundred, after a thousand, then ten thousand, and so infinitely on. By which the Efficacy of the Creator's Word is apparently Evident, Crescite et Multiplicamini, encrease and multiply. And by how much the oftner the medicine is dissolved, by so much the more it encreases in Virtue and Power, which otherwise without any more solutions, would remain in its simple or single State of imperfection; Here is a Celestial

and Divine Fountain set Open, which no man is able to draw dry, nor can it be wholy exhausted, should the World endure to External Generations. (Hermes Trismegistus, 1692)

The necessity for similarity is repeatedly stressed, since, given the spiritual nature of this substance, its helpfulness must depend upon the analogy of its dynamic with the functioning of the person whom it was to heal.

Thus, Paracelsus avers that

never has a hot disease been cured by coldness, nor a cold one by heat. But it has happened that likes have healed likes. (Paracelsus, 1928: 494)

and Man is:

heaven and earth, and the lower spheres, the four elements and whatever is within them, wherefore he is properly called by name of microcosmos for he is the whole world. (Paracelsus, 1928: 361)

Thus scorpio cures its scorpio, realgar its realgar, mercurius its mercurius. . . . (Paracelsus, 1928: 361)

Hence

Since all of this exists also in the external world the physician must learn upon the illnesses of the visible things their similarity of their coming into being and being dispersed. By virtue of the spagyric art he ought to reduce the bodies to their stuff of origin. Thus he finds out from what substance a particular illness comes. Once he has established all stuffs of origin he knows about all illnesses. (Paracelsus, 1928: 75)

And for the doctor who thus knows 'the health and disease of the elements and knows alchemy' (Jung, 1941: para. 27), 'there is no sickness against which some remedy has not been created and established to drive it out and cure it' (Paracelsus, 1951: p. 77).

We can see in these quotations that Paracelsus and the alchemists envisioned the existence of a psychophysical and spiritual analogon to human dynamics inherent in the various substances of the outer world. Their 'spiritual' *quintessentia* could be extracted and, by virtue of their similarity to the human situation, they were expected to reconnect the human psychosomatic entity with its corresponding unconditioned archetypal source ground and, thereby, to heal that which is ill or arrested in its development.

Trained as he was in terms of nineteenth-century positivistic medical viewpoints, Jung was puzzled by such statements. He could not conceive of the possibility of such transmaterial principles as a-priori constituents of matter. Thus he explained the alchemist's descriptions in terms of projections upon matter, which needed to be 'taken back' and be recognized exclusively as aspects of the human psyche. Even though he noted that the alchemists repeatedly affirmed that the processes in question involve psychical transformation *as well as* physical substance dynamics, Jung remarked that:

> if the adept really concocted such potions in his retort, he must surely have chosen his ingredients on account of their magical significance. He worked, accordingly, with *ideas*, with psychological processes, but referred to them under the name of the corresponding substances. . . . It never occurred to the mind of the alchemist to cast any doubt whatsoever on this *intellectual monstrosity* [sic]. (Jung, 1955–6: paras 704, 695)

Some among you may, however, have already recognized the remarkable resemblance between that alchemist's 'intellectual monstrosity' and the frame of reference of homeopathy, with which Jung was largely unfamiliar, as I can testify from personal conversations with him. For traditional medicine, homeopathy represents as much of an 'intellectual monstrosity' as does alchemy, and for the same reason: it works with 'substance which is not substance' and considers psychological, psychophysical and somatic dynamics to be equivalent to and corresponding, hence 'similar', to outer world substances.

HOMEOPATHY

It would lead too far afield to discuss the basic paradigmatic differences between the approach of homeopathy and of orthodox medicine which has relegated the latter to the status of 'alternative medicine'. Suffice it to say that, basing itself upon pure observation and clinical experience, homeopathy utilizes a dynamic for which the seventeenth-century thought system, as it still prevails in official medicine, can find no rational explanation or theoretical model. Moreover, since homeopathy bases its indications upon the strictly individual criteria of the particular given situation and patient, the current methods of statistical 'proof' are as little workable as they are for the evaluation of the effectiveness of psychotherapy and psycho-analysis. In view of 'official' medicine's insistence upon a plausible theoretical model, which still takes precedence over unbiased observation, and the relative inapplicability of statistical methods for its evaluation, homeopathy is still considered unacceptable by mainstream medical practice.

Nevertheless there is on record already a vast array of studies that have verified the efficacy of the homeopathic method. (The most significant recent examples are listed in the References.)

Homeopathy is based on the fact, experimentally established and clinically verified, that any medicine will cure that particular kind of disease the symptoms of which happen to be most similar to those symptoms which it produces upon healthy persons when consistently ingested. Such systematic testing of drugs on large numbers of average healthy humans (not animals), for the sake of eliciting their typical bodily, mental and emotional symptoms, is fundamental for the practice of homeopathy. (It is called 'proving', from the German word 'prüfen'.) However, such similarity must include the specific Gestalt-totality of the disorder rather than mere fortuitous details.

For instance, the disorder brought about by inhaling onion (*Allium cepa*) duplicates the initial phase of a head cold. However, a similar state is also brought about by the initial toxic effects of arsenic. Hence, onion and arsenic, in appropriate dosage, are expected to, and indeed do, abolish a cold when taken during the early phase. However, these substances are not arbitrarily interchangeable. For the substance to work, the 'fit' between remedy and patient must be highly specific.

Suppose a patient evidences the symptoms of a cold and wants to avoid cold air because it makes him feel worse. Onion would be an ineffective remedy in this case, because the nasal irritation it produces is aggravated by warmth not by cold. In fact, it is usually made to feel better by cold, and this patient seeks heat, not cold. Now an arsenic irritation, which also duplicates the initial phases of a head cold, behaves in the opposite fashion from onion: arsenic is assuaged by warmth. Since we have a patient who seeks heat, arsenic, not onion, would be the most appropriate remedy, the best 'fit'. (These drugs are not the only ones that would apply and for the later phases still others are to be considered. For simplicity's sake I limit my examples to only two substances.)

The dynamics of the right remedy must include not merely the temperature preferences but all the physical, emotional, and psychological characteristics that constitute the particular phenomenologically descriptive field of the patient's given condition and states, even the seemingly most irrelevant. An actual case, of course, involves many more variables than the two we have chosen above. So this process of matching the substance with the personal and constitutional idiosyncrasies of the patient must be continued with each variable – whether mental, emotional or physical. The correspondence between remedy and patient has to be highly personal, constitutionally specific, and exactly matched to the descriptive phenomena in the field.

For example – again simplified – given a particular somatic state such as perhaps an intestinal disorder, an attenuated preparation of windflower (*Pulsatilia*) is more likely to be effective with people of an overtly mild, timid and yielding disposition than it is with those of an angry, aggressive, irascible temper. The latter type would be more likely to respond to a particular form of strychnine (*nux vomica*), while another strychnine compound, the St Ignatius bean, corresponds to psychological states of grief, bereavement, and abandonment. Gold, to mention another example, influences primarily heart and circulatory functioning and affects personalities of serious, over-responsible and depressive, even suicidal tendencies.

Hence, every substance field represents a Gestalt-pattern of circumscribed personality traits, temperament, and emotional propensities in unison with biological response patterns and disorders that it has the potential to induce and heal.

Every existing substance, when subject to the proving experiment, exhibits a similarity, hence also a healing capacity for some human (or animal) disturbed state. And, in view of the immense number of still unproven substances (the homeopathic materia medica at present contains approximately a thousand or fifteen hundred proven medicines, out of a practically infinite number of still unproven potential medicines, each with its own specific characteristics), we may well assume that for every possibility of human affliction, there exists a healing substance 'out there'. We confront here the amazing fact that psychobiological response patterns that are aspects of the human life-drama are duplicated in the structural and life activity of the earth's substances. The psychosomatic totalities of ill persons and medicines appear as similar field patterns, mutually inclusive of human organism and non-human, 'external' and supposedly 'inanimate' substances.

However, the further 'intellectual monstrosity' that makes homeopathy so unbelievable to the minds of the orthodox scientist is its use of dosages that have been attenuated past the point where it seems obvious that no molecule of the original drug could still be present.

As was to be expected, it turned out that when the toxic effects of medicines were added to the already existing similar disease state, the drugs selected on the basis of similarity frequently caused initial aggravations of the condition they were supposed to cure. Guided by some intuition or stroke of genius, Hahnemann, the discoverer of homeopathy, in order, as he thought then, to reduce dosage, proceeded to dilute his medicines in a way that differed from the usual. Instead of ordinary dilution he proceeded stepwise in phases of repeated one to ten or one to a hundred attenuations, while at each step succussing the resulting solution a hundred times. Eventually on the basis of trial and error he came to repeating this process thirty times, insisting upon thorough (hundred times) succussive shaking for each step. Each of these 'dilution steps' is called a 'potency'. Hahnemann and his followers found that, on the average, a thirtieth potency produced the smoothest curative effect, without undue previous aggravation of symptoms. This runs in the face of the fact, fortunately as yet unknown to Hahnemann, that, according to Avogadro's number, the probability of any molecule of the original medicine still being present in such a dilution of 1:100 to the thirtieth power, is about nil. No material or chemical effect can be expected from such a dilution. Nevertheless it happens that these preparations are extremely effective, provided they are prepared in the step-by-step succussion fashion described, and administered according to the simile principle. When the simile principle is disregarded, or the attenuations have not been carried out by stepwise succussion, ordinary dilutions are ineffective. On the other hand, when diluted and thoroughly succussed in stepwise 1:10 or 1:100 succession, the continuing presence of 'something' in dilutions that exceed Avogadro's limit has been demonstrated by biological, biochemical, and nuclear magnetic resonance methods (Coulter, 1981: 52–63).

Moreover, the strangest aspect of this phenomenology bears out the thesis of the *Tractatus aureus*: while the intensity of the potentially toxic substance effect gradually diminishes in dilutions from the concentrated strength to the thirtieth step, the energetic effect increases when the attenuation is carried further into the ultramolecular realm beyond the thirtieth, to the two-hundredth, thousandth, ten-thousandth up to hundred-thousandth and millionth step. Such high potencies can cause quite an uproar in delicate conditions, and can even be dangerous when administered injudiciously. Apparently, what we deal with here is not a dilution in the ordinary sense, but another, as yet unknown dispersion of the substance which, while 'dematerializing' on the molecular level, preserves and even intensifies its specific characteristics in terms of dynamics.

At first, the pathology-inducing 'proving' experiments were conducted with the usual, material dosages of the medicinal substances. Later, however, not only the therapeutic applications but also the provings were carried out with potentized, 'dematerialized' dosages until symptoms were produced. Surprising as it may seem, in that 'non-material' form the same typical proving symptoms are elicited as with the crude material. However, again in line with the *Tractatus aureus*, the process of stepwise 'potentization' activates dynamic effects upon the living organism by substances hitherto considered 'harmless' or medically 'inert' such as club moss, chamomile, ordinary table salt, or inert substances like insoluble quartz or metallic gold.

The nature of such highly attenuated, indeed really dematerialized 'substances' might be likened to spirit, information, or meaning in matter. It points to a border area where material and non-material dynamic, mind and matter, psyche and soma seem to overlap and appear like varying expressions of basic, encompassing arche-typal themes. The operative reality of such encompassing ground-themes, which in a symbolic fashion depict a 'personality', 'spirit' or 'anima' of substance, has emerged from extended clinical experience.

Evidently, the formal patterns underlying or expressing themselves in human dynamics, emotions, conflicts, thought forms and organic functioning correspond to formal and functional elements that also underlie the make-up of the building stones of our planet as well as of its inhabitants. These patterns underlie activity and form. They are creative, archetypal principles of order and meaning that, in differing manifestational 'code' forms, embody corresponding functional complex systems on the level of mineral, plant, animal and human body-and-awareness systems. For every human life-theme played out as complex and somatic pattern there is, apparently, a mirroring energy field that biopsychologically encodes that complex in the substancebody of the earth. Their nature might be considered psyche-like, not psychological but psychoid. Hence, also on the human level, they operate through the psychoid system and always involve somatic as well as psychic effects. These field patterns can be evoked psychically, as we know from work in our consulting rooms. But they can also be evoked via the 'essences' distilled out of substance, via 'substance that is not substance', the insubstantial or substanceless homeopathic high potency.

Just as mental and psychological form patterns can, by synchronicity, constellate analogous material events, so also can dense 'material' substance be 'thinned out' and dematerialized into directive principles of order and form, by the process of potentization. In both directions the functional connection or essential unity between 'inner' and 'outer' dynamic rests upon the principle of analogy, metaphor or similarity. Clinically, this similarity of the substance 'personality' to that of the patient serves as therapeutic indication for its use.

TRANSFERENCE IMPLICATIONS

Before we look at clinical illustrations of the unique way homeopathy depicts and affects these fundamental 'spirit-personalities' we have to consider the effect upon the transference of the therapist's suggesting or offering medication.

Owing to legal restrictions or because of their insufficient familiarity with the Homeopathic Materia Medica many therapists wishing to use homeopathy may have to refer to a qualified homeopathic practitioner rather than dispense remedies themselves. For them the transference implications will probably be not very different from those to be expected when they refer a client out for diagnostic consultation or for psychotropic medication. The analysand might fear that the therapist may want to get rid of him, that he is too heavy a burden for the therapist, too difficult a case or a 'bad' patient. Conversely, there may also result a split transference when the patient plays the medicine against the analytic process and feels that the medicine is to do the whole job now instead of his or her own work on himself or herself.

For the psychoanalyst who undertakes to dispense the medicine himself, the transference problems arise from the partial shift of archetypal role from that of the relatively neutral observer and partner in the search to the medical model of the director of treatment or all-knowing guru. Needless to say, all the above contingencies, particularly the abandonment, authority, and guru complexes, including those of the therapist himself or herself, as well as the therapist's counter-transferential anxiety, impatience, and authority needs will have to be carefully evaluated and worked through. They will also have to be weighted as to appropriate timing and whether the hoped-for benefit of the intervention of giving a medicine balances the problems it may raise at that particular point of the process.

At times a remedy might have to be temporarily or permanently withheld for the sake of more psychological work. On the other hand, a stalled phase of the treatment might be moved into positive activity by the medicine with transference issues hitherto repressed or denied brought into the open. Thus the unblocking effect on the psychoid level may further more effective psychoanalytic work, as was the case in the instances described below.

I shall now give illustrations of the unique way homeopathy depicts these functional 'spirit-personalities' of its spagyric medicines and how these viewpoints have been applied in clinical situations. For reasons of space I can give only a cursory description which focuses upon the psychological personality patterns. In actual clinical use the corresponding typical somatic features must be equally considered.

CASES

Our first patient was a 25-year-old woman with a severe depression and dis-orientation of the reality function. She was passively inert, yet full of impatience and fury about imaginary enemies, with obsessive flights of ideas and illusory notions – i.e. that her hands or other parts of her body wanted to talk to her or disturb her. She was not interested in any school or job activities, because she wanted to 'save' her energies; she complained about constant tiredness and a weakness that supposedly prevented any activity, about feelings of emptiness and a sense of being unreal. She felt that she could not control what 'happened' to her, that parts of her body were separate, hence she was afraid that inadvertently she might commit acts of violence. For that reason she avoided human contact. Her appearance and dress and hair were neglected, and looked dirty in spite of a washing compulsion.

In school she had been diagnosed as 'learning disabled' and put into special classes. She was 'helped' with her homework by her father, a professional writer who never failed to show his intellectual superiority, and thus she never learned to trust her own abilities. From everybody she sensed contempt and concluded that there was no point in trying to assert herself and to relate to people except by withdrawing.

After three years of mainly reductive analysis and some therapeutic regression she was relatively well able to understand her problems. She discovered that she was convinced that there was nobody in the world who would understand her, that there was no point in making any effort, since 'it all would come to nothing anyway'. These feelings centred around her sense of having been neglected and held in contempt by her father who, while purportedly 'helping' her, made it always quite clear that he preferred her extroverted, cheerful and socially successful older brother. According to her memories, father also had the need to show off and to prove to his children, especially to her, how powerful and smart he was, and how wrong and stupid she was.

As she assimilated these insights the obsessive aspects of her condition began to improve. However, her depressions and hopelessness as well as the lethargy remained unchanged.

Eventually she brought dreams: In one she was trying to drive her own damaged car, but feared that it might be injured in the effort. In another she tried to connect with a woman whom she associatively described as a well-adapted social person, but felt that her body or her mother did not allow it. Those dreams I took as speaking not only of her identity with the ineffectual mother but also as referring to a resistance from the Hyle (mother, car, body). This I considered a possible call for substance support. The similar medicine would have to reflect the self-image of an angry, even wrathful and embittered, but also discouraged, humiliated and insulted 'down and out' person who could not come to herself in consequence of feeling a 'nerd', peddler or beggar, worthless, put down and ridiculed, having lost the game before it even started, hence having no chance in life. These features are reflected in the pictures of *Psorinum*, a medicine derived from potentizing the content of a scabies vesicle, the 'beggar's filth'. Its substance picture may be likened to a spirit or 'demon' of self-contempt, humiliation and neglectful disregard of self and body and of one's human dignity, reflected and materialized in the scabies eruption – a neglect of one's way of meeting the world (skin as the surface where inner meets outer).

One dose of the thousandth centesimal potency brought about a dramatic change. The patient now brought a dream in which she enjoyed walking and watching a beautiful spring morning's sunrise. Her posture straightened. She began to pay attention to the way she dressed and, quite spontaneously, got an attractive haircut. Her mood level improved and a first sense of humour began to appear. But, most importantly, a shift occurred in the accessibility of the negative transference. Up to that time, she had remained relatively lethargic and withdrawn, at best merely acknowledging interpretations but isolating herself from interaction with the therapist behind a wall of passive aggression – in the habitual style she had developed in dealing with her father-complex. Now, she began to come out of this lethargic cocoon and started to challenge interpretations and even began actively to express resistance. Eventually she allowed her bottled-up anger to show in verbal fights with the therapist. She had a chance to discover that her furious and at times obsessive anger and invectives did not kill the relationship as she had feared it would have done with her father. Aggressive libido thus found a channel that moved from depression to assertion, and self-assurance, expressed in her being able to pull herself together and to apply herself to systematic work. Upon eventual repetition of the dose, she developed an active interest in, and a cooperative attitude towards, psychological self-understanding and some months after the first dose she decided to go back to college. Analysis continued for several more years, now mostly focused upon the working out of relationship problems.

The next example is that of a middle-aged divorced man. He was the son of an alcholic father and a paranoid, psychotic mother. As a child he felt he had to take care of his mother, yet was often abused, beaten, and almost tortured by her, while having the reality of the situation whitewashed. On entering therapy he was suicidal, given to extremes of mood swings and at times prone to hallucinatory states and psychotic transference projections of both the sociopathic neglectful father and the abusive mother. He tended alternatingly to feel himself as a hateful evil and then a victimized 'good boy' and was either excessively dependent and clinging or closed off and unable to communicate. He wanted to be a 'good father' and take care of his own children and then hated to be bothered by them.

In therapy he was unable to remember sessions from one week to the next, although he kept obsessive and copious reports. These functioned more as if to evacuate and/or accumulate them away into a safer, non-human object and to attempt to destroy the therapist's intentions as his mother's wild envy had nearly destroyed him. Because of splitting and a fragmentary pre-ego he could not hear interpretations or begin to observe the part-aspects of his psyche. The same ground had to be gone over again and again without resulting in any capacity to assimilate insights. Over several years the therapist came to feel that the patient's discriminatory and metabolizing capacities were submerged beyond reach in an insufficiently psychologized affect and drive level. Hence the help of a *medicamentum spagyricum* was called for.

For months, however, the client refused to consider a homeopathic consultation as if it would threaten his alternate tight control and avoidance of the analyst and therapeutic process. He said he never went to doctors. Specific protests involving his poverty and a hopelessness regarding 'unnecessary treatment' were interpreted in terms of the therapy, and eventually he was able to imagine his resistance to medication in terms of an identification with what he perceived was his mother's aversion to any helpful intervention. He was also suspicious of a male consultant, who might, like his father, blandly dismiss his concerns, as well as of the 'magical' qualities of homeopathy, which resonated in his consciousness alongside his father's sociopathic and alcoholic escapades. At length his psyche intervened through the body with an unusually nasty allergy attack. Now he agreed to see the consultant, but with a controlling proviso by which he defended himself against the doctor/father and expressed his combination of trust and hostility in relation to the now perhaps ineffectual but safer analyst/mother. His terms were that he would take the medication from the consultant into his therapy session and take it there.

After the consultation, about which he continued to voice suspicion, he finally swallowed the tiny pills with an air of casual disdain that seemed to express an identification with the blithe, omnipotent dismissal of his father complex. However, his allergy improved dramatically within the hour, and he was amazed and able for the first time in the therapy to express gratitude, since the source of the valued help was at a sufficient distance from the therapist.

In view of the man's tendency to extremes of dissociated splitting the first medicine chosen was *anacardium orientale* in the two-hundredth potency. *Anacardium* is a nut from the mountains of Eastern India. It has an external coating of an oil which is black, caustic and 'bad', but the heart of the nut is sweet. The personality may be called malicious, but with a sweet heart. Dissociation, splitness and separation up to the extreme of schizophrenia are part of its characteristic proving picture. A symptom, mentioned in its proving and clinically typical, is a sense of two wills, one bad, one good; for instance, the description reads: 'a deeply religious person feeling impelled to hate and curse god, or feeling impelled to do what one hates and does not want to do', as in this case our patient's alternating and mutually opposed urges.

The effect of this medicine was quite dramatic. In addition to temporarily easing his allergy, the dissociative splitting and obsessive defences eased considerably. However, the pathology dramatically shifted to the somatic level which he began now to be able to experience consciously. He began to suffer attacks of bronchial asthma and severe rheumatic pains and swelling of joints. Affect now came to the fore by being focused upon his body. Now he could allow himself to feel pain and fear that were observable because they were projected upon his physical condition: he imagined and felt threatened damage from the negative mother as nature – external factors like heat or cold or the weather. He felt quite dependent upon the therapist whom he called almost daily, sometimes several times a day, to report on his physical condition or his fears. Nonetheless he was also still fixed in his habitual patterns and avoided trying new initiatives and ways of relating, even refusing to call the homeopathic consultant when it would have been appropriate. This behaviour now felt more like refusal-resistances and harboured the beginnings of a coalescing core of selfhood.

At this stage a further medicine, carbonate of calcium, was chosen on the basis of its similarity, this time to this person's basic psychosomatic constitutional personality 'picture'. The criteria for the choice were given by his physical typology: short and squat, obese and flabby body build, sensitivity to external climatic factors, particularly wet and cold; and on the other by his basic temperamental habitus: slow, systematic and stubborn, clinging, defensive and one-track-minded – albeit in the track of his current mood.

The carbonate of calcium is prepared from the middle layers of the inner, snow-white part of the oyster shell. Rather than a chemically 'pure' product the oyster calcium is 'live' inasmuch as the limestone rocks are sedimentary rocks derived from ancient sedimentation of oyster-like animal life. The essence of calcium, hence is 'oyster-like'. The form principle of the oyster is underwater life of a soft gelatinous inner core, capable of producing a pearl in its centre around an injuring foreign element. This soft core is surrounded and protected by the hard lime-stone armour of the closed shell. The oyster immovably and 'determinedly' clings to any available fixed support. In this sense then carbonate of calcium presents itself in the organism like a builder of solid ground amidst the flow of waters. The human corollary or its main theme is protection of the individual physical and mental structure against external and internal influences that might dissolve and overwhelm it.

Calcium's tendency is to build up stable organizations out of a yet unorganized inner world and, at the same time, to protect against external influences which may be too strong, without excluding them altogether. Organically, this expresses itself in a square, stocky or even plumpish body build and psychologically in a determined or even stubborn disposition with an urge for independence, self-realization and self-support.

Calcium people are generally slow, practical and economical, conscientious, responsible, even over-responsible workers, who steadily plod along. They are reliable partners, but hate to be dependent, they are satisfied to build patiently and drag stone upon stone in their work. Work is very important to them but is not competitive or ambitious. They are loyal and duty-bound, often dominated by a perfectionistic superego, full of 'shoulds' and 'don'ts'. When the activity of this field pattern is disturbed or traumatized its polar opposite is constellated. Then, like our patient, these types may lack initiative, be too easily frightened, and apprehensive, looking for support, be too open to influences from their surroundings, too easily affected, hypersensitive or too armoured and isolated in order to compensate for their lack of ability to meet a challenge by initiative – thus, becoming stubborn and obstinate. (Physiologically that same defencelessness and failure of adaptability and of meeting challenges, we find as hypersensitivity to rough weather, coldness, dampness and the lack of stamina and endurance.) This will result in dependency, passivity, withdrawal and loss of social relationships.

This medicine, given in two-hundredth and later, thousandth potencies, not only completely healed his physical symptoms and discomforts but also enabled him to become accessible to analytic exploration and interpretation. As the analysis proceeded, the patient was able to develop empathy for his genuine suffering and some differentiation from his obsessions. While accepting that he had a 'psychotic pocket' he even began to develop a sense of humour. Analysis continued for many years and resulted in an increasingly satisfactory work and relationship to life.

CONCLUSION

The alchemist's spagyric process laboured toward the creation of the *lapis* by aiming at a reduction or approximation of substance to the prima materia, namely the informational field that underlies and 'condenses' itself into what we experience as substance. The homeopathic method is a modern form of this process. As the aboriginal, unconditioned, archetypal 'purity' of the prima materia is approached, its ordering effect is mobilized for normalizing the corresponding areas of human encoding. In terms of psychological work we speak of the effects of the constellated Self. When, as in psychotic and borderline cases, the way to psychic cognition is barred, it may be opened through the 'substance that is not a substance', the spirit or *quintessentia* of substance.

In the cases I described, as in most instances, the 'spagyric medicine' helps remove psychoid fixations which hinder the progress of analytical therapy. When the consequences of serious childhood damage, emotional and physical abuse, rape, incest, war, concentration-camp and prison-camp experiences, drug addiction, or other inveterate conditioning have become imprinted somatically, they create stubbornly resistant dissociations and repetition compulsions. In these instances the therapeutic approach stands to benefit from addressing itself also, or perhaps even primarily, to the biologic-psychoid substratum, the 'subtle' body fields.

Nevertheless, psychoanalysis remains essential also in these cases and the importance of the psychotherapist is not diminished. Even though the simillimum will be helpful in removing a blockage of revitalizing energy, and aid the development of an adequate ego sense capable of witnessing and confronting the instinctual unconscious, it is not, of itself, capable of removing the underlying personality problems. Moreover, to the extent that adequate cognitional and integrative capacities happen to be available, the reliance on a medicine can he counterproductive: the notion that the medicine could solve one's difficulties of relationship to one's selfhood and to others may interfere with the maturational process. On the other hand, when insufficient ego strength and cognitional capacities are the main problems then the homeopathic medicine can make the psychological work easier and more effective. But even then, with borderlines and others, psychotherapy has to be continued. Basic life decisions, ethical and interpersonal relationship problems and difficulties as well as one's relationship to one's complexes, to one's creativity and to the transpersonal dimension require the psychological differentiation and the agonizing work of the ego in confronting the unconscious, as the second step towards the achievement of the *unio mentalis*.

ACKNOWLEDGEMENTS

My thanks are due to Sylvia Brenton Perera, my companion and colleague, for her help in reading this chapter and offering editorial comment and criticism, and for the clinical material of one of her analytic clients for whom I became the homeopathic consultant.

NOTE

This chapter first appeared in *Journal of Analytical Psychology*, JAP 1996, Vol. 41, no. 3, 369–386, and is copyright of Blackwell Publishers.

REFERENCES

Coulter, H. J. (1981) *Homeopathic Science and Modern Medicine.* Berkeley, CA: North Atlantic Books.

Hermes Trismegistus (1692) *The Golden Work of Hermes Trismegistus [Tractatus aureus].* Translated out of Hebrew into Arabick, then into Greek, afterwards into Latin; and now done out of Latin into English, Claused and largely commented upon by William Salmon Professor of Physick. Printed for J. Harris and T. Hawkins. (Privately mimeographed, Chapter VII, p. 51.)

Jung, C. G. (1921) 'Definitions', *Collected Works*, Vol. 6. London: Routledge & Kegan Paul.

Jung, C. G. (1941). 'Paracelsus the physician', *Collected Works*, Vol. 15. London: Routledge & Kegan Paul.

Jung, C. G. (1955–6). *Mysterium Coniunctionis*, *Collected Works*, Vol. 14. London: Routledge & Kegan Paul.

Paracelsus (1928). *Sämtliche Werke*, Vol. 2, transl. B. Aschner. Jena: Gustav Fischer.

Paracelsus (1951). *Selected Writings*, Edited by J. Jacobi; transl. N. Guterman. Princeton, NJ: Princeton University Press.

Paracelsus *Opus Paramirum*, Vol. 1. Edited by K. Sudhoff.

Homeopathic studies

Benzecri, P. (1991) 'Comparaison entre quatre méthodes de sevrage après une thérapeutique anxiolytique'. *Cahiers de l'Analyse des Donndes*, Vol. 16, no. 4, 389–402.

Haidvogel, M. (1992) 'Klinische Studien zum Wirkungsnachweis der Homoopathie'. *Der Kinderarzt*, Vol. 23, no. 9, 1477–1484.

Jenaer, M., Marichal, B., Wassenhoven, M. van, Vandenbrouke, P. and Hervieux, L. (1993) *Traité théorique et pratique d'immunotherapie à doses infinitesimales: Science de la reequilibration du système immunitaire*. Limoges: Editions Roger Jollois.

King, G. (1988) *Experimental Investigations for the Purpose of Scientific Proving of the Efficacy of Homeopathic Preparations: A Literature Review of Publications from English-speaking Countries*. Inaugural dissertation, Tierärztliche Hochschule, Hanover.

Kleijnen, P. and Knipschield, G. ter Reid (1991) 'Clinical trials of homeopathy'. *British Medical Journal*, Vol. 302, no. 3, 316–323. (Includes studies on homeopathy and mental illness.)

Reilly, D., Taylor, M., Beattie, N. *et al.* (1994) 'Is evidence for homeopathy reproducible?' *Lancet*, Vol. 344, 1601–1606.

Resch, G. and Gutmann, V. (1987) *Wissenschaftliche Grundlagen der Homöopathie*. Berg-am-Starberger: O-Verlag.

Righetti, M. (1988) *Forschung in der Homöopathie: Grundlage, Problematik und Ergebnisse*. Gottingen: Burgdorf Verlag.

Zimmermann, G. (1993) 'Die Homöopathie und die theoretische Physik: Ein Gesprach mit Univ. Professor Dr H. Pietschmann, Institut für Theoretische Physik der Universität Wien'. *Osterreichische Apotheker Zeitung*, Vol. 47, no. 40, 75–77.

(b) The demonization of the body in analysis

Robert Withers

The analytic session has lapsed into silence. I am lost in my own thoughts for a few moments. When I turn back I find my client is writhing, as if in agony, on the couch. The muscles in her legs are clenched and contorted, her breathing rapid. I notice her eyes are frightened and glazed as she turns her head from side to side. By now, three years into the analysis, I recognize the signs. She is caught in a flashback, reliving a terrifying experience from an appalling childhood.

I wonder whether to intervene with what has become one of my stock responses.

'Are you having a flashback?' or
'Where are you now?'

But before I can decide what to say she starts to plead in a low voice.

'I want you to speak now.'
'To distract you from what's happening in the flashback?'

She turns, catches my eye for an instant (I sit beside her) and holds me with a despairing smile.

'I'm afraid I'll get lost in it.'

I know she is talking about a fear of madness, of being unable to stop reliving the past and return to the here and now of the session. At times she can use the sound of my voice to do that. At other times though, it can become woven into the flashback itself. I also know from experience if she does not speak about what is happening to her, she is likely to self-harm when she gets home, and try to anaesthetize herself against the nightmares that will wake her up by drinking too much. She may also miss sessions or contemplate suicide in an attempt to avoid the maelstrom of emotion that has been stirred up.

'Try to talk about it' I say.
'There aren't any words. Just blackness . . .'

Nevertheless as she starts to speak, haltingly at first, a picture begins to emerge and the flashback starts to turn to memory. At first there are likely to be bodily sensations. Perhaps the sense of holding herself rocking beneath her cot in the hospital feeling abandoned by her parents. Or the smells, which she eventually identifies as her father's sweat and semen mixed with her own blood and shit and then pieces over the coming months into a memory of abuse.

The words recounting these experiences act as a thread linking her present to the past, herself to me and eventually, it is to be hoped, the fragments of herself together. At times, however, the fear becomes too great, the words cease and a stillness comes over her. She has cut the thread and found the imaginary safe place to which she retreated in childhood from the terror, the pain and the rage. She lies calm and emotionless while tears stream down my face. In her mind she is back in a world of squirrels and rabbits, where people are kind – for a while.

Little has changed since Freud's day. Perhaps today analysts would make more use of the transference and countertransference than he did. The flashback to feeling abandoned in the hospital might be linked to unmanageable feelings around an impending break; the analyst's tears to her own uncried ones – and so on. Certainly tracking the transference significance of the flashbacks has been useful in ameliorating the danger of her becoming overwhelmed by them. In that sense the transference can act like a homeopathic version of the original trauma, a place where unmanageable feelings can be worked through. But despite this shift in emphasis, the essence of the analytic method with a patient like this remains remarkably similar to that employed by Freud in the early days of 'the talking cure' (see Freud and Breuer, 1893–6). It is frightening, time-consuming, hard work for both parties. It is nevertheless, potentially at least, immensely rewarding as feelings and experiences, which previously expressed themselves only in borderline or somatic symptoms begin to become contained and symbolized in words, thoughts, dreams and memories, for the first time.

Later on in the same day I am sitting with a patient who has come to see me from time to time for homeopathic treatment since the days before I trained to be an analyst. Her first son suffered from cerebral palsy shortly after birth. His doctors gave him little chance of ever doing much more than sitting up – let alone walking or talking. She attributes the fact that he has grown into a fairly normal young man largely to my homeopathic treatment. Today she is coming to see me because she is finding it hard to cope with her second, six-year-old son (by a different man). In the course of our session she remarks that she thinks some of her difficulties may be related to the fact that the boy's father effectively raped her two weeks after the birth.

I prescribe staphis agria 10M for her, a homeopathic remedy which is so dilute it does not chemically exist, and another remedy for her son. It is normal homeopathic practice to see members of the same family. A month later she returns saying she is still finding her son difficult, though much less of a 'little demon'. She herself feels more whole and able to cope. 'It is as if the remedy has stitched me up.' Of course she has the past experience of my help with her older son to bolster the hope that the remedies I have given will work. My feeling though is that her six-year-old may eventually need psychotherapy (but not with me). Nevertheless, it is fair to say that the symptomatic relief that she herself feels at this early stage is something it may have taken years of analytic work to achieve. She appears to feel more emotionally whole after the remedy despite not having really talked through the emotional effects of being raped by the boy's father. I, however, am left with a nagging sense of unease to accompany the gratification of having somehow helped her feel better.

That sense of unease contrasts with Edward Whitmont's apparent confidence in homeopathy in his article above.

> When the consequences of serious childhood damage, emotional and physical abuse, rape, incest, war, concentration-camp and prison-camp experiences, drug addiction, or other inveterate conditioning have become imprinted somatically, they create stubbornly resistant dissociations and repetition compulsions. In these instances the therapeutic approach stands to benefit from addressing itself also, or perhaps even primarily, to the biologic-psychoid substratum, the 'subtle' body fields.

He writes; and leaves us in no doubt that he regards homeopathy as a highly effective way of working with those body fields (p. 233). Despite Whitmont's claims to the contrary, however, the existence of such body fields remains highly speculative. Nor is there any scientifically acceptable evidence that homeopathy can act physically upon them (Linde *et al.*, 1997). There is therefore a danger of contributing to homeopathy's marginalization by appealing to energy fields to explain its effects. As I hope to show, however, there is another way of understanding at least some of its effects, which does not rely on the magical or the scientifically unproven. But before going on to consider this, I wish to pause to examine Whitmont's central project in the above article.

WORKING WITH ANALYTIC IMPASSE

Put at its simplest, that project seems to me to be to propose that analysts consider using homeopathy in situations where potentially important analytic material is not psychologically accessible. Under these circumstances he suggests that homeopathic remedies can help make such material symbolizable and hence available for analysis. Without it, conventional analytic methods are, he believes, of only limited value and liable to reach an impasse. 'In order to modify the pathology of the psychoid', he says, 'psychotherapy is in need of complementary modalities of a precognitional [i.e. non-symbolic] nature.' He goes on to offer two cases to illustrate this point.

The search for ways of overcoming the problem of analytic impasse is of considerable therapeutic importance. I will return to consider the viability of Whitmont's particular solution to the problem in the course of this article, when I have laid the groundwork to do so more effectively. In the meantime I would like to acknowledge my debt to him for pioneering a Jungian approach to homeopathy.

I found this invaluable in my own academic research into the psychology of homeopathy (Withers, 1979a, 1979b), and a source of inspiration in my eventual decision to train as an analyst.

My first case above illustrates, however, that conventional analytic methods need not be as limited in treating the somatically imprinted effects of serious childhood damage as he thinks. Relatively early on in the course of our work together for instance, the chronic fatigue, from which my client originally suffered, lifted significantly without recourse to any complementary therapy.

Whitmont might reply that not every analytic patient is able to flash back to traumatic material so readily. Although this is true, it is worth noting that that did not happen in this case until we had moved from once- to four-times-a-week analysis. It seems, then, as though the secure holding offered by a full analytic relationship may have been necessary for it to occur. It also seems though that Whitmont may have been too categorical in dismissing the clinical benefits of the analytic method in such cases.

UNDERSTANDING HOMEOPATHY ANALYTICALLY

If Whitmont too readily dismisses the clinical potential of analysis, he is also I believe at times too quick to dismiss its explanatory power. Thus he regards Jung's attempts to understand alchemy in terms of the projection of the contents of the unconscious onto matter, as due to the limitations of his 'nineteenth-century positivistic medical viewpoint' (p. 223). But I hope to illustrate that a combination of this Jungian formulation with some of Bion's concepts (Bion, 1953), can help illuminate the operation of homeopathy – without necessitating the upheaval of contemporary Western science.

Whitmont's first case, it will be recalled, is of a woman in her mid-twenties who seems to be suffering from severe depression and a borderline condition. The analysis reaches an impasse following a limited therapeutic regression and an intellectual understanding of the origin of her symptoms, which nevertheless leaves her depressed, lethargic and hopeless. 'These feelings centred around her sense of being neglected and held in contempt by her father . . .', he writes (p. 229). Rephrasing this we could say she was unable to manage her father's contempt, and that her symptoms stemmed from the *toxic* effect of internalizing this (Bion, 1953). Whitmont gave her back an image of that contempt in a safe (*detoxified*) form – a remedy made of potentized pus from the scabies vesicle. She probably knew what substance he was giving her. So it is easy to imagine what a powerful emotional effect taking the remedy could have had. But, even if he had withheld its name, she would still have believed she was taking the safe form of a substance that could cause her emotional and physical condition by the homeopathic principle. Such a substance would thus constitute an ideal *container* for the *projection* of the emotions at the heart of her pathology. Once projected there she only had to believe in the safety of the remedy she was given, and trust Whitmont's knowledge of homeopathy, in order to take those projections back in a symbolically *detoxified* and therefore therapeutic form. The fact that there was less than a one in a billion chance of encountering even a single molecule of the original pus in the remedy is thus irrelevant. On this view its therapeutic effect was due to a psychological process of projection, transformation and reintrojection, which only appears magical because it was largely unconscious.

This could be considered an example of Bion's concept of the transformation of beta into alpha elements (Bion, 1953). The remedy then would act as a container, via projection, of previously uncontained and therefore toxic beta elements. Homeopathic potentization would represent their detoxification into alpha elements. Taking the remedy would enable their internalization in that form by the patient (Bion, 1953). Symptom relief could then follow (see Withers, 2001). This formulation could be regarded as the offspring of a Jung/Bion marriage, and a variant of Fordham's theory of deintegration/reintegration (see, for example, Fordham, 1957).

At the same time as these psychological effects of the remedy, there appear to have been parallel deintegrative and reintegrative processes at work in the actual dynamics of the transference and countertransference. Once more, however, these seem to have been largely unconscious and go unremarked by Whitmont. Nevertheless, it is striking how like the patient's all-knowing father he must have seemed to her when he made the shift from analyst to homeopath. As he himself says, this change involves

> . . . the partial shift of archetypal role from that of relatively neutral observer and partner in the search to the medical model of director of treatment or all-knowing guru.

So he both adopted the role of the all-knowing father, and gave her back an image of herself (in remedy form) as contemptible. Unlike her real father, however, Whitmont seems to have been able to tolerate the hostility unleashed when he assumed that position. The fact that their relationship was able to withstand it was, as he says, probably crucial in helping her turn her anger outward into the world rather than inwards into depression. But once more, it is not necessary to envisage a physical action of the remedy here in order to account for this process. To use a phrase attributed to Plaut (1956), Whitmont had 'incarnated the archetype' of the father. And it seems likely that the emergence of this emotionally charged theme into their relationship produced a significant therapeutic effect. Thus in my view Whitmont has underestimated the contribution that analysis can make to understanding the effects of both the remedy, and the therapeutic dynamics.

One question that naturally arises at this point is the extent to which homeopathy in general can be understood in terms of such psychological mechanisms. Whatever its physical effects, it certainly seems likely that psychological factors constitute a far larger part of its action than is generally recognized (see Withers, 2001). All homeopathic remedies are chosen on the basis of their ability to mimic symptoms and psychological states. So they should all be capable in principle of facilitating the transformation of beta into alpha elements along the lines described above. Untransformed, of course, it is, in Bion's view, these beta elements that give rise to the psychosomatic and borderline symptoms under discussion (Bion, 1953, 1959).

It also seems relevant that remedies are dispensed on pills of milk sugar (lactose). The mother's offering of breast milk in response to her infant's cries of hunger is the early prototype of these processes of containment and transformation. So it is conceivable that taking the remedy triggers a body memory of these early experiences, and this too contributes to its therapeutic effect. Whatever the truth of these speculations, it seems clear that homeopathy is capable of evoking powerful psychological forces that need not remain entirely shrouded in mystery.

IMPASSE REVISITED

This, however, gives rise to a potentially embarrassing question for analysts. Like Whitmont I have noticed that homeopathy can quite often relieve symptoms more quickly than analysis. My homeopathic case above illustrates as much. But how can this be, if homeopathy itself is acting largely or wholly psychologically? Part of the answer to this question will be apparent from the preceding discussion. But I believe that further consideration of Whitmont's case reveals there may be an additional factor at work.

It seems likely from his account, that one thing that held up his patient's analysis was her fear of re-experiencing unbearable feelings of worthlessness in the transference. I have already pointed out above how the change from analyst to homeopath could have reactivated those feelings. Paradoxically, however, they could have simultaneously been diminished by the administration of the remedy, because *any therapeutic change could now be attributed to that remedy rather than the analyst*. In this way, uncontained feelings of envy towards him, which were blocking the analysis, could have been bypassed.

The work of Herbert Rosenfeld (1987) linking analytic impasse to envy is of special relevance here. He points out that at times in a conventional analysis it may feel more bearable to remain stuck than allow the analyst to promote therapeutic change. That way the unbearable envy of the analyst's apparent creativity in contrast to the patient's apparent emptiness is avoided. It should now be possible to understand why homeopathy may in practice permit symptomatic relief in certain cases of analytic impasse.

There are, however, potential dangers as well as benefits in this amalgamation of homeopathic and analytic practices. I will be in a better position to discuss these when I have briefly clarified some important differences between the two disciplines.

HOMEOPATHY

The differences between analysis and homeopathy can easily become obscured in a case such as Whitmont's where the two have already been amalgamated. I think it is fair to say, however, that homeopathic patients are far more likely to present with physical or mixed emotional/physical symptoms than analytic ones. Where they do present emotionally, as in my homeopathic case above, they tend to do so in a way that avoids not just envy but any regressive emotional involvement with the therapist. My patient for instance was typical in that she reported crying after taking her staphis agria but did not cry in a session with me.

People who choose homeopathy may therefore self-select partly on the basis of a wish to avoid dependent relationships. They depend instead on their remedy, which thus acts like a transitional object (Winnicott, 1951). Practitioners who choose homeopathy likewise may prefer to avoid the perceived dangers of close relationships. Appointments, for instance, occur typically only monthly.[1]

I have also often noticed alarm in homeopathic supervisees when signs of strong emotion emerge in a session. The typical reaction is to wish to refer the patient straight on to a psychotherapist. This apparent fear of strong emotions often seems to be reciprocated in the patient. Certainly from an analytic point of view, the patient who somatizes often does so to avoid feeling painful emotions or thinking about their implications (see, for example, Taylor (1985) on alexithymia). A shared fear of emotion may then underlie both parties' choice of homeopathy as a means of treatment.

Homeopathic theory is philosophically idealistic, however, despite its therapeutic reliance on remedies and fear of strong feelings. Emotion, spirit and mind are conceived as at the centre of the person, with the body on the periphery (Kent, 1911; Vithoulkas, 1980). But paradoxically there is very little therapeutic attempt to work directly with these psychological elements. They are usually simply regarded as especially important factors in determining remedy choice and worked on through the remedies.

ANALYSIS

All this contrasts strongly with analytic theory and practice. Despite its therapeutic emphasis on the mind, for instance, there are strong philosophically materialistic strands present in both Freudian and Jungian analysis. These are evident in Freud's 'Project towards a physiological psychology' (1896) as well as post-Jungian conceptions of the archetypes as innate genetically determined biological structures (see, for example, Stevens, Controversy Eight in the present volume).

---

1   See Duckworth and Stone (Controversy Ten in the present volume) for a related discussion.

Most significantly perhaps, whereas homeopaths and their patients appear to defend against regression and emotional relating, analysts and theirs appear to defend against the body and physical relating. Thus there is a taboo on touch, and analytic theory places the somatic in the most inaccessible pre-symbolic (psychoid) part of the person. In part this is no more than common sense. Who for instance would expect to effectively treat a sore throat with psychotherapy? The successful homeopathic treatment of such a sore throat with a high potency remedy of course brings even this common sense into question. So does the operation of the placebo effect (see, for example, Peters, 2001). But even leaving these instances aside, there are good reasons to suppose that the positioning of the body as taboo in psychotherapy is also partly defensive in origin.

In contrast to homeopaths, analysts and their patients seem to share a yearning for an intimate dependent relationship (see Duckworth and Stone, Controversy Ten in the present volume). The price of that intimacy, however, seems to be the exclusion of the body from the analytic relationship. Presumably in this way some of the dangers of both sexual acting out and 'malignant regression' (Bateman and Holmes, 1995: 162) are reduced. It was these dangers that in part led Freud to abandon the massage technique that accompanied the treatment of his early analytic cases (see Jones, 1961). They also led to Breuer's famous difficulties with Anna O and his eventual abandonment of psychoanalysis (Jones, 1961). My first case above indicates an additional reason for what could be called this analytic 'demonization of the body', however. It has to do with dissociation as a defence against trauma.

That patient, it will be recalled, retreated to an imaginary safe place when she experienced her environment as unbearably traumatic. She did this by dissociating from her body. As she flashed back to the original trauma, it was in her body that she first re-experienced it. The body thus became the site of 'demonic' experience as well as a potential source of healing from it. That duality can be seen in a dream of hers in which some unidentified people were trying to give her a baby with a squirrel's head. The dream image seems to have depicted the reunion of mind (squirrel – representing the imaginary safe place) with body (represented by the baby). This dream occurred after she had relived a particularly traumatic piece of abuse, and it indicates her horror at having to face the monstrous consequences of that abuse emotionally, in order to heal from it.

Myths such as that of Theseus and the Minotaur seem to depict the same journey of the soul back from a state of dissociation to one of wholeness through facing the terror of the original trauma. The patient's ego here is in the place of the hero, Theseus. The analyst, like Ariadne, holds the thread of words that helps him negotiate the labyrinth. The demonic Minotaur hidden at its heart is half-bull, half-man – the product of Queen Pasiphaë's intercourse with a white bull (Graves, 1955). This bull seems to represent those unacceptable human desires (including incestuous wishes) that must be sacrificed in order to live in society, as well as the events that occur when they are not. The labyrinth itself could be regarded in part as an expression of a confusional defence thrown up to hide that (real or imagined) incest and its consequences – but also as a healthy response to the decision to attempt to overcome the defensive split between mind and body by confronting the trauma. It (the labyrinth) may thus serve to reduce the risk of breakdown by regulating the amount of reality to which consciousness is exposed.

Naturally the trauma at the heart of the labyrinth need not always be incest. In the precocious split of mind from body identified by Winnicott (1949) as the precursor of the false self, that trauma may have been the experience of disruptions to the state of 'going on being' in early infancy; while in certain schizoid individuals (see, for example, Guntrip, 1968: 35) the very existence of appetites in the here and now may be experienced as traumatic. In all these cases, however, where a person identifies with a 'head ego', it tends to be the body that is feared as the apparent site of trauma. And this may contribute to attracting people to analysis, as a therapy that shares this phobia of the body and identification with the mind. It is hardly surprising under these circumstances if that fear at times overcomes the psyche-soma's drive towards reintegration, and analytic work becomes stuck. A final consideration of the wisdom of Whitmont's project should now be possible.

RETURN TO WHITMONT'S PROJECT

In the admittedly oversimplified account above, the analytic journey could be described as centripetal. That is, it is a movement of consciousness towards a confrontation with psyche-somatic reality. This contrasts with the centrifugal homeopathic journey described by Whitmont.[2] There a remedy is given to liberate parts of the ego from the bodily drives (body psychoid) with which they have become merged. From the analytic point of view therefore, there is a danger that the symptomatic relief afforded by homeopathy may be achieved at the expense of consciously working material through. When my homeopathic patient cried after taking her staphis agria, for instance, she did so without consciously knowing what she was crying about. Arguably though, the patient may feel this loss of consciousness is a price worth paying if it helps overcome genuine intractable analytic impasse, and affords some symptom relief.

Many apparent cases of impasse however may actually be surmountable analytically. Fordham (1957), Rosenfeld (1987), Bollas (1987) and others have all attempted to find ways of dealing with previously unanalysable material. They generally involve the analyst working closely on feelings engendered within the therapeutic relationship. But if even these methods fail, I do not personally see any reason for objecting to the use of homeopathy or other therapies to complement analytic work along the lines suggested by Whitmont. In some ways the situation would then be similar to working analytically with patients on psychotropic medication, even though these act more chemically.

---

2   This formulation also seems to accord with Erich Neumann's (1954) notion of 'centroversion'.

It should be noted, however, that even psychiatrically trained analysts do not tend to medicate their own patients. I believe there are many good reasons for this, which apply equally to complementary therapy. The increased danger of malignant regression and sexual acting out when analysts work physically with their patients has already been touched on. And working homeopathically usually does involve examining patients, enquiring after their physical symptoms and giving them physical remedies – even if these act mainly psychologically. Such physical involvement could make the regressive pull, already strong in many analytic relationships, overwhelming. The potential for analytic abuse of power and the adoption of a kind of therapeutic omnipotence would thus be increased, as would the risk of breakdown in the patient. For these reasons I believe there are dangers in analysts treating their own patients with complementary medicine, which generally outweigh the potential therapeutic benefits.

IMPASSE IN COMPLEMENTARY THERAPY

On the other hand there are certain cases of what could be termed 'complementary impasse' that seem to stem from the emergence of problematic emotional material in the complementary therapy relationship. This can often be resolved through the application of relatively simple analytic insight. The centripetal nature of the homeopathic journey lessens the risk of regression in such cases, although it can occur if the therapeutic relationship starts to evolve into a primarily psycho-therapeutic one. For this reason it is generally preferable for the complementary therapist to refer the patient on to a colleague before this happens, even if he or she is analytically qualified. Presumably it is the fear of such an occurrence that accounts for the homeopathic mistrust of emotion remarked on above.

CONCLUSION

In this paper I have considered Edward Whitmont's proposal that analysts make use of homeopathy or other forms of complementary therapy in cases that seem intractable to ordinary analytic methods. I have concluded firstly that many such cases may not in fact be as intractable as they appear. Secondly that analysis itself can help make sense of both the action of homeopathic remedies and the effects of the therapeutic dynamics in many homeopathic (and other complementary therapy) cases. To that extent I have questioned Whitmont's formulation of homeopathy, which relies on a scientifically unsubstantiated appeal to 'subtle body fields'. Despite these reservations, however, I have argued that there is nothing intrinsically problematic in Whitmont's proposals, provided the analyst does not conduct both the analysis and the complementary treatment himself. In such cases the dangers of acting out, serious regression or even breakdown are in my opinion usually too great to justify the potential therapeutic benefits. I have gone on to point out some other possibilities for cooperation between analysis and complementary therapy, particularly in the use of basic analytic insight to help resolve certain cases of 'complementary impasse'.

Finally there are one or two loose ends I would like to attempt to tie up. I am aware that the presentation of my homeopathic vignettes at the start of this paper left some unanswered questions. Do I really believe that it might be possible to explain these cases, and especially the child's recovery from cerebral palsy, psychologically? And why did I feel uneasy when my homeopathic patient felt better?

I am not sure I can fully answer either of these questions. Part of my unease was no doubt due to the apparently magical nature of my homeopathic intervention, but also, I suspect, to the unequivocally positive transference I received. Did this mean that somebody else, the boy's father for instance, had to receive an equally strong negative transference? The answer to the other question I will have to leave open. I do recall, however, that the boy's mother was receiving counselling (with someone else) at the same time as I treated her son homeopathically for his cerebral palsy. And I often wonder what role, if any, that counselling may have had in *his* eventual recovery (see, for example, Mannoni, 1970).

REFERENCES

Bateman, A. and Holmes, J. (1995) *Introduction to Psychoanalysis*. London: Routledge.

Bion, W. (1953) 'A theory of thinking'. *International Journal of Psycho-analysis*, Vol. 53; also in *Second Thoughts*. London: Heinemann, 1967.

Bion, W. (1959) 'Attacks on linking', *International Journal of Psycho-analysis*, Vol. 40; also in *Second Thoughts*. London: Heinemann, 1967.

Bollas, C. (1987) *The Shadow of the Object: Psychoanalysis of the Unthought Known*. London: Free Association Books.

Fordham, M. (1957) 'Notes on the transference', in *New Developments in Analytical Psychology*. London: Routledge.

Freud, S. (1895) *Project for a Scientific Psychology*. Standard Edition, Vol. 18, London: Hogarth.

Freud, S. and Breuer, J. (1893–6) *Studies on Hysteria*. Standard Edition, Vol. 2. London: Hogarth.

Graves, R. (1955) *The Greek Myths*, Harmondsworth, UK: Penguin.

Guntrip H. (1968) *Schizoid Phenomena, Object Relations and the Self*. London: Hogarth Press. (Page reference from London: Karnac Books, 1992 edition.)

Jones, E. (1961) *The Life and Works of Sigmund Freud*, New York: Basic Books.

Kent J. (1911) *Lectures on Homoeopathic Philosophy*. Philadelphia PA: Boericke and Tafel.

Linde, K. *et al.* (1997) 'Are the clinical effects of homeopathy placebo effects? A meta-analysis of placebo controlled trials', *Lancet*, no. 350, 834–843.

Mannoni, M. (1970) *The Child, His Illness and the Others*. London: Tavistock.

Neumann, E. (1954) *Origins and History of Consciousness*. London: Routledge & Kegan Paul.

Peters, D. (2001) *Understanding the Placebo Effect in Complementary Medicine*. Edinburgh: Churchill-Livingstone.

Plaut, F. (1956) 'The transference in analytical psychology'. *British Journal of Medical Psychology*, Vol. 29, no. 1.

Rosenfeld, H. (1987) *Impasse and Interpretation*. London: Tavistock.

Taylor, G. (1985) *Psychosomatic Medicine and Contemporary Psychoanalysis*. Madison, CT: International Universities Press.

Vithoulkas, G. (1980) *The Science of Homeopathy*. New York: Grove Press.

Winnicott, D. (1949) 'Mind and its relation to the psyche-soma'. *International Journal of Psycho-analysis*. Also in *Through Paediatrics to Psychoanalysis*. London: Hogarth Press, 1987.

Winnicott, D. (1951) 'Transitional objects and transitional phenomena'. *International Journal of Psycho-analysis*, Vol. 34 (1953). Also in *Through Paediatrics to Psychoanalysis*. London: Hogarth Press, 1987.

Withers, R. (1979a) 'Towards a psychology of homoeopathy'. M.Phil. Thesis, University of Sussex.

Withers, R. (1979b) 'Towards a psychology of homoeopathy and the high potencies'. *The British Homoeopathic Journal*, vol. LXVIII, no.3.

Withers, R. (2001) 'Psychoanalysis, complementary medicine and the placebo' in D. Peters (Ed.), *Understanding the Placebo Effect in Complementary Medicine*, Edinburgh: Churchill Livingstone.

The contemporary status of archetypal theory

CONTROVERSY EIGHT

The contemporary status
of archetypal theory

Introduction

This controversy raises crucial questions about the epistemological basis of analysis. Should we ground our work in the 'hard sciences' of biology, ethology and genetics, or are our theories and practices best understood in the light of the 'soft sciences' of linguistics, sociology and cultural studies? If some synthesis of these two is possible and desirable, what form should that take? These are far-ranging questions with important implications reaching beyond the field of analytical psychology itself deep into the 'crisis of modernity'. Anthony Stevens and Paul Kugler discuss the issues from contrasting perspectives in relation to the status of archetypal theory.

Stevens argues that the future of analytical psychology is under threat as its practices and assumptions are increasingly scrutinized and challenged. The best chance of securing its future lies, he believes, in aligning archetypal theory to the hard sciences of genetics, ethology and the emerging field of evolutionary psychology. Far from constituting an appeal to nineteenth-century essentialism, as opponents claim, recent advances in these disciplines provide analytical psychology with vital support. To ignore that support is to risk our demise as a living therapeutic system and our transformation into a primarily intellectual disembodied discipline.

Paul Kugler argues for a 'co-evolutionary' approach to archetypal theory. He acknowledges that evolutionary factors have affected hard-wired aspects of our psyches, but these have remained essentially unchanged for over ten thousand years. During that time our life-styles have changed massively. Understanding the impact of these changes on our psyches is therefore impossible on the basis of an appeal to evolutionary factors alone. Instead we need to explore how these evolutionary factors have interacted with the cultural changes that language has made possible. Those changes are he argues best understood in the light of the soft sciences. To ignore the effect of language, he implies, is to ignore what is essentially human in archetypal psychology.

(a) Archetypal theory: the evolutionary dimension

Anthony Stevens

THEMES AND VARIATIONS

With his theory of archetypes operating as components of the collective unconscious, Jung sought to define the living bedrock of human psychology. Virtually alone among eminent psychologists of the twentieth century, he rejected the *tabula rasa* theory of human psychological development, wholeheartedly embracing the notion that evolutionary pressures had determined the basic structures and functions of the human psyche. Practically all other psychologists and psychoanalysts, as well as sociologists and anthropologists, focused on the myriad ways that individuals differed from one another and attempted to account for these differences in terms of the cultural and social influences they had been subjected to in the course of growing up. In opposition to this view, Jung held that a truly scientific psychology must start from what human beings had in common before the study of individual differences could proceed with any hope of reaching meaningful or valid conclusions.

This inevitably brought him into conflict with Sigmund Freud. Whereas Freud insisted that the unconscious mind was entirely personal and peculiar to the individual and made up of repressed wishes and traumatic memories, Jung maintained that there existed an additional phylogenetic layer (the 'collective unconscious'), which incorporated the entire psychic potential of humankind. Support for this notion came from the studies Jung conducted with his colleagues at the Burghölzli Hospital in Zurich into the delusions and hallucinations of schizophrenic patients. They were able to demonstrate that these contained motifs and images that also occurred in myths, religions, and fairy tales from all over the world (Jung, 1956). Jung concluded that there must exist a dynamic substratum, common to all humanity, on the basis of which each individual builds his or her own experience of life, developing a unique array of psychological characteristics. In other words, the archetypes of the collective unconscious provided the basic themes of human life on which each individual worked out his or her own sets of variations.

Of all Jung's ideas, none has proved more controversial than his theory of a collective unconscious of which the archetypes function as dynamic components. Yet it is a hypothesis that has been rediscovered and reproposed by specialists in a number of different disciplines (for example, Chomsky's 'deep structures', Piaget's 'innate schemata', Lévi-Strauss's structuralist view of the unconscious as a 'universe of rules', and the ethological concept of 'innate releasing mechanisms' responsible for typical 'patterns of behaviour'. See also Gray, 1996; Stevens, 1999). 'I have chosen the term "collective"', he wrote, 'because this part of the unconscious is not individual but universal; in contrast to the personal psyche, it has contents and modes of behaviour that are more or less the same everywhere and in all individuals' (Jung, 1959: 3–4).

Jung related this 'common psychic substrate of a suprapersonal nature' to the structure of the brain: 'every man is born with a brain that is profoundly differentiated, and this makes him capable of very various mental functions, which are neither ontologically developed [n]or acquired. . . . This particular circumstance explains, for example, the remarkable analogies presented by the unconscious in the most remotely separated races and peoples' (Jung, 1953: 269–270). Hence the extraordinary correspondence of cultural artefacts occurring throughout the world. 'The universal similarity of human brains leads us then to admit the existence of a certain psychic function, identical with itself in all individuals; we call it the collective psyche' (Jung, 1953: 270).

With hindsight, this seems such a reasonable position to adopt that future generations will find it hard to understand why Jung's proposal encountered as much opposition as it did. In addition to the entrenched antagonism of academics wedded to the Standard Social Science Model (the SSSM, which is deeply hostile to the idea that biology or innate structures could have a part to play in human psychology), Jung also suffered a blistering from the Freudians, who, usurping the high scientific ground, dismissed him as a crank and a mystic. It is ironic that now, with the dawn of a new century, Jung's theory of archetypes, first proposed and termed 'primordial images' nearly a hundred years ago, is being rehabilitated by the new disciplines of evolutionary psychology and evolutionary psychiatry, while Freud's scientific credentials have been seriously impugned (Esterson, 1993; Webster, 1997; Macmillan, 1997; Wilcocks, 1997).

ARCHETYPES AND EVOLUTIONARY THEORY

Freud and Jung both shared the highest regard for Charles Darwin and believed that their psychological theories were compatible with his theory of evolution. Unfortunately, in both cases, theirs was a mongrel form of Darwinism, as much generated by the ideas of Jean Baptiste Lamarck (that characteristics acquired by one generation could be inherited by the next) and of Ernst Haeckel (that ontogeny repeats phylogeny) as by Darwin's notion of the evolution of species through natural selection. Acceptance of Jung's theory of archetypes, however, like acceptance of the notion of 'innate strategies' postulated by present-day evolutionary psychologists, does not require the adoption of a Lamarckian or a Haeckelian stance: archetypes can be conceived as innate neuropsychic structures which evolved by natural selection to accomplish certain specific goals (e.g., to form attachments, seek sexual partners, and form alliances within small groups), and this is compatible with the position that Jung adopted from 1947 onwards (Jung, 1947/1960).

What becomes fixed in the genetic structure is the *predisposition* to the kinds of experience which Jung described as archetypal, not the experiences themselves. Jung eventually acquitted himself of the charge of Lamarckism when he announced, in 1947, a clear theoretical distinction between the deeply unconscious and therefore unknowable *archetype-as-such* (similar to Kant's *das Ding-an-sich*) and the archetypal images, ideas and behaviours that the archetype-as-such gives rise to (Jung, 1947/1960: 213). This position is fully in accord with modern biological usage and is no more Lamarckian or Haeckelian than maintaining that children are innately disposed to acquire speech (Chomsky, 1965), or to run on two legs.

Jung specifically distanced himself from the position which critics then and since have accused him of adopting: 'Again and again', he wrote, 'I encounter the mistaken notion that an archetype is determined in regard to its content, in other words that it is a kind of unconscious idea (if such an expression be permissible). It is necessary to point out once more that archetypes are not determined as to their content, but only as regards their form, and then only to a very limited degree. A primordial image is determined as to its content only when it has become conscious and is therefore filled out with the material of conscious experience' (Jung, 1959: 79).

Though Jung remained all his life primarily interested in the psychic manifestations of archetypes, he nevertheless understood that a strictly scientific approach would make more headway if it concentrated on their behavioural manifestations. As he himself insisted, the archetype 'is not meant to denote an inherited idea, but rather an inherited mode of functioning, corresponding to the inborn way in which the chick emerges from the egg, the bird builds its nest, a certain kind of wasp stings the motor ganglion of the caterpillar, and eels find their way to the Bermudas. In other words, it is a "pattern of behaviour". *This aspect of the archetype, the purely biological one, is the proper concern of scientific psychology*' (Jung, 1977b: 518; italics added). For Jung, archetypes and instincts were inextricably linked, the archetype providing information concerning the *meaningful* nature of the typical stimulus characteristics by which instinctive energies were activated and towards which they were directed.

Repeatedly, Jung stressed that the archetype was not an arid, intellectual concept but a living, empirical entity, charged not only with meaningfulness but also with *feeling*. 'It would be an unpardonable sin of omission', he wrote, 'were we to overlook the *feeling-value* (Jung's italics) of the archetype. This is extremely important both theoretically and therapeutically' (1960: 209). Psychology, he maintained, is the only science that has to take 'feeling-value' into account, for feeling 'forms the link between psychic events on the one hand, and meaning and life on the other' (Jung, 1977a: 260). In other words, the archetype is 'a piece of life', 'a living system of reactions and aptitudes' (1960: 157) and it is connected with the living individual by the bridge of emotion' (Jung, 1977a: 257).

In *Archetype: A Natural History of the Self* (Stevens, 1982), I drew attention to the many striking parallels which exist between the concepts of analytical psychology and those of ethology (the branch of behavioural science that studies animals in their natural habitats) and argued that both disciplines were studying the same archetypal phenomena, but from opposite ends. Jungian psychology focused on their introverted psychic manifestations while ethology examined their extraverted behavioural expression. I attempted to demonstrate how these two approaches complemented one another in such fundamental areas as bonding between parents and children, sexual desire and gender differences, courtship and mating, cooperation and hostility between individuals and groups, and the development of the individual through the course of the human life-cycle. I went on to argue that if Jungians wished to place analytical psychology on a sound epistemological basis they would do well to draw closer to the ethologists and become aware of the discoveries which were being made, not only in the observation of animal behaviour but in the cross-cultural studies of human communities throughout the world (Eibl-Eibesfeldt, 1971; Ekman, 1973; Fox, 1975; Murdock, 1945).

Since then, evolutionary psychologists and psychiatrists on both sides of the Atlantic have detected and announced the presence of neuropsychic propensities which are virtually indistinguishable from archetypes. Gilbert (1994), refers to them as 'mentalities', Gardner (1988) as 'master programmes' or 'propensity states', while Wenegrat (1984) borrows the sociobiological term 'genetically transmitted response strategies'. Buss (1995) refers to 'evolved psychological mechanisms', Nesse (1987) to 'prepared tendencies', and Cosmides and Tooby (1989) to 'multiple mental modules'. These evolved propensities or modules are held responsible for psychosocial goals and strategies that are shared by all members of the species, whether they be healthy or ill. As Jung put it, 'The collective unconscious contains the whole spiritual heritage of mankind's evolution, born anew in the brain structure of every individual' (Jung, 1960b: 158). 'Ultimately, every individual life is at the same time the eternal life of the species' (Jung, 1958a: 89).

The reaffirmation of Jung's original insights by contemporary evolutionary psychologists is of great significance for all psychotherapeutic disciplines: a theoretical basis begins to emerge for a science of human development and for a systematic approach to human psychology (Stevens, 1998c). *Psychopathology* can then be understood to occur when 'archetypal' strategies malfunction as a result of environmental insults or deficiencies at critical stages of development. A sound theoretical basis in terms of which hypotheses can be formulated will enable these insults and deficiencies to be empirically investigated and defined (Stevens and Price, 2000a, 2000b). Though Jung is seldom mentioned by evolutionary psychologists, his primacy in introducing the archetypal hypothesis into psychology must be acknowledged: it is one of the truly seminal ideas of the twentieth century.

NEO-JUNGIAN REVISIONISM

It is understandable that, given the academic prejudices that persisted for most of the twentieth century, Jung's archetypal theory should have been out of favour for so long. What is more difficult to appreciate is the readiness with which many practitioners, who identify themselves as Jungians, have sought to deny the biological implications of Jung's thinking. On the face of it, this is extraordinary. For, at a time when evolutionary psychology is providing overwhelming support for Jung's position, Jungians themselves have displayed a desire to retreat from it. There must be a number of reasons to account for this.

In the first place, many are hostile to what they see as the intrusion of biology into psychology because they caricature it as 'reductive'. Darwinism has a bad reputation among those reared in the humanities, not because of Darwin and his ideas *per se*, but because of what 'social Darwinists' in general, and Adolf Hitler in particular, made of them. As a result they perceive any attempt to rehabilitate the biological roots of Jung's hypothesis as antipathetic to the liberal causes that neo-Jungians espouse – such as sexual and racial equality. However, to adopt an evolutionary view of the collective unconscious does not subvert such causes. On the contrary, it puts attempts to further them on a firm epistemological base, for the archetypal structures of which the collective unconscious is composed are common to us all, irrespective of race, geographical location, or creed, by virtue of our shared evolutionary history.

One important factor is the kind of education most Jungians have before becoming analysts. Unlike Jung himself, few of them have received a medical or biological training. As a consequence, Jungian discourse has become increasingly *dis-embodied*, as if the physiological correlates of psychic events were of little or no account. *Individuation* – the life task of becoming as whole and complete a human being as one's circumstances allow – is conceived to be a wholly spiritual process in which all biological contributions (except for the maintenance of life itself) are ignored as irrelevant. This is in marked contrast to Jung's own position: 'We keep forgetting that we are primates and that we have to make allowances for these primitive layers in our psyche', he wrote. 'Individuation is not only an upward but a downward process. Without any body, there is no mind and therefore no individuation' (McGuire and Hull, 1977). Apart from myself, only a tiny minority of writers have taken Jung's injunction seriously. These include Card (1990), Routh (1981), Walters (1993), and McDowell (1999).

Instead of receiving a grounding in biology, most contemporary Jungians are products of university departments in which the SSSM has continued to enjoy the status of holy writ. As a result, they have been afflicted by a form of 'cognitive dissonance' (Festinger, 1957): for when they came to study Jungian theory they were forced to reconcile what they had been taught to see as the extreme plasticity of human psychology with Jung's notion of an innately structured psyche. To resolve this paradox most felt a need to distance themselves from Jung's evolutionary perspective in order to redefine archetypal theory in a form compatible with the anti-biological consensus of the social scientists. This revisionist under-taking has proceeded so far that it has become a tenet of neo-Jungian orthodoxy. It is symptomatic of this trend that in 1998 the editors of the *Journal of Analytical Psychology*, the most widely read international quarterly of Jungian theory and practice, felt it appropriate to publish a long article by a Finnish philosopher, Petteri Pietikainen, arguing that Jungians should cease to see archetypes as 'biologically inherited supra-individual predispositions of the collective unconscious', and instead conceive them as 'culturally determined functionary forms'. Such a proposal was tantamount to advocating a complete regression to pre-Jungian *tabula rasa* psychology and pre-Darwinian life science, and yet it was considered worthy of receiving the careful consideration by the international Jungian community. Responding to Pietikainen's suggestion in the same issue (Stevens, 1998a), I argued that to adopt it would be to strike a blow at the epistemological foundations of Jungian psychology.

CAN ANALYTICAL PSYCHOLOGY SURVIVE?

Attacks on Jung, such as those launched by Richard Noll (1994; 1997) and rebutted by Sonu Shamdasami (1998) and myself (Stevens, 1999) follow similar onslaughts on the reputation of Sigmund Freud (Crews, 1994; Esterson, 1993; Lakoff and Coyne, 1993; Macmillan, 1997; Webster, 1997; Wilcocks, 1997). If the founding fathers of analytic psychotherapy are shown to have feet of clay (Storr, 1996) and their basic premises are discredited, what is to prevent the entire psychotherapeutic edifice from collapsing?

At a time when all forms of depth psychology are being subjected to critical reassessment, and when fewer clients are chasing more analysts, we have entered a post-apostolic era in which our colleagues can no longer enjoy direct or indirect contact with the personality of Jung. Increasingly the lay public as well as govern-ment agencies and insurance companies are going to enquire why analytical psychologists hold to the principles, theories, beliefs and practices that they do. The justification, 'Dr Jung said it was so', will no longer be enough. People are going to demand proof. An essential issue for analytical psychology at this time in its history, therefore, is epistemological. And this is why it is important, at a time when evolutionary theory is beginning to play a central role in psychological and psychiatric thinking, to stress and not to compromise the biological basis of, and the contemporary parallels to, archetypal theory.

If archetypal theory is to survive in its Jungian form, Jungians will have to keep abreast of current thinking in evolutionary psychology and psychiatry as well as having a nodding acquaintance with the postmodern epistemologists, the coherent phenomenologists, and all the other enthusiasts of the new historicist, anti-essentialist type. Of all current thinkers, the evolutionary psychologists are making by far the most significant and lasting contribution. 'Constructivism', on the other hand, represents an academic fashion, which, like behaviourism, Marxism and associationism, will pass: for it can itself be 'deconstructed' and be exposed as *tabula rasa* theory making a final, forlorn attempt to swim against the tide of history.

As I believe the constructivists will discover, the introduction of evolutionary concepts into psychology represents a paradigm shift which will have a profound influence on theory and practice in the century ahead. No psychological system will survive unless it can adapt to Darwin's great insight into the nature and processes of our evolutionary history. It provides the indispensable paradigm of the life sciences. Both Jung and Freud understood this. To drag analytical psychology out of this paradigm, as some neo-Jungians would have us do, would be to ascend into the misty uplands of postmodernist discourse and, to misquote Prospero, transform analytical psychology into the baseless fabric of Jung's vision, its actors melted into air, into thin air, and, like this insubstantial pageant faded, leave not a rack behind.

THE *UNUS MUNDUS*

That the different schools of therapy, founded on the assumptions of their charismatic leaders, have developed into exclusive and mutually hostile 'sects' is because these assumptions have largely escaped objective verification. But this state of affairs cannot last. As research into psychotherapeutic practice proceeds and we learn more about 'what works for whom' (Roth and Fonagy, 1996), differences between the various schools will be eroded and a new theoretical synthesis will emerge. To this new paradigm, Jung's evolutionary-archetypal perspective is capable of providing a rich nucleus round which all theoretical approaches could muster. Already, there is general agreement among evolutionary psychologists and psychiatrists that, as a species, our behaviour is directed to certain biosocial goals. These have been defined as *care-eliciting* and *care-giving* (attachment behaviour), *mate-selection* (sexual attraction, courtship, and mate retention), *alliance formation* (affiliation, friendship, and reciprocal behaviour), and *ranking behaviour* (competition for resources, dominance and submissive behaviour, and gaining and maintaining status). What is most striking about this list is that each of these fundamental goals has historically provided the primary area of concern for the major schools of analysis: thus, care-eliciting, care-giving, and alliance formation have provided the primary material for Klein, Winnicott, and Bowlby, mate-selection and sex for Freud, rank behaviour for Adler, and goal-directed behaviour in the service of self-actualization for Jung. With the unifying perspective that evolutionary psychology offers, the empirical study of the basic programmes running in the unconscious at last becomes a scientific possibility.

This might seem to be a wholly welcome development, yet many analysts will wish to resist it, sensing in it a move towards 'biologism', 'adaptationism' and 'Darwinian fundamentalism'. Some have even argued that analysis should altogether abandon any attempt to think of itself as a scientific discipline but rather aspire to be a branch of the humanities, like literary criticism or biblical exegesis (from which the term hermeneutics is derived). To many this has seemed an attractive proposal, but, unfortunately, it overlooks the fact that analysts of all schools make statements about human psychology, its basic characteristics, the pathological consequences of certain childhood events, and the therapeutic outcome of analytic interventions which are susceptible to scientific validation or refutation. The only honourable escape from this dilemma would be for analysts to give up all claims to psychopathological explanation and therapeutic effectiveness in order to become a mere branch of 'cultural studies'. This, in my view, would represent a fundamental betrayal of its *raison d'être*.

To stress the biological validity of archetypal theory is not to argue that archetypes function as rigidly determined imperatives. As Jung himself put it, the archetype is 'an inherited *tendency* of the human mind to form representations that vary a great deal without losing their basic pattern' (Jung, 1977a: 228; Jung's italics). To examine the biological implications of these 'basic patterns' is not to endorse Richard Dawkins' (1976) view – or the sociobiological view – of human beings as robots blindly programmed by selfish genes seeking their own reproductive success. Genes provide us with programmes of cognition, feeling and behaviour which are designed to achieve certain biosocial goals, but what we make of them is determined by our personal histories and our conscious capacity for choice. What is fallacious about the position adopted by Dawkins and the sociobiologists is that it leaves out the psychological level of experience altogether. Our care-giving propensities evolved to ensure that we look after our children. But we can just as readily employ them to obtain gratification from looking after our pets, cars, houses and gardens and our bodies through dieting and going to the gym. Men using sexual fantasies for their personal gratification are not getting their genes into the next generation: they are making use of a genetically prescribed programme whose ultimate purpose is mating and procreation. Whether or not a man makes use of this programme to achieve the biosocial goal to which it is directed is largely up to him. He may prefer to become a monk.

Far from putting a reductive trip on Jungian psychology and strapping it down to some neo-Darwinian bandwagon, evolutionary psychology is making a richly creative contribution by 'amplifying' the heuristic and empirical implications of the archetypal hypothesis. There is no conflict between the evolutionary approach and the free expression of our hermeneutic capacities. Indeed, this is the wonder of the whole Darwinian epic. That what was originally a clump of replicating molecules in the primordial soup should become capable of writing Shakespearian sonnets, building Chartres Cathedral, composing *Don Giovanni*, painting the Sistine Chapel, putting a man on the moon, and devising analytical psychology. It is creative use of our evolved capacities that makes these achievements possible. Biology is an indispensable part of the process. But biological imperatives are themselves expressions of some supraordinate pattern or set of principles. Jung shared the Schopenhauerian intuition that ultimate reality is a unity – the *unus mundus* of the medieval philosophers – an underlying order in the universe which transcends the Cartesian division between mind and body as well as our human categories of space, time and causality. Jung's final position was that archetypal structures precondition all psychophysical events: they are not only fundamental to the existence of all living organisms but are continuous with structures controlling the behaviour of inorganic matter as well. He considered that the physicist's investigation of matter and the psychologist's investigation of mind were different ways of approaching the same underlying reality – a view strongly supported by the physicist and Nobel laureate, Wolfgang Pauli. Since archetypes precondition all existence, they are manifest in the spiritual achievements of art, science, and religion, as well as in the organization of organic and inorganic matter.

AN EXPANDED VIEW OF THE SELF

It is because of Jung's appreciation of the evolutionary significance of archetypes that analytical psychology adopts a broader therapeutic perspective than any other school of analysis. Like the evolutionary psychiatrist, the Jungian analyst looks beyond the personal predicament of the patient and relates it to the story of humankind, viewing mental distress not as an 'illness' to be conquered but as the adaptive response of a potentially healthy organism struggling to meet the demands of life. To view symptom formation as an adaptive process is to make a contribution of priceless value, for it creates *therapeutic optimism* (Stevens, 1998c). Every human being is richly endowed with the archetypal potential of the species. This means that, however disordered, one-sided, or constricted an individual's psychological development may be, the *potential* for further growth and better adaptation is nevertheless *there*, implicit in the psychophysical structure of the organism. As a result, patients can be helped to grow beyond the defective or inadequate form of adjustment that their personal history has permitted.

This is perhaps the most important conceptual contribution that the evolutionary approach has to make: it grants an expanded view of the self. Jung conceived of the Self (preferring to use the initial capital to stress the difference between his concept and the everyday use of the term) as the central nucleus of the entire personality. It contains the archetypal endowment of the individual and coordinates and implements the programme for the life-cycle from the cradle to the grave. The Self is not just the sum total of one's personal life experiences, as the object-relations theorists and self-psychologists maintain, but the product of many millions of years of development. Within each one of us the vast potential of humanity is contained. This provides an added dimension to the *individuation* process: it is about integrating ontogeny with phylogeny, uniting one's personal experience with the potential experience of humanity. It means making the most of the mentalities with which evolution has equipped us and bringing them to fulfilment in our lives.

Success in this endeavour will depend on the therapist's skill in releasing the unused creative potential in the patient's personality. A model for this is provided by classical Jungian analysis, which seeks to mobilize archetypal components of the phylogenetic psyche (which Jung called the two-million-year-old Self) by encouraging patients to dream, to fantasize, to paint, to open themselves to relationships with new friends and acquaintances, and to find new ways of relating to old ones, as well as becoming conscious of the complexes, strategies and conflicts that have been controlling their lives in the past.

In particular, the evolutionary dimension has re-evoked the central importance of symbol-formation in the therapeutic process. Freud believed symbols to be purely private and pathological, insisting that only *repressed* material was symbolized. Jung took a wholly different view, maintaining that we possess an innate symbol-forming propensity which exists as a healthy, creative, and integral part of our total psychic equipment. Although possessing a flexible capacity for local and personal variations, this symbolizing ability proceeds on an archetypal basis, which gives rise to characteristic symbolic manifestations (Jung and von Franz, 1964; Kast, 1992; Stevens, 1998b). In adopting this position, Jung again fell foul of the Standard Social Science Model, with its *tabula rasa* view of the mind as a general-purpose learning mechanism free of all content other than what 'culture' put into it. But as the SSSM disintegrates, the view is fast gaining ground that the human capacity to use symbols, perceive meanings, create myths and religions, evolved as the result of selection pressures encountered by our species in the environment of evolutionary adaptedness (Burkert, 1996; Mithen, 1996; Stevens, 1998b). By making use of the essentially adaptive function of symbols arising in the course of an analysis, the skilled therapist can help to mobilize the patient's unlived potential and promote a better adjustment to social reality. This has, in fact, been the main procedure used by classical Jungian analysts since the 1920s. The evolutionary perspective now opens up this richly creative process to a much greater population of therapists from differing backgrounds and traditions.

Whatever upheavals may be in store for us as a result of theoretical revisions, outcome studies, clinical audits, and research on the biochemistry of the brain, the primary duty of the psychotherapist will remain the same: to put empathy, knowledge, and professional skill at the service of the patient. Above all, the psychotherapeutic quest is a quest for *meaning*. In the 1930s, Jung wrote: 'About a third of my cases are not suffering from any clearly definable neurosis, but from the senselessness and aimlessness of their lives. I should not object if this were called the general neurosis of our age' (1954: 14). Neurosis, he said, in the nearest he came to a definition, is the suffering of a soul that has not found its meaning. A major factor bringing patients into therapy is a need to make sense of their lives.

From early childhood a human being is an exploratory organism, forever seeking to impose meaning on events. The development of conscious awareness of ourselves is constructed out of meanings. This is the fundamental datum of the individuation process, for archetypes are meaning-creating imperatives. As a consequence, 'meaning is something that always demonstrates itself and is experienced on its own merits' (1958b: 360). Through use of active imagination, dream interpretation, transference interpretation, and, most essentially, the medium of the therapeutic relationship itself, it is the therapist's task to endorse and facilitate the patient's basic need to discover his or her own constellations of meaning.

In the past, biology would have been considered wholly irrelevant to this process. Until very recently, workers in neuroscience and in artificial intelligence have sustained the fantasy that forms of intelligence and language could be devised on the basis of pure logic without having to postulate anything so messy as 'meaning'. The realization has now dawned that this cannot be the case and scientists have begun to accept meaning as a fundamental concept in biology (Bruner, 1990). Meaning, it seems, is something that nature cannot do without, and this may help to explain how it is that dreaming, remembering, and consciousness have emerged as the massive biological achievements that they are.

REFERENCES

Bruner, J. (1990) *Acts of Meaning*. Cambridge, MA: Harvard University Press.

Burkert, W. (1996) *Creation of the Sacred: Tracks of Biology in Early Religions*. Cambridge, MA: Harvard University Press.

Buss, D. M. (1995) 'Evolutionary psychology: a new paradigm for psychological science'. *Psychological Enquiry*, Vol.6, no. 1, 1–30.

Card, C. R. (1990) *The Archetypal Hypothesis of Jung and Pauli and its Relevance to Physics and Epistemology*. Unpublished paper, the Department of Physics and Astronomy, University of Victoria, British Columbia.

Chomsky, N. (1965) *Aspects of the Theory of Syntax*. Cambridge, MA: MIT Press.

Cosmides, L. and Tooby, J. (1989) 'Evolutionary psychology and the generation of culture, part 1: case study: a computational theory of social exchange', *Ethology and Sociobiology*, Vol. 10, 51–97.

Crews, F. (1994) 'The revenge of the repressed'. *New York Review of Books*, part I, 17 November 1994, 54–60; part II, 1 December 1994, 49–58.

Dawkins, R. (1976) *The Selfish Gene*. Oxford: Oxford University Press.

Eibl-Eibesfeldt, I. (1971) *Love and Hate*. London: Methuen.

Ekman, P. (1973) 'Cross-cultural studies of facial expression', in *Darwin and Facial Expression: A Century of Research in Review*, edited by P. Ekman, pp. 169–222. New York: Academic Press.

Esterson, A. (1993) *Seductive Mirage: An Exploration of the Work of Sigmund Freud*. Chicago: Open Court.

Festinger, L. (1957) *The Theory of Cognitive Dissonance*. Evanston, IL: Row, Peterson.

Fox, R. (1975) 'Primate kin and human kinship', in *Biosocial Anthropology*, edited by R. Fox, pp.9–35. London: Malaby Press.

Gardner, R. (1988) 'Psychic syndromes as infrastructure for intra-specific communication', in M. R. A. Chance (Ed.), *Social Fabrics of the Mind*. Hove, UK: Lawrence Erlbaum Associates.

Gilbert, P. (1989) *Human Nature and Suffering*. Hove, UK: Lawrence Erlbaum Associates.

Gilbert, P. (1995) 'Biopsychosocial approaches and evolutionary theory as aids to interaction in clinical psychology and psychotherapy', *Clinical Psychology and Psychotherapy*, Vol. 2, 134–156.

Gray, R. M. (1996) *Archetypal Explorations: An Integrative Approach to Human Behaviour*. London: Routledge.

Jung, C. G. (1947/1960) 'On the nature of the psyche'. *Collected Works*, Vol. 8, pp. 159–234. London: Routledge & Kegan Paul.

Jung, C. G. (1953) 'The structure of the unconscious'. *Collected Works*, Vol. 7, pp. 263–292. London: Routledge & Kegan Paul.

Jung, C. G. (1954) 'The practical use of dream-analysis'. *Collected Works*, Vol. 16, pp.139–161.

Jung, C. G. (1956) *Symbols of Transformation*, Foreword to the second Swiss edition. *Collected Works*, Vol. 5, pp. xxviii–xxix. London: Routledge & Kegan Paul.

Jung, C. G. (1958a) 'Psychology and religion'. *Collected Works*, Vol. 11, pp. 3–105. London: Routledge & Kegan Paul.

Jung, C. G. (1958b) 'Answer to Job'. *Collected Works*, Vol. 11, pp. 357–470. London: Routledge & Kegan Paul.

Jung, C. G. (1959) 'The concept of the collective unconscious'. *Collected Works*, Vol. 9i, pp. 42–53.

Jung, C. G. (1977a) 'Symbols and the interpretation of dreams'. *Collected Works*, Vol. 18, pp. 185–264. London: Routledge & Kegan Paul.

Jung, C. G. (1977b) 'Foreword to Harding: Womens' Mysteries'. *Collected Works*, Vol. 18, pp. 518–520. London: Routledge & Kegan Paul.

Jung, C. G. and von Franz, M.-L. (Eds) (1964) *Man and His Symbols*. London: Aldus Books.

Kast, Verena (1992) *The Dynamics of Symbols: Fundamentals of Jungian Psychotherapy* (translated by Susan A. Schwarz). New York: Fromm International.

Lakoff, R. T. and Coyne, J.C. (1993) *Father Knows Best: The Use and Abuse of Power in Freud's Case of 'Dora'*. New York: Teachers College Press.

Macmillan, M. (1997) *Freud Evaluated: The Completed Arc*. Cambridge, MA: MIT Press.

McDowell, M. J. (1999) 'Relating to the mystery: a biological view of analytical psychology' *Quadrant: Journal of the C. G. Jung Foundation for Analytical Psychology*, Vol. 29, no. 1, 12–32. New York.

McGuire, W. and Hull, R. F. C. (1977) *C. G. Jung Speaking*. Princeton, NJ: Princeton University Press.

Mithen, S. (1996) *The Prehistory of the Mind: The Cognitive Origins of Art, Religion and Science*. London: Thames & Hudson.

Murdock, G. P. (1945) 'The common denominator of culture', in R. Linton (Ed.), *The Science of Man in the World Crisis*. New York: Cambridge University Press.

Nesse, R. M. (1987) 'An evolutionary perspective on panic disorder and agoraphobia'. *Ethology and Sociobiology*, Vol. 8, no. 3s, 73–84.

Noll, R. (1994) *The Jung Cult: Origins of a Charismatic Movement*. Princeton, NJ: Princeton University Press.

Noll, R. (1997) *The Aryan Christ: The Secret Life of Carl Jung*. New York: Random House.

Pietikainen, P. (1998) 'Archetypes as symbolic forms'. *Journal of Analytical Psychology*, Vol. 43, no. 3, 325–343.

Roth, A. and Fonagy, P. (1996) *What Works for Whom? A Critical Review of Psychotherapy Research*. New York: Guilford Press.

Routh, V. (1981) *Jungian Psychology and Evolutionary Theory: An Enquiry into the Relation of Psyche to Phylogenesis*. Unpublished dissertation submitted at Brunel University, Uxbridge, Middlesex.

Shamdasani, S. (1998) *Cult Fictions: C. G. Jung and the Founding of Analytical Psychology*. London: Routledge.

Stevens, A. (1982) *Archetype: A Natural History of the Self*. London: Routledge & Kegan Paul.

Stevens, A. (1998a) 'Response to P. Pietikainen'. *The Journal of Analytical Psychology*, Vol. 43. no. 3, 345–355.

Stevens, A. (1998b) *Ariadne's Clue: A Guide to the Symbols of Humankind*. London: Allen Lane.

Stevens, A. (1998c) *An Intelligent Person's Guide to Psychotherapy*. London: Duckworth.

Stevens, A. (1999) *On Jung* (second edition). London: Penguin.

Stevens, A. and Price, J. (2000a) *Evolutionary Psychiatry: A New Beginning* (second edition). London: Routledge.

Stevens, A. and Price, J. (2000b) *Prophets, Cults and Madness*. London: Duckworth.

Storr, A. (1996) *Feet of Clay: A Study of Gurus*. London: HarperCollins.

Walters, S. (1993) 'Archetypes and algorithms: Evolutionary psychology and Carl Jung's theory of the collective unconscious'. Unpublished paper received from the Department of Psychology, Simon Fraser University, Burnaby, British Columbia.

Webster, R. (1997) *Why Freud Was Wrong: Sin, Science and Psychoanalysis*. London: HarperCollins.

Wenegrat, B. (1985) *Sociobiology and Mental Disorder*. Menlo Park, CA: Addison-Wesley.

Wilcocks, R. (1994) *Maelzel's Chess Player: Sigmund Freud and the Rhetoric of Deceit*. Lanham, MD: Rowman & Littlefield.

(b) Psyche, language and biology: the argument for a co-evolutionary approach

Paul Kugler

One of the major challenges confronting depth psychology today is formulating a theoretical understanding of how archetypes relate to biology, culture and language. This is no small task. Each one of these complicated areas of study is a challenge. Formulating how they interact over time in the development of human nature is even more challenging. This essay will explore the evolutionary process through which archetypal components of human nature emerge out of the interaction of biology with language and culture.[1]

In recent years the very notion of human nature and its 'essential' or archetypal aspects has become the focus of an intense debate between two competing theoretical perspectives. On one side of the debate are the social constructivists who focus on the role language and culture plays in 'constructing' our sense of reality, as well as the archetypal aspects of the human psyche. On the other side of the debate, the evolutionary psychologists emphasize the role of evolution and human biology. In each perspective, the function and ontological status of the archetype differs significantly. Social constructivists view 'the archetype' as a linguistic construct, a metaphoric by-product of language, while evolutionary psychologists construe archetypes as genetically determined entities, rooted in biology and driven by the evolutionary process. In the following essay we will review key elements of this language/biology debate with respect to a theory of archetypes and attempt in the process to formulate a new understanding of *how language and culture interact with biology in the natural history of the human psyche*.

---

1 Hogenson, George (1999), "Evolution, psychology and the emergence of the psyche", Paper delivered at The National Conference of Jungian Analysts, Santa Fe, New Mexico, October 18, 1999.

POSTMODERNISM AND SOCIAL CONSTRUCTIVISM

During the past few decades a revolution in thought has taken place in the social sciences. This has variously been referred to as the language turn in philosophy, postmodernism in the arts and constructivism in the social sciences (Wittgenstein, 1958; Derrida, 1974; Foucault, 1967; Adams, 1996; Goldberg, 1994; Hauke, 2000; Kugler, 1990a, 1990b; Moore, 1999; Teicholz, 1999). The common element in all these movements has been an intense focus on the roles language and culture play in the construction of our theories as well as our identities.

The language turn in philosophy has led to the realization that theory of any kind, be it literary, philosophical, clinical, or scientific, does not allow for a transparent view to the so-called empirical world. Our theories and their explanatory terms (for example, archetype) have no location outside of language, neither objective nor empirical, and can never be a ground, only a mediator. The reader of any *text* – fictional or scientific – is suspended between the literal and metaphoric significances of the text's 'root' metaphors, unable to maintain a stable connection between the various meanings of the root metaphor and a single unambiguous referent. This inevitably leads to a *linguistic relativity* and a *semantic indeterminacy* with respect to any textual formulation.

Our theories and descriptions of the personality are not only influenced by the linguistic medium being used, but also subject to what Jung calls our personal equation. The social constructivists emphasize not only the language-locked features of theory, but also the enormous diversity of psychological phenomena to be found in cultures around the world and throughout history. Cultural differences are explained in terms of *differences* in local conditions, linguistic constraints and history. From this perspective, it is not the world, nor its properties that are constructed, but rather, *the vocabularies in whose terms we know them*. The vocabularies (scientific, mathematical, rational, psychological, mythological, fictional, etc.) used to describe the world and its properties are constructed by human beings living in a specific geographical place, at a particular moment in history, embedded in a cultural context, speaking one of many possible languages, at a certain age in their human life-cycle. All these factors produce subtle effects on our descriptions of the world. As any one of these factors shifts, our understanding of the properties shifts as well.

To help develop a better appreciation of the import role language plays in structuring the psyche, let us turn for a moment to the ontogenetic implications of language acquisition in psychic development.

THE BIRTH OF THE MEMETIC FUNCTION

In the psychological life of a child few events have greater significance than the acquisition of language. The development of the capacity for psychic representation occurs in the infant between six and eighteen months. At this age the child develops the capacity to separate from and recognize its own image as other. For example, the infant who has previously shown no sign of recognition when looking in a mirror, or in a mirroring relationship, suddenly begins to smile in seeing its reflected image for the child has developed the capacity to recognize its own representation (Lacan, 1977; Kugler, 1987). The achievement of this originary reflexivity differentiates the psychic image of the child from its physical body. Prior to this stage, the child lacks the capacity to distinguish the subjective from the objective, the representational from the biological. Desire and its object are indistinguishable. If there is hunger, it is not the child's hunger for the infant is incapable of conceiving a 'self' separate from its biological desire. But during the mirror stage, this unity of experience is split and *the child develops the capacity to differentiate the psychic image from biological experience.*

Through the process of developing the capacity for representation and replication, first on the level of psychic images and later on the level of language proper, a self becomes divided from itself and in the process capable of self-reflection. The importance of the creation of a divided subject, an ego/Self structure, capable of self-reflection cannot be overemphasized (Kugler, 1993). For in acquiring linguistic competence, the infant learns to speak to the world through a network of collectively determined symbols, a system of unconscious meanings organized in advance of any individual ego (Lacan 1977; Kugler, 1982, 1983–4).

FROM IMAGO TO WORD: A SECOND ONTOLOGICAL RUPTURE

The differentiation between the biological infant and the psychic image with which the infant identifies is only the anticipation of a far more profound differentiation of the psyche that will occur during language acquisition. The later process of acquiring language replaces the mirror image of the body with a linguistic image, the first person pronoun. With the acquisition of language comes a second ontological rupture, this time between word and body, between description and event. During the mirror stage the human subject becomes possible when neurological development allows the infant to distinguish objects, and the human subject becomes actual when the child develops the capacity for representation and replication. The realization that *human subjectivity is constructed through the reflexive creation of representations*, leads to the awareness that we are in language and creating metaphors of ourselves, as well as of our understanding of ourselves, all the time.

The human subject is something constructed through metaphorizing in every dimension of our psychic existence and does not come into being without the participation of an elaborate linguistic environment. For without the capacity for the self to represent itself, either as an image or as a word, and thereby look back at itself from another perspective, the construction of personality and its characteristic capacity for representation and self-reflection would be impossible (Kugler,

1987; Lacan 1977). Let us turn now to the phylogenetic significance of language development in the evolution of the psyche, and in particular, to Darwin and the recent advances in evolutionary psychology.

THE DARWINIAN REVIVAL

The current revival of interest in Darwin can be traced back to the early 1960s when William Hamilton, a rather shy postgraduate student at the London School of Economics, began to question Darwin's theory of group selection. If altruism benefited the species or the group in which a person lived, it would be favoured, Darwin argued, by natural selection. Groups in which people sacrificed themselves for the common good, would be more cohesive and, therefore, more successful than other groups. Darwin's theory of group selection had remained largely unquestioned until the 1960s. Hamilton argued that within any group, altruists would tend to be exploited by non-altruists who would then end up with the majority of the resources. This in turn should make the non-altruists better able to reproduce and survive longer. Eventually, he argued, the altruists would become extinct. If this is the case, *Hamilton wondered, how could genes which produce altruistic behaviour survive and be passed down from generation to generation*?

As a child Hamilton had often helped his mother with honey bees she kept in hives near their home. While struggling to understand Darwin's theory of group selection, he remembered being stung as a child when he would go too near a hive. Worker bees would sense possible danger, fly out and sting the intruder. A barb on the end of the bee's stinger lodges in the intruder's flesh and as the bee tries to fly away it dies, tearing off the back portion of its body. A successful sting by a worker bee protecting the colony is certain death. Hamilton wondered how Darwinian evolution could possibly account for such a suicidal form of adaptation, especially when none of the worker bee's genes were passed on to subsequent generations?

ADOPTING THE GENE'S PERSPECTIVE

Hamilton explained the lethal altruistic behaviour in terms of the bee's reproductive system. Worker bees do not mate, leaving all the reproduction to the queen. What Hamilton realized, however, was that all the worker bees come from the same mother and, therefore, share the same percentage of her genes. Hamilton theorized that from the point of view of the genes, it did not matter if an individual organism lived or died, but that a copy of the genes lived on. In the case of the worker bee that stung him, copies of the same genes continued to live in all the other bees in the hive. By shifting the evolutionary perspective from an individual organism to the gene itself, Hamilton was able to formulate his notion of 'inclusive fitness' or ' kin selection', arguing that *what is of prime importance in evolution is the survival of the genes, not the individual* (Hamilton, 1963, 1995). This shift in perspective from the individual organism to the gene reoriented evolutionary theory and set the stage for the modern revival of interest in Darwin's theories.

One of the most influential books in the neo-Darwinian movement is Richard Dawkins' *The Selfish Gene* (1976). The main theme of his book is based on Hamilton's idea that the gene is selfish, more concerned with its own survival than that of the individual. Dawkins' book was controversial at the time, promoting the idea that humans are 'survival machines', 'robot vehicles blindly programmed to preserve the selfish molecules known as genes' (Preface to *The Selfish Gene*). When Dawkins' selfish gene theory was first put forward over twenty-five years ago as a modern upgrade of Darwin's natural selection, it was considered radical. Today in the field of evolutionary psychology the idea that genes will do anything necessary to reproduce themselves in the next generation has become orthodoxy in many quarters (Dawkins, 1976; Barkow *et al.*, 1992; Dennet, 1995).[2] These neo-Darwinians insist that underneath all the broad cultural variations the essential structure of human minds is identical.

For many of the new Darwinians the most significant evolution of the human brain took place prior to the invention of agriculture during the neolithic period (Tooby and Cosmides, 1990b; Pinker, 1994, 1997; Stevens and Price, 1996; Stevens 1999). On the genetic level evolutionary change is very slow. It has only been 10,000 years since the neolithic revolution and humans first began growing their own food and building cities. From the perspective of evolutionary psychology not enough time has elapsed since the Pleistocene period for human behaviour to have changed in genetic terms. Consequently, the minds of contemporary humans must reflect structural adaptations evolved to meet challenges faced by our hunter-gatherer ancestors. Anthony Stevens and John Price theorize that the archetypal structures of today's psyche are adapted to the environment of the Pleistocene period. To understand a person's current mental behaviour, including their psychopathology, the clinician needs, in part, to understand the behaviour in terms of adaptations evolved to meet the challenges of the Pleistocene environment (Stevens and Price, 1996; Stevens, 1982, 1999). Stevens' theory that archetypes-as-such have evolved through the biological process of adaptation and natural selection is predicated on several assumptions: (1) the process of evolution is the same for all species, (2) the role of learning, language, culture and consciousness plays only a minor role in the evolutionary equation and (3) archetypes are embedded in the genetic code of human biology. But what if human evolution is fundamentally different from the biologically driven process found in all other species? Is it possible that in acquiring the capacity for symbolic representation our species crossed the animal/human divide and forever altered its evolutionary process?

2 'Evolutionary psychology' as used here refers to a particular approach to evolution championed by John Tooby, an anthropologist, and his wife, Leda Cosmides, a psychologist. Together they run the Center for Evolutionary Psychology at the University of California at Santa Barbara.

BIOLOGY AND LANGUAGE: A CO-EVOLUTIONARY PROCESS

> . . . the major structural and functional innovations that make human brains capable of unprecedented mental feats evolved in response to the use of something as abstract and virtual as the power of words . . . the first use of symbolic reference by some distant ancestors changed how natural selection processes have affected hominid brain evolution ever since. (Deacon, 1997)

In recent years an alternative to Darwinian evolution has begun to take shape (Deacon, 1997; Durham, 1991; Blackmore, 1999; Hogenson, 1999; Mithen, 1996). Rather than focus on the biological similarities in evolution between humans and other species, this approach emphasizes, instead, what makes human evolution different – the role of language and culture in the evolutionary process.

The great evolutionary leap forward for humans came with the development of symbolic representation and language. While certain other species have evolved a limited ability to communicate (for example, apes, chimpanzees, parrots, and dolphins) the differences between human languages with its *symbolic capacity* and all other natural modes of communicating are great (Deacon, 1997). But why, we might ask, is the development of language and its capacity for symbolic representation so important from an evolutionary point of view? Where the gene replicates biological information and passes it on physically to the next generation, language allows for the *production and reproduction of a new kind of information*, psychic and cultural information that can also be duplicated and passed on to other members of the species. The development of this productive and memetic capacity constitutes the emergence in human evolution of a second means for transmitting information across generations. Prior to the capacity for human language, learning could not be duplicated on a symbolic level. But as soon as language develops, so too does the ability to disseminate the products of learning.

But how might this cultural and linguistic process of disseminating intergenerational information dynamically interact with the process of genetic evolution? Consider, for a moment, the dramatic increase in the average height of humans over the past two centuries. How much of this change in human biology can be attributed to genetic transformations in our species? According to Daniel Dennett, a staunch Darwinian, little if any at all can be accounted for through changes in the biological evolution of human genetics (Dennett, 1995). During the period in which the dramatic growth change has occurred, only about ten generations have elapsed. Even if there were significant evolutionary forces in the natural environment supporting such an adaptive change, the time frame in genetic terms is far too little to account for such a dramatic change in physical height. What has changed significantly, however, during this same time period has been human living conditions, medical care, public health practices, farming techniques and dietary habits. These cultural innovations produced significant alterations in the human phenotype over the past two hundred years.

Dennett, so moved by the power of cultural innovation in the evolutionary process, concedes: 'Anyone who worries about "genetic determinism" should be reminded that virtually all the differences discernible between the people of, say Plato's day and the people living today – their physical talents, proclivities, attitudes, prospects – must be due to cultural changes, since fewer than two hundred generations separate us from Plato. Environmental changes due to cultural innovations change the landscape of phenotypic expression so much, and so fast, however, that they can in principle change the genetic selection pressures rapidly – the Baldwin Effect is a simple instance of such a change in selection pressure due to widespread behavioral innovation' (Dennett, 1995).

THE BALDWIN EFFECT

The Baldwin Effect is named after one of its discoverers, James Baldwin, a leading nineteenth-century American child psychologist. The Baldwin Effect was simultaneously discovered by two other nineteenth-century evolutionists, Conway L. Morgan and H. F. Osborn.[3] An early proponent of evolution, Baldwin was concerned about an evolutionary theory that left mind out of the equation. He proceeded to demonstrate that humans could alter or guide the *further evolution of their species by solving environmental problems during their lifetime, thereby making these problems easier to solve in the future and altering the conditions of competition for their offspring.*

Baldwin's theory is contained in his essay 'A new factor in evolution' in which he concludes: 'Evolution is, therefore, not more biological than psychological' (Baldwin, 1896; Hogenson, 1999). The Baldwin Effect is an important contribution to evolutionary theory, introducing mind and psychology into the evolutionary process without falling victim to the problems that plagued Lamarck and his theory of direct intergenerational transmission of acquired characteristics.

George Hogenson, a Jungian analyst and philosopher, has written a seminal essay on 'Evolution, psychology and the emergence of the psyche' in which he documents the influence of Baldwin and Morgan on Jung's theory of archetypes. Through a carefully researched analysis of the references Jung draws on in his early formulation of the relation between archetype and instinct, Hogenson convincingly demonstrates the influence of Baldwin and Morgan on Jung's theory. Where Freud was clearly a Lamarckian, Jung did not subscribe to the theory of direct intergenerational transmission of acquired characteristics. Jung was influenced, instead, by Baldwin's and Morgan's efforts to understand the role of psychology and learning in human evolution.[4]

---

3   For more information on the significance of James Baldwin in the history of evolutionary theory see Hogenson (1999) and Richards (1987, especially pp. 480–503).
4   Hogenson's research challenges Anthony Stevens' claim that Jung was influenced by Lamarck. See Stevens, 1982: 12–18.

Hogenson integrates Baldwin's early theoretical work with current advances in cognitive psychology and the neurosciences. Since the early 1980s a revolution has occurred in our ability to research certain evolutionary questions as a result of the development of powerful new computers. Researchers are now able to simulate with computers complex evolutionary processes that in nature would require far too much time to complete in a laboratory setting. In 1987, Geoffrey Hinton and Steven Nowland published a groundbreaking paper describing the use of computer simulation to research how learning affects human evolution. Hinton and Nowlan demonstrated that if an organism could set some of its genetic variables through a learning factor, it adapted better than did an organism that relied entirely on random variation and natural selection (Hogenson, 1999). Hinton and Nowlan's computer experiment and many subsequent variations on it (Hutchins and Hazlehurst, 1990; Hendricks-Jansen, H., 1996; Hogenson, 1999; Pinker, 1997) further demonstrate that language and cultural innovation have become such powerful forces in evolution that they are now capable of modifying many of the earlier genetically driven processes of biological transformation.

IMITATION AND THE PROCESS OF REPLICATION

Susan Blackmore, a British psychologist, has developed a new theory of evolution based on folding Baldwin's insights back into a more traditional Darwinian framework. Blackmore's theory builds upon Dawkins' earlier concept of the meme, the cultural equivalent of the gene (Dawkins, 1976). The meme is defined as the smallest unit of cultural information capable of being replicated and passed on to subsequent generations according to the laws of natural selection and survival of the fittest. The development of the capacity for imitation, according to Blackmore, sets our ancestors apart from all other species. Once imitation has developed, a second, much faster means for disseminating information enters the evolutionary process. The replication and transmission of memes between humans changes the environment in which genes are selected, and in doing so forces them to build better and better meme-spreading apparatus. The primary function of language, according to Blackmore, is to spread memes and in so doing dramatically alter biological evolution.

The application of Darwin's natural selection to cover any kind of replication in which copies are made and transmitted to other members of the species, poses certain problems. For example, psychologists know only too well that we unconsciously imitate others, especially our parents, and through this process transmit certain patterns of behaviour from one generation to the next. The capacity to unconsciously imitate and pass on discrete elements of information to other members of the species is, for Blackmore, the key factor in human evolution. While I would agree that the ability to reproduce psychic and cultural information is critical in the development of the child ontogenetically, as well as the species phylo- genetically, I question the assumption that the genetic process of biological replication is being 'duplicated' on the psychic and cultural levels. Evolutionary geneticists have known for many years that natural selection works only if there is a low rate of mutation. For Blackmore to apply Darwin's laws of natural selection to the cultural and psychological realms the *duplication must have a high degree of fidelity*, i.e. the quality of the copying and transmission must be extremely good. Just here the problem arises: memes appear to have a low degree of fidelity. When memes are transmitted there is considerably more 'noise' (mutation) than is found in the process of genetic transmission. Consider, for a moment, the process by which the child imitates and introjects the parent. *The child's psychic image of the parent (a meme, in Blackmore's theory) is not an exact replication of the actual parent.* It was precisely this low fidelity that originally led Jung to refer to psychic images as imagos, rather than representations. Blackmore, however, must subscribe to the assumption that psychic and cultural images (memes) are high-fidelity copies in order to successfully apply Darwin's theory of natural selection and survival of the fittest. I would propose, instead, that the low fidelity encountered in the transmission of psychic and cultural information reflects the fact that *productive as well as reproductive processes* are taking place. It is through the productive process that creativity enters this second line of intergenerational transmission. The creative moment arises out of the low fidelity and enters the evolutionary process precisely in *the difference between the original and the reproduction.*[5]

THE EMERGENT PROPERTIES OF ARCHETYPES

Language acquisition with its capacity to produce and reproduce information is an essential factor in the evolution of modern humans. Our evolution differs from other species because it has been dependent on two lines of transmission of species-specific information, not one. Once the capacity for symbolic representation develops, first through images and then through words, there is introduced into the evolutionary process a new means for disseminating intergenerational information. Hogenson theorizes that *archetypes are properties that have emerged out of the dynamic relationship between biology and language.* This is a bold and important claim which attempts to account for the emergence of archetypal properties out of the dynamic relationship between human biology and the newly evolved capacity for symbolic representation. In 1989 Lionel Corbett and I adopted a similar position in the context of a discussion of 'The Origin and Evolution of the Self' (Corbett and Kugler, 1989). There we addressed the importance of explaining *the emergent properties of the self* without appealing to structuring principles outside the system (personality) itself, for example, using biology to explain psychology. In

---

5   For a review of the history of this problem in Western thought, see my essay 'Psychic imaging: a bridge between subject and object' (Kugler, 1997).

physiologically based psychology, there has been a tradition to look for 'smart' microscopic cells to explain macroscopic psychological events. This approach has always had its problems. The model inevitably regresses to either genetics, the physical environment, or innate metaphysical first principles, without ever accounting for the structurality of the microscopic cells (e.g. the structurality of the genetic code). Psychology's theoretical challenge is to explain how macroscopic psychic regularities emerge out of microscopic physiological elements such that the psychological regularities exhibit a certain degree of autonomy. The regularities of the personality (archetypes) form the basis for the laws of psychology, just as biological regularities form the basis for the laws of physiology, and physical regularities form the basis for the laws of physics.

The regularity of archetypes at the psychological level has its own unique lawfulness.[6] As we scale up from physics to biology to psychology, each successive level is sustained by regularities that are manifest on the scale below. For example, in physics the regularities of the nucleus as described by quantum electrodynamics form important boundary conditions for the behaviour that *emerges* as we scale up to the next level, the electron level. At this level the behaviour of electrons are influenced by the structural properties, the boundary conditions, provided by the nucleus. However, and this is the important point, the behaviour of electrons is not explainable, nor reducible, to the structural properties of the previous level, the nucleus. At the electron level a new set of regularities appears describable by its own set of laws, Schrödinger's wave mechanics or Heisenberg's matrix mechanics. Beyond the electron level emerge the regularities describable by the laws of classical mechanics. At each level the scale below provides a stable set of constraints or 'boundary conditions' for the dynamics on the next larger level. As we scale up through the biological and psychological levels of experience, the regularities that manifest are similarly influenced by the more micro scales, but are not reducible to them (Turvey and Kugler, 1987). My theoretical understanding of archetypes is congruent with Hogenson's position that archetypes are not located in the genetic structure of human biology (Stevens, 1999), but rather are *properties that have emerged out of the dynamic relationship between biology and language.*

CROSSING THE ANIMAL/HUMAN DIVIDE

Our theories of evolution have come a long way since Darwin's early biologically driven model based on variation and natural selection. Where other species evolve along biological lines, humans evolve through a co-evolutionary spiral involving biology, language and culture. Cultural artefacts and human language have only been around a brief period of time in biological terms, and yet our species has used

6   Where rules run into the problem of representationalism and the regress problem of embodiment, laws avoid this dilemma.

this newly acquired symbolic ability to transform our planet as well as our biology. The key software innovations that propelled the human species over the animal/human divide and into the co-evolutionary spiral were the abilities to construct metaphors and imagine.[7] Once these capacities for *psychic production and reproduction developed human evolution forever altered its course, becoming an interactive dynamic between the forces of biology, language and culture.*

NOTE

I wish to express my thanks to Peter Kugler for his help in clarifying my understanding of the self-organization of complex living systems.

REFERENCES

Adams, Michael (1996) *The Multicultural Imagination*. London: Routledge.

Baldwin, J. M. (1896/1996). 'A new factor in evolution'. In R. K. Belew and M. Mitchel (Eds), *Adaptive Individuals in Evolving Populations: Models and Algorithms* (pp. 59–80). Reading, MA: Addison-Wesley.

Barkow, J.M., Cosmides, L. and Tooby, J. (Eds) (1992) *The Adapted Mind: Evolutionary Psychology and the Generation of Culture*. New York: Oxford University Press.

Blackmore, S. (1999) *The Meme Machine*. Oxford: Oxford University Press.

Corbett, Lionel and Kugler, Paul (1989) 'The Self in Jung and Kohut', in Arnold Goldberg (Ed.), *Dimensions of Self Experience*. Hillsdale, NJ: Analytic Press.

Dawkins, Richard (1976) *The Selfish Gene*. Oxford: Oxford University Press.

Dawkins, Richard (1998) *Unweaving the Rainbow*. Boston: Mariner Books.

Dennett, D. C. (1995) *Darwin's Dangerous Idea: Evolution and the Meanings of Life*. New York: Simon & Schuster.

Derrida, J. (1974) *Of Grammatology*, trans. G. Spivak. Baltimore, MD: Johns Hopkins University Press.

Durham, William (1991) *Coevolution*. Stanford, CA: Stanford University Press.

Fodor, Jerry (1983) *The Modularity of Mind*. Cambridge, MA: MIT Press.

Foucault, Michael (1967) *Madness and Civilization*, trans. R. Howard. London: Tavistock.

Goldberg, David (1994) *Multi-Culturalism: A Critical Reader*. Oxford: Blackwell.

Gould, S. J. (1997) 'Evolution: the pleasures of pluralism'. *New York Review of Books*, June 26, 47–52.

Hamilton, W. D. (1963) 'The evolution of altruistic behavior'. *American Naturalist*, Vol. 97, 354–356.

7 'Perhaps it was the step from constrained virtual reality, where the brain simulates a model of what the sense organs are telling it, to unconstrained virtual reality, in which the brain simulates things that are not actually there at the time – imagination, daydreaming, "what if?" calculations about hypothetical futures. . . . We can get outside the universe. I mean in the sense of putting a model inside our skulls' (Dawkins, 1998: 311–312).

Hamilton, W. D. (1995) *Narrow Roads of Gene Land: 1, The Evolution of Social Behavior*. Oxford: Oxford University Press.

Hauke, Christopher (2000) *Jung and the Postmodern*. London: Routledge.

Hendricks-Jansen, H. (1996). *Catching Ourselves in the Act: Situated Activity, Interactive Emergence, Evolutiuon, and Human Thought*. Cambridge, MA: MIT Press.

Hogenson, George (1999) 'Evolution, psychology and the emergence of the psyche'. Paper delivered at The National Conference of Jungian Analysts, Santa Fe, New Mexico, October 18, 1999. Published as 'The Baldwin effect: a neglected influence on C. G. Jung's evolutionary thinking'. *Journal of Analytical Psychology*, Vol. 46, 591–611, (2001).

Hutchins, E. and Hazelhurst, B. (1990) 'Learning in the cultural process', In C. G. Langton, C. Taylor, J. D. Farmer and S. Rasmussen (Eds), *Artificial Life II* (pp. 689–706). Redwood City, CA: Addison-Wesley.

Kugler, Paul (1982) *The Alchemy of Discourse: An Archetypal Approach to Language*. Lewisburg, PA: Bucknell University Press.

Kugler, Paul (1983–4) 'Involuntary poetics'. *The New Literary History: A Journal of Theory and Interpretation*, Vol. XV, pp. 491–501.

Kugler, Paul (1987) 'Jacques Lacan: postmodern depth psychology and the birth of the self-reflexive subject', in Polly Young-Eisendrath and James Hall (Eds), *The Book of the Self*. New York: New York University Press.

Kugler, Paul (1990a) 'The unconscious in a postmodern depth psychology', in K. Barnaby and P. Acierno (Eds), *C. G. Jung and the Humanities*. Princeton, NJ: Princeton University Press.

Kugler, Paul (1990b) 'Clinical authority: some thoughts out of season'. *Quadrant: The Journal of Contemporary Jungian Thought*, Vol. XXIII, no. 2. Norwood, NJ: Ablex Publishing.

Kugler, Paul (1993) 'The "subject" of dreams' *Journal of the Association for the Study of Dreams*, Vol. 3, no. 2, 123–136.

Kugler, Paul (1997) 'Psychic imaging: a bridge between subject and object', in P. Young-Eisendrath and D. Dawson (Eds), *The Cambridge Companion to Jung*. Cambridge: Cambridge University Press.

Lacan, Jacques (1977) *Ecrits: A Selection*, trans. Alan Sheridan. New York: W. W. Norton.

Mithen, Steven (1996) *The Prehistory of the Mind*. London: Thames & Hudson.

Moore, Richard (1999) *The Creation of Reality in Psychoanalysis*. Hillsdale, NJ: Analytic Press.

Pinker, S. (1994) *The Language Instinct*. New York: HarperCollins.

Pinker, S. (1997) *How the Mind Works*. New York: W. W. Norton.

Richards, Robert (1987) *Darwin and the Emergence of Evolutionary Theories of Mind*. Chicago, IL: University of Chicago Press.

Rosen, David (Ed.) (1999) *Evolution of the Psyche*. Westport, CT: Praeger.

Stevens, A. (1982) *Archetypes*. London: Routledge.

Stevens, A. (1999) *Ariadne's Clue: A Guide to the Symbols of Humankind*. Princeton, NJ: Princeton University Press.

Stevens, A. and Price, J. (1996) *Evolutionary Psychiatry: A New Beginning*. London: Routledge.

Teicholz, Judith (1999) *Kohut, Loewald and the Postmoderns*. Hillsdale, NJ: Analytic Press.

Tooby, J. and Cosmides, L. (1990a) 'On the universality of human nature and the uniqueness of the individual'. *Journal of Personality*, Vol. 58, no. 1, 17–67.

Tooby, J. and Cosmides, L. (1990b) 'The past explains the present: emotional adaptations and the structure of ancestral environments'. *Ethology and Sociobiology*, Vol. 11, 375–424.

Turvey, M. and Kugler, Peter (1987) *Information, Natural Law and the Self-assembly of Rhythmic Movement*. Hillsdale, NJ: Lawrence Erlbaum Associates.

Wittgenstein, L. (1958) *Philosophical Investigations*, trans. G. E. M Anscombe. London: Macmillan.

Reflections on the anima and culture

Introduction

In this chapter contrasting attitudes to Jungian ideas of the feminine are explored. Joy Schaverien starts from the assumption that there is something problematic in Jung's formulations – feminist perspectives make her wary of an implicit essentialism in his position. At times she argues, Jung tends to confuse the influence of culture with that of biology and this results in an unjustified elevation of elements of his theories beyond the cultural context in which they were formulated. Her chapter thus develops themes raised in the preceding chapter, and contrasts strongly with Anthony Stevens' position. Despite these reservations she maintains the clinical importance of Jung's ideas, however. She uses a case to illustrate how disowned parts of a man's self can be split off and projected into 'the feminine'. But in order to preserve this valuable core of the Jungian corpus, she argues that a critical stance towards some of his more culture-bound assumptions should be adopted.

Ann Shearer by contrast is content to start by positing the existence of an innate archetype of the feminine and seeing where this leads. She accepts that notions of this archetype may well reflect elements of the patriarchy within which they were conceived – but wonders whether we can usefully or effectively separate the two. She does take issue with Jung's proscriptive use of notions of the archetypal feminine, and also outlines the role of his personal history in toning his feeling responses to both anima and animus. Having expressed these reservations, however, she moves into a playful exploration of the feminine, the masculine and the relationship between them, in a way that she hopes will open up understanding of both self and others. She goes on for instance to posit the existence of an archetypally female (Athenian) consciousness connected to care and relating and contrasts this with a male (Apollonian) one connected to the search for abstract truth. Schaverien might well respond that the cultural assumptions underlying such formulations could prove restrictive if they are not questioned.

(a) The psychological feminine and contrasexuality in analytical psychology

Joy Schaverien

Jung's erudite knowledge of, and interest, in cultures other than his own is the reason that his writings are of interest in so many different spheres of human endeavour. Critically appraised, Jung's insights continue to offer a valuable means of understanding the human psyche. However, some of the views he expressed pose a challenge to present-day analytical psychologists. When considering the feminine in analytical psychology we are inevitably confronted by the contradictions in his attitude. The concept of contrasexuality is at the centre of Jung's understanding of the human psyche. However, this is not simple because, whilst some of Jung's most poetic insights refer to the concept of anima, his most androcentric passages are written in discussion of animus. Jungian analysts and theorists are therefore confronted with a problem that, if not addressed, leaves us open to justified criticism from colleagues. Jung's theories cannot be applied unquestioningly in a post-feminist era, yet it would be a considerable loss to dismiss the potential that is offered by this means of conceptualizing the psyche. In this paper it is my intention to discuss some of the problems which a Jungian approach to the feminine evokes but also to affirm its validity through a brief clinical example.

It is important to read Jung in order to distinguish the wealth of valuable insights from attitudes that are clearly unacceptable; only then is it possible to revision some of his work. One area where this is called for is his writing on gender and particularly the psychological feminine. Here I am making a distinction between what may be regarded as the 'feminine' in the psyche of both men and women and 'female psychology' – i.e. the psychology of women (Wehr, 1987). In an attempt to distinguish its positive aspects from cultural bias it is necessary to outline some of the theory that is the basis of any discussion of analytical psychology.

THE COLLECTIVE UNCONSCIOUS AND ARCHETYPES

Central in Jungian terminology is the collective unconscious. This is considered to be a layer in the psyche that underlies the personal unconscious. It is sometimes likened to geological strata where, as one layer is revealed, it is discovered to be founded on another and yet another (Jacobi, 1942). The collective unconscious is the deepest and least accessible of these layers; it is the foundation of all the others. Jung writes that it can never be fully known nor depotentiated and he suggests that all we can hope for is to gain a conscious attitude in relation to it (Jung, 1959a: 3).

The collective unconscious is expressed through archetypes. These are instinctual patterns that have no form in their own right; they are neither tangible nor visible but rather structure sense perceptions. They are also the underlying pattern from which images take form in dreams, myth and art. Archetypes are often attributed human form and characterized by figures such as the 'hero' and the 'great mother'. They may manifest themselves in psychological types, which centre around generational aspects of the personality, such as 'senex', where someone who is very young may have an elderly outlook on life, or 'puer', the 'Peter Pan' character who does not grow up.

Taken too literally, archetypes can be viewed as really existing, rather than as a form of cultural or psychological patterning. Then, regarded as fixed, they can be applied to defend an essentialist position. This means that certain characteristics may be attributed as innate in women or in certain ethnic groups. A recent issue of the *Journal of Analytical Psychology* (Vol. 43, no. 3, July 1998) carried a debate about whether archetypes are a biological 'given' or social construction. This draws heated argument on both sides and is relevant when discussing 'the feminine' in analytical psychology.

In Jung's view the psyche is made up of opposites; this means that any conscious attitude is compensated by an unconscious one. The opposites manifest themselves in culture as well as in the psychological development of the individual. They may be characterized by extremes such as hot and cold, light and dark, day and night and, most significantly for this discussion, by masculine and feminine. The idea is that the psyche unconsciously splits off rejected aspects of the personality, projects them and then regards them as 'other'. Within the analytic encounter these may become manifest in a number of ways, within the transference, in dreams or in behaviour and the aim is to use this understanding to integrate them within the personality. Schwartz-Salant (1989) has drawn parallels with projective identification.

However, there is a problem because, in classical Jungian theory, black and dark are attributed to the unconscious state, whilst white and light are seen as conscious. This can be misused, sometimes unconsciously, perpetuating cultural divisions. If this theory is applied uncritically an implicit racism may be transmitted in the wider culture of society as well as in the consulting room. Awareness of this has developed since Dalal (1988) had the courage to point out the racism in some of Jung's writings and, furthermore, it is now known that archetypal theory appealed to the Nazis (Samuels, 1993). There is a similar difficulty with the feminine element in the psyche. This too is attributed to the dark unconscious state, whilst the masculine is associated with light and consciousness. The problem is that, in the language of opposites, there is always an 'other' who may become the unthinking repository for unwanted projections. Despite all these difficulties archetypal theory remains an authentic way of understanding the psyche. Therefore renewed awareness is needed if it is still to be applied in clinical practice or in cultural theory.

ANIMA AND ANIMUS

Anima and animus are manifestations of archetypal motifs which attribute gendered status to the opposites. The anima is a representation of the female element in the male psyche and the animus is the representation of the male element in the female psyche. In Jung's writings the feminine is equated with Eros and the masculine with Logos (Jung, 1959b: 14). There are aspects of both in women and men which, if they are unconscious, will be projected and attached to a figure of the opposite sex. Thus the unconscious in a man may be characterized by the appearance in his 'dreams, visions or fantasies' of a female or 'anima' figure. This is often an idealized archetypal image, perhaps a beautiful young woman or a wise old woman. The point about such inner figures is that they are a manifestation of some aspect of the self, even if at first they appear somewhat alien, they lead towards a resolution of a projected part of the personality and to individuation.

The anima is very often attached to the mother imago. 'Every mother and every beloved is forced to become the carrier and embodiment of this omnipresent and ageless image which corresponds to the deepest reality in a man' (Jung, 1959b: 12–13). Although often considered as a soul image, Jung found this term too vague and preferred anima, which was more specific (Jung, 1959b: 13–14). The anima accounts, in part at least, for the incestuous dynamic that may be experienced in the transference. The projection of the anima may lead to idealization, or else an intense hatred propelled by fear of intimacy. This may be particularly intense for a man working with a female therapist (Schaverien, 1995, 1997). It seems that, in writing of 'anima' Jung was struggling to express an image for his own psychological and spiritual aspirations, as well as those of many of his male patients. This is conveyed with a great deal of subtlety and sensitivity in his writings. The anima is often a romantic temptress which seemed, and still seems, to offer a means of expressing the soul of man. This would indicate that the idea offers an understanding of some 'innate' element in the male psyche. However, if this were to be accepted then there is a problem in the shift from anima to animus.

When Jung writes of animus he displays himself as an unquestioning, dominant member of a patriarchal society, as a man with certain clearly defined expectations of the respective social roles of men and women. The essentialist view of the archetypes as 'innate' is revealed in its more negative aspect. Anima is a sympathetic portrayal of the inner world of a man but animus is much less agreeable; it is presented as a stereotyped view of the 'other', an outer world construction. Although Jung speculates that the animus in women is similar to the anima in man, he is less eloquent, even perhaps a little reluctant, when discussing it. He writes: 'if the anima is an archetype that is found in men, it is reasonable to suppose that an equivalent archetype must be present in woman. For just as the man is compensated by woman so the woman is compensated by man' (Jung, 1959b: 14). So it seems he is a little uncertain about this. Wehr (1987) has suggested that this is because Jung, as a man, was discussing experiences which were not his own. Furthermore he often confused men's anima projections with female psychology and so he confused inner world insights with a socially constructed view of gender difference (Wehr, 1987).

Animus possession in women produces the aggressive uncooperative mate of the man. This is evident when Jung writes of women, who are unconsciously identified with the masculine element in the psyche: 'No matter how friendly and obliging a woman's Eros may be, no logic on earth can shake her if she is ridden by the animus' (Jung, 1959b: 15). If there was any doubt about it he compounds the outer world view point by writing that, 'Often the man has the feeling . . . that only seduction or a beating or rape would have the necessary power of persuasion' (Jung, 1959b: 15). Here Jung slips from the inner world into the outer world and what was a creative metaphor for the inner world, the psyche of man, becomes something rather more sinister in his attitude to women. The idealized anima figure has now got out of control and, in the real world, behaves in ways that provokes a 'non-idealizing' reaction. The shadow is revealed and, what is more appalling to the present-day reader, here is the traditional justification for violence by men towards women; the woman is blamed.

Unconscious possession by either anima or animus results in behaviours, which are undesirable; however, both seem to be attributed to negative aspects of the feminine. Surprisingly it is also the feminine that is denigrated in men's behaviour. Jung writes: 'men can argue in a very womanish way too, when they are anima-possessed and have thus been transformed into the animus of their own anima' (Jung, 1959b: 15). Thus it is the masculine woman or the man who is feminine in his attitude that are denigrated. If we take this view uncritically we could be into an argument which supports the idea that there is something innately bad about masculine women or feminine men.

My reason for reiterating these passages is that they are among the worst of Jung's excesses, and characteristic of the problem that we have to confront when applying Jungian concepts within a feminist frame. If that was all there was to the theory we could leave it – forget it exists – but it is not all there is to it and this becomes evident within the very same chapter in *Aion* (1959b). Here Jung makes it clear that the purpose of understanding the opposite elements, within the individual psyche, is to develop a conscious attitude and to recognize and subsequently integrate the projections within the personality: 'the autonomy of the collective unconscious expresses itself in the figures of anima and animus. They personify those of its contents which, when withdrawn from projection, can be integrated into consciousness' (Jung, 1959b: 20).

Combined with the theory of contrasexuality, which will be described later in the chapter, I find this a helpful way of understanding the psyche. This is the dilemma; there are so many significant insights in Jung's writing that, if we dismiss him for his misogyny, there is the danger of ejecting the alchemist's gold with the murky waters in which it is disguised. I turn now to some of the wider discussion of these themes.

BIOLOGY AND CULTURE

Stoller's distinction between sex and gender offers a helpful clarification. Stoller (1968) establishes that sex is biological. It is determined by physical conditions, i.e.: chromosomes, genitalia, hormonal states and secondary sexual characteristics. These biological differences are denoted by the terms male and female. He emphasizes that 'There are elements of both in many humans but the male has a preponderance of masculinity and the female has a preponderance of femininity' (Stoller, 1968: 9). Gender is psychological or cultural rather than biological and this is denoted by the terms masculinity and femininity. 'Gender identity' and 'gender role' are conditioned by both the above and develop, beginning at birth, into a 'core gender identity' (Stoller, 1968: 29–30). Stoller (1968, 1975) argues, based on a wealth of clinical evidence, that the establishment of gender identity is reinforced by the environment. Therefore, 'gender identity and gender role' are affected by both biological and environmental factors.

In many ways this is consonant with Jung's account of contrasexuality in *The Psychology of the Transference* (Jung, 1946). This is the crossover between the unconscious masculine elements in the female psyche and unconscious feminine elements in the male psyche. Thus contrasexuality lends itself to a creative attitude to healthy gender confusion in normal development. In analysis the aim is to bring these unconscious elements into consciousness and eventually to integrate them within the psyche.

ESSENTIALISM

At one time the idea that biology was destiny was taken as a 'given'. However, over the last few decades debates in feminism have centred on the distinction between biology and culture and questioned whether men and women are 'essentially', that is 'naturally' different. 'Essentialist theories' consider that the experience of the world is determined by biology before culture (Brennan, 1989: 7). These assume that women are the weaker sex and that they are naturally more nurturant and intuitive than men (Brennan, 1989: 7). Feminism set out to challenge such beliefs. However, during the early days of these debates, it seems analytical psychologists paid little attention to feminism and feminists paid little attention to Jungians (Rigsby, 1994). Many classical Jungian texts could be classed as essentialist assuming that the differences between women and men were innate.

Within feminism debates which have developed since the first challenges to essentialism are characterized on the one hand by Anglo-American feminists and on the other by French feminists. Much of the feminist debate regarding sexual difference centres on the interpretation of the Lacanian Symbolic. The Symbolic is not about symbolism in the traditionally understood form but rather about the speaking subject. It is about the move towards the 'other'. French feminists, particularly Irigaray (1974), engaging with the challenge of Lacan, argue that women and men are different and, 'seeing in it positive value, attempt to establish the nature of the difference' (Brennan, 1989: 2). Although sometimes seen as essentialist, their writings are an attempt to acknowledge difference without taking on an essentialist position (Whitford, 1989). They are trying to find a language appropriate to female experience without resorting to the arguments about the difference being innate.

In considering the psychological feminine in analytical psychology these issues are inevitably brought into focus. Difference in the experiences of women and men, culturally and socially, will affect their relationships and their approach to analysis. In the view of the other in the Lacanian sense there is a potential connection with Jung's opposites, which are also about 'otherness'. However, the Lacanian view is very different from the Jungian one. These debates are complex and I cannot give them sufficient space here to do justice to them, but they are relevant when considering the feminine in analytical psychology (see Schaverien, 1995, 1998).

JUNG AND FEMINISM

So if Jung is essentialist what can we do about it in our practice? Rigsby (1994) has pointed out that Jungians often reject feminist arguments and feminists very often ignore Jung; there is frequently avoidance from both of addressing these problematic areas. However, if Jung's work is to continue to be useful clinically it is necessary to open these issues for debate in an attempt to revision some of the theory.

Wehr writes, 'Had he [Jung] located both discussions [of anima and animus] within the context of patriarchy's influence on men and women's sense of self, both would be improved' (Wehr, 1987: 104). She proposes that: 'Even though in some ways he was unable to see through his own projections he did come up with a remarkable model for understanding men's feelings about women' (Wehr, 1987: 117). Wehr writes that there is a real difficulty in resolving a critical attitude to his sexism whilst maintaining a regard for his 'very real contribution to human self-understanding' (Wehr, 1987: 124).

Young-Eisendrath (1984), and Young-Eisendrath and Weidemann (1987) have given accounts of the ways in which these theories can be understood and applied within a feminist frame of reference. Young-Eisendrath (1984) working with heterosexual couples, directly confronts the negative image of the Hag and the apparently more positive image of the Hero, to offer an understanding of the woman who is denigrated in relationship by her male partner. Through case example she shows how it is the inability of the couple to communicate with each other and integrate anima/animus projections which causes both to feel resentful, misunderstood and unable to relate to each other. Transformation of the psychological state of both may occur when the projections become conscious and so are withdrawn. In working with individuals we can see similar patterns played out in the transference/countertransference dynamic.

In a collection of papers (Schwartz-Salant and Stein, 1992) anima and animus are addressed from a number of different perspectives. Young-Eisendrath (1992) writes that she finds the concept most useful clinically when applied to Jung's theory of contrasexuality which 'invites a psychological analysis of the other arising in one's own subjectivity. This is extremely useful in clarifying gender differences . . . providing . . . we revise our theory of gender so that it is relative and contextualized' (Young-Eisendrath, 1992: 175–176). She argues that there is no self-evident or neutral truth about gender: 'gender has no ahistorical, universal meanings' (Young-Eisendrath, 1992: 159). This is a point made in a different way by Hopcke (1991) who has analysed the contradictory attitudes to homosexuality in the writings of Jung and his followers. He argues for a less fixed attitude to sexual orientation which could be understood to be the result of a 'personal and archetypal confluence of the masculine, feminine, and androgyne' (Hopcke, 1991: 187). Significantly he proposes that sexual orientation may be fluid and changing in different phases of life.

Before giving a brief clinical example I turn to Jung's own description of contrasexuality as it shows how complicated are the multitude of projections experienced within an analytic encounter. As already discussed, contrasexuality is the crossover between the unconscious masculine elements in the female psyche and unconscious feminine elements in the male psyche. This is a complicated set of relationships, which manifest themselves in the transference/countertransference relationship, in the following ways which Jung reminds us are not linear, nor sequential (Jung, 1946: 59). These are:

(a) 'An uncomplicated personal relationship. [This we know as the real relationship.]
(b) A relationship of the man to his anima and of the woman to her animus. [A relationship to the other in the self.]
(c) A relationship of anima to animus and vice versa. [The unconscious relationship.]
(d) A relationship of the woman's animus to the man . . . and of the man's anima to the woman . . . ' [The relationship to the unconscious in the Other.] (Jung, 1946: 59; the words in brackets mine)

All analytic relationships become a mixture of these elements whether in the same gender pairing or in cross-gender pairs. Jung writes:

> . . . Anima and animus are projected upon their human counterparts and thus create by suggestion a primitive relationship . . . But in so far as anima and animus undoubtedly represent the contrasexual components of the personality,

their . . . character does not point back towards the group but 'forwards' to the integration of personality, i.e., to individuation. (Jung, 1946: 68)

This is the point about understanding of these elements in the psyche: the aim is their integration as part of the individuation process. I conclude this paper with a brief clinical example. Elsewhere I have given examples of idealized and positive anima projections (Schaverien, 1991, 1998). The example, which follows, is rather different; instead of showing how anima leads to soul, this example illustrates an earlier stage; it shows the need for contrasexuality in the psyche and the problem of too fixed a view of gender identity.

CLINICAL VIGNETTE

In this brief vignette from a relatively early stage in analysis it is possible to see the effects of one-sided development. The psychological feminine is split off. It is projected and experienced as alien and persecutory and so it is attacked. My countertransference experience is recorded in brackets, interspersed with the text.

Mr X, in his fifties, is male and knows it; we could say that he suffers from gender certainty. In the first session after a break he is stirred up and anxious. He has been attending weekly for 9 months and now, after some hesitation, he is going to talk about his sexuality. He begins by saying, 'If I had all the money I have spent on prostitutes I would be rich.' He then proceeds to tell of sexual exploits with women/girls. [As this progresses I start to feel increasingly uncomfortable. I am very aware of myself as a woman in his presence and, what is more, one whom he pays for her services.]

He tells how, when he was young, people seemed to think he used women. He says that it was a bit like rape; but of course they wanted it. He then justifies his actions with an explanation based on biology. Familiar with the behaviour of animals, he says that the bulls know when a cow is ready. 'Young bulls will try anything whilst old bulls won't bother unless the cow is ready. It is the same with men; 'when you walk down the street you feel it if a woman is ready. It is painful, I sense it in my loins and I would rather it didn't happen. What can you do?' [This essentialist viewpoint is presented to justify his experience. It is innate and therefore something that men cannot resist. I briefly wonder if he considers that I am ready. I feel threatened.]

He then uses the same argument to justify his interest in a young girl. 'She wiggles her arse – she is asking for it and what can a man do? I would be in real trouble.' [I am starting to feel distaste for this man. I am also aware, because he has told me before: that this is what he feared if he talked to me about these feelings. He is revealing himself as incapable of considering the feelings of the other person. The only interest he has here is in his own bodily sensations. He seems very angry and as if he is being attacked by this behaviour from someone who is barely more than a child. Perhaps we could understand this girl to be a representation of a negative anima figure or as a rejected part of himself. [I suggest to him that the girl might be unaware of the effect she is having on him.] He seems to ignore this but then goes on to talk about how his wife humiliates him. [It seems that he uses physical sexual activity to maintain the split in his self-perception. It is a distraction from his sense of inadequacy.]

I cannot expand on this case here but the point, that I hope is evident from this passage, is that Mr X is completely out of touch with his feminine side. He is clearly terrified of his own vulnerability and of the perceived power of women in relation to him. He sees the feminine, embodied in women, as totally 'other'. He evokes the 'innate' view of instinct to defend his position. His essentialist view of gender difference is fixed; and based on his biological sex, as well as his social role. However, if we view this brief vignette more closely it is possible to see that he feels excluded from something a bit mysterious. In a way he is tormented by being shut out of the feminine world and so feels threatened by it. His traditional position gives him some solace but it does not really work.

In the next session he suggested that perhaps it is time that he left his therapy. When I suggested that this was because of the last session he admitted that he felt ashamed. [I had felt very worried and had actually hoped that he would leave during the intervening week. But when he suggested doing so my feeling was immediately transformed into understanding of his predicament. Then I was in touch with him and so able to interpret his fear that, after his confession in the last session, he assumed that I would want him to leave.]

Once this was out in the open he was able to admit his vulnerability which might be understood to be linked to the feminine in his own psyche. Imaginally he could be understood to be the rapist but also the female victim of the rape. This fitted with his history of having suffered abuse. Now the feminine element in the psyche began to be befriended and, as I did not reject him, he was able to accept the victim as a part of his own personality. Thus a psychological transformation began to take place.

This is an extreme example and the countertransference reveals that the contrasexual elements were initially unconscious. Whilst Mr X was talking from the position of a man, cut off from the psychological feminine, I was transfixed in the feminine position. As victim I was only able to consider rejecting him. [I am not suggesting that the feminine position is always that of victim, but in this man's inner world, at this particular time, that was the case.] Once he was able to take a more fluid view of the situation, movement was possible. As I was permitted to see his vulnerability the power in the relationship became more equal and I was no longer transfixed; then I no longer felt like rejecting him. This shows how important it is that the analyst does not act too quickly on countertransference responses. Staying with his polarized view of sexual difference permitted his gentler self to emerge. The psychological feminine, which had been split off, was now available in the analytic encounter.

CONCLUSION

In this chapter I have attempted to give a sense of the problems in Jung's attitude to the feminine but I hope also to have shown that the reason for a critical approach is because of the immense legacy of his insights. If we merely dismiss him for some of his less acceptable views the loss would be ours. It is up to analytical psychologists today to be thankful for the wealth of theory that he has given us and to take a critical approach to his oeuvre and so it will continue to be applicable into the twenty first century.

REFERENCES

Brennan, T. (ed.) (1989) *Between Feminism and Psychoanalysis*. London: Routledge.

Dalal, F. (1988) 'The racism of Jung'. *Race & Class*, Vol. XXIX, no. 3, 1–22.

Hopcke R. H. (1991) *Jung, Jungians and Homosexuality*. Boston: Shambala.

Irigaray, L. (1974) *The Speculum of the Other Woman*, translated by Gillian C. Bell. New York: Cornell University Press.

Jacobi, Y. (1942) *The Psychology of C. G. Jung*. London: Routledge & Kegan Paul.

Jung C. G. (1946) *The Psychology of the Transference. Collected Works*, Vol. 16. Princeton, NJ: Bollingen.

Jung C. G. (1956) *Symbols of Transformation Collected Works*, Vol. 5. Princeton, NJ: Bollingen.

Jung C. G. (1959a) *The Archetypes and the Collective Unconscious. Collected Works*, Vol. 9, Part 1. Princeton, NJ: Bollingen.

Jung C. G. (1959b) *Aion. Collected Works*, Vol. 9, Part 11. Princeton, NJ: Bollingen.

Rigsby, R, K. (1994) 'Jung, archetypalists, and fear of feminism'. *Continuum*, Vol. 3, 35–58.

Samuels, A. (1985) *Jung and the Post-Jungians*. London: Routledge & Kegan Paul.

Samuels, A. (1989) 'Countertransference and the mundus imaginalis', Chapter 9 in *The Plural Psyche: Personality, Morality and the Father*. London: Routledge.

Samuels, A. (1993) *The Political Psyche*. London: Routledge.

Schaverien, J. (1991) *The Revealing Image: Analytical Art Psychotherapy in Theory and Practice*. London: Jessica Kingsley, 1999.

Schaverien, J. (1995) *Desire and the Female Therapist: Engendered Gazes in Psychotherapy and Art Therapy*. London: Routledge.

Schaverien, J. (1997) 'Men who leave too soon: reflections on the erotic transference and countertransference'. *British Journal of Psychotherapy*, Vol. 14, no. 1, 3–16.

Schaverien, J. (1998) 'Jung, the transference and the psychological feminine', in I. B. Seu and M. C. Heenan (Eds), *Feminism and Psychotherapy: Reflections on Contemporary Theories and Practices*. London: Sage.

Schwartz-Salant, N. (1989) *The Borderline Personality: Vision and Healing*. Wilmette, IL: Chiron.

Schwartz-Salant, N. and Stein, M. (Eds) (1992) *Gender and Soul in Psychotherapy*. Wilmette, IL: Chiron.

Stoller, R. J. (1968) *Sex and Gender*. London: Hogarth Press.

Stoller, R. J. (1975) *The Transexual Experiment*. London: Hogarth Press.

Young-Eisendrath, P. (1984) *Hags and Heroes: A Feminist Approach to Jungian Psychotherapy with Couples*. Toronto: Inner City Books.

Young-Eisendrath, P. (1992) 'Gender, animus and related topics', in N. Schwartz-Salant and M. Stein (Eds), *Gender and Soul in Psychotherapy*. Wilmette, IL: Chiron.

Young-Eisendrath, P. and Weideman, F. (1987) *Female Authority: Empowering Women through Psychotherapy*. New York: Guilford Press.

Wehr, D. S. (1987) *Jung & Feminism: Liberating Archetypes*. London: Routledge.

Whitford, M. (1989) 'Rereading Irigaray', in T. Brennan (Ed.), *Between Feminism & Psychoanalysis*. London: Routledge.

Wright, E. (Ed.) (1992) *Feminism and Psychoanalysis: A Critical Dictionary*. Oxford: Blackwell.

(b) Jung and the feminine

Ann Shearer

Has any aspect of Jung's work raised more discussion or drawn more heat, anger, disappointment and passionate defence than the theories he spins around the core of 'the feminine'? They fascinate us, it seems. They confuse us. They animate us! They can focus the collective weight of a century and more of unprecedented upheaval in relationships between Western women and men; they can touch the most private parts of the psyche in search of individual identity. We cannot leave them alone, forever elaborating from this perspective or that; they are a-buzz with -isms. We are drawn by them into elaborations we may not have intended at all – of dreams, of mythologies, of the theory of archetypes itself; clear thought is veiled into a haze. These theories work on us, in fact, very much as Jung tells us that animus and anima will. This congruence seems to me extraordinary. I feel I have hardly begun to grasp and be grasped by what it means.

By the yardstick of painstaking contemporary differentiations between sex and gender, Jung of course hardly scores highly. But I find it hard to get too exercised about this, especially when the jury is still so far out on sexual differences and their psychological consequences that two Jungian authors between the same covers can offer such very different interpretations of their significance (Young-Eisendrath, 1992; Zinkin, 1992). More than this: when 'the patriarchy' has had its way with us for 4,000 years or so, it seems somewhat academic to wonder whether something called 'the feminine' is innate or the product of that culture. My own interest has been rather more pragmatic: to accept that there have been energies imaged as 'feminine' throughout these 'patriarchal' times and to explore their historical expressions for clues about both collective patterns and contemporary lives (Shearer, 1998). First causes I can allow to guard their mysteries.

> Whence all creation had its origin
> He, whether he fashioned it or whether he did not,
> He who surveys it from the highest heaven
> He knows – or maybe even he does not.
> $\qquad$ (*Rig Veda*, X, 129)

So what does it mean to people here and now at the start of the twenty-first century to have a fantasy of 'the feminine within' (or 'anima') or to experience being (or being called) 'feminine'? To ask such questions – and they do seem to be ones which a great number of Western women and men are asking, an expression of a collective psychic situation – neither depends on nor implies any pre-set definition or concept of the term. Rather the reverse: it is in the explorations that the images and energies which connect the personal to the archetypal will emerge, and that connection, far from constraining, must surely bring a sense of expansion, of becoming more ample, to the individual. We have only to let our mind's eye conjure all the variety it can of images summoned by that one word 'feminine' to glimpse the hugeness of the finally unknowable realm on which our psychic life rests, the 'riverbed along which the current of psychic life has always flowed' (Jung, 1956: para. 337).

So to posit an archetype of 'the feminine', innate and irreducible, may open the way to exploration rather than closing possibilities of experience. To allow for the archetype at work in us may lift us beyond the limitation of our time, environment and personal experience. 'Archetypes are not disseminated only by tradition, language and migration', as Jung says, 'but can re-arise spontaneously, at any time, at any place, and without any outside influence. This means that there are present in every psyche forms which are unconscious but nonetheless active – living dispositions . . . that preform and continually influence our thoughts and feelings and actions' (1954a: paras. 153–4).

Let us not imagine either that our contemporary perceptions around this notion of 'the feminine' are necessarily fuller than those which went before. In fact, as Ginette Paris valuably points out, in contemporary tendencies to worship at the altar of the Great Mother we may be falling into a monotheism rather than engaging with the very different aspects of the feminine to which we are invited by the multiplicity of female divinities of the past (1986: 197–199). Athene is not Artemis, nor Hestia neither.

As a very different tradition also tells us, The Daughters are not The Mother. Consider, for instance, the placing of this very exercise as Controversy Nine in the present series. Nine: the measure of the human being, having to do also with contemplation, with truth, with the Three Worlds, always reproducing itself in its multiples, related to the Great Goddess, to fertility and death – and later to the masculine too, balancing the spiritual and the material. In the *I Ching* – so often the contemporary basis of restricted images of 'the Feminine' as the receptive, earth, mother and so on – the ninth Hexagram is Hsiao Ch'u: the Taming Power of the Small. The image: the wind drives across heaven, amassing clouds; the Gentle, the Eldest Daughter, exercises her influence on the Creative masculine. A limited influence, so the commentaries tell us: only the promise of the blessing of rain.

Well, some might think at this point, no wonder Jung so valued the *I Ching!* Patriarchy rules, even the next generation of the feminine is limited to influence rather than direct power. The Gentle, indeed! But in the early commentaries, the nature of the Eldest Daughter is also vehemence; she is the force that can get threefold value in the market. And while the middle daughter is The Clinging, and the youngest is The Joyous, the former also means fire, sun, lightning, coats of mail, helmets, lances, weapons and the latter means smashing, breaking apart, dropping off, bursting open (Wilhelm, 1968: 227–279).

There is a wealth of invitation to play in such imagery, it seems to me, and playing may be an essential route to imagining the 'feminine' more fully. 'The discriminating intellect', as Jung says, 'naturally keeps on trying to establish (the archetypes') singleness of meaning and thus misses the essential point: for what we can above all establish as the one thing consistent with their nature is their manifold meaning, their almost limitless wealth of reference, which makes any unilateral formulation impossible' (1954b: para 80).

As I understand it, then, there is nothing at all in Jung's theory of archetypes to restrict our exploration of 'the feminine' – and even, if that is our inclination, of whether it exists or not. No, the point at which I throw the book across the room is when Jung corsets his own vision by eliding the imagery of 'the feminine' as anima with 'the feminine' as woman's psychology. It is not his characterization of 'the feminine' itself that irks me – for it seems to me that the world could do with a great deal more of Eros, of that attention to the relatedness of people and things, whichever name we put to it. It is rather the proscriptive use he makes of this characterization for women's lives. The difficulties created when man's inner image and experience of 'the feminine' embodied as woman is taken to be objective definition of actual women's reality are well-rehearsed (e.g. Goldberg, 1976; Wehr, 1988). Jung's repeated insistence on anima as an inevitably 'unconscious', 'inferior', 'caricatured' and 'second-rate' version of the feminine, which could help preserve distinctions between her and actual women, in fact only compounds the problem when they are conflated in this way.

So, of course, does his often-remarked animus against the animus. And so the monstrous regiment of 'animus-hounds' snarls its way through the pages, as 'woman' betrays her 'true nature' by, say, interesting herself in 'commerce, politics, technology and science' rather than in the realm of 'psychic relatedness' and falls into that 'lunatic logic' which drives the rational mind to 'the white heat of frenzy' (Jung, 1934: para. 330; 1963a: para. 228). And just as Jung sees the negative effects of animus primarily in terms of their effect on men, rather than on the women who must bear them, so it is men rather than women who are primarily served by its positive manifestations. Animus may, for instance, '(bring) forth creative seeds which have the power to fertilise the feminine side of the man', or bring woman a measure of spirit that she needs 'in order to pass it on to her son' (1934: 336; 1963a: 233). No inconsistencies here: 'Man's foremost interest should be his work' he said towards the end of his life. 'But a woman – man is her work and her business' (McGuire and Hull, 1980: 236).

Well, as Jung himself insisted, 'every psychology . . . has the character of a subjective confession. . . . Even when I deal with empirical data I am necessarily speaking about myself' (1929: 774). He knew the legacy of his own early experience of his parents: 'The feeling I associated with "woman" was for a long time that of innate unreliability. "Father", on the other hand, meant reliability and – power-lessness. That is the handicap I started off with' (1963b: 23). Not hard to see, perhaps, in his perception of his mother – loving by day, and by night 'archaic and ruthless, ruthless as truth and nature' – the genesis of his fascination with the anima; nor to sense, in his profound disappointment with a father who could not engage in truth with the faith he mouthed, a forerunner of his animosity towards the animus, that 'second-rate man', carrier of empty opinion, producer of 'an inexhaustible supply of illogical arguments and false explanations' (1963b: 70–74; 1931: 338).

That Jung was a man of his time, place and class, influenced by his own early experiences, will not be surprising to depth psychologists. What seems to me far more remarkable is how far he went beyond the understandings of his intellectual era. It was only in the year of his birth, for instance, that the dual roles of egg and sperm in human generation were finally described, the female part until then being completely denied by many. A quarter of a century later, in the year that Freud bombed with *The Interpretation of Dreams*, the hot best-seller was Dr Paul Moebius's *On the Physiological Inferiority of Women*, which demonstrated once for all that the inferior size of a woman's brain must conclusively debar her from participating in 'the masculine world' (Hillman, 1972: 295–296). And then Jung asserts – in an intellectual climate whose roots stretch back through medieval scholasticism to classical philosophy – that in each man, *superior et nobilior*, there is a 'feminine' element which he dishonours at his peril! At a time too when so many influential thinkers were warning of the dangers of the 'man–woman' hybrid which would result if women went to university (Showalter, 1987: 222–223), we can at least salute Jung's perception that there was a 'masculine' element of everywoman which could be neither denied nor ignored.

That was then. But although the content of the story has changed, has its essential form really altered? For women and men to grapple with what we mean by 'masculine' and 'feminine', and with what each means in and to the life of self and other, seems a given of our human nature. The fact of our two sexes has carried images and stories of the Other – the not-I, the one who also defines me – over countless generations and places. It still does: it is not books with titles like 'Women are from Venus and so are Men' or 'Men are from Mars and Women Likewise' that flow from the popular psychology shelves.

So who am I, and who is that Other, and where are we different and same? We are faced with the questioning from the first moment of consciousness. 'This at *last* is bone of my bones and flesh of my flesh', cries Adam when Eve is finally drawn – unlike the rest of creation, or even his first wife, Lilith – from his very substance; 'she shall be called Woman because she was taken out of Man'. Is this the state of Paradise to which we long to return, this knowing no difference between the substance of self and that of Other? We tell stories of it, imagining the infancy of the individual from this tale of the infancy of the world. But what we know more surely is that at the very moment of consciousness, the apple once bitten, that blissful state is forever lost: sew fig leaves as they will, Adam and Eve must live for ever with the sense of their naked Otherness and the bitter distance between each other and God. Adam now knows that it is because he has heeded his wife that he is condemned to toil an accursed ground; Eve knows the agonizing consequences of her inescapable desire for her husband. That terrible condemnation of humankind to suffering and exile from the Self and the Other, and the concomitant longing for re-union, seem to me to be the fundamental human situation that Jung addresses through his theory of the contrasexual archetype. That is why it has such a continuing energy, such a power to move us, far beyond the individual content that he brought to it in his day and we do in ours.

When the anima first imaged herself to Jung, it was no small sense of separation with which he was living. His parting from Freud had left him disorientated. He had reached a fundamental and uncomfortable question: 'What is your myth – the myth in which you live?' He had no answer. And then – in a form which he associated with his eldest daughter! – came the first appearance of the anima: the dream of the green stone table and the white dove which transformed into the little girl who spoke to him of the twelve dead (Bennet, 1982: 75; Jung, 1963b: 195). Almost a year later, he took 'the decisive step': 'I let myself drop'. In only his second attempt to reach the bottom, he found himself on the edge of 'a cosmic abyss'. There he met Elijah and the blind Salome, that first personification of what he was later to call Eros. The fantasies continued. But what, Jung asked himself, was he really doing? Then came the voice of that 'woman within' and the speculation on 'anima' and 'the soul' (1963b: 205–206, 210–211).

Not easy for us, perhaps, in these familiar sequences, to imagine the experience of that descent into the 'seething life' of the unconscious, the threat posed by those 'nonsensical' fantasies, the fear of madness. We, after all, have Jung's maps to guide us, as well as those of many other depth psychologists. But if Salome was blind 'because she does not see the meaning of things', neither at that time did Jung himself. Without Freud's version of the relationship between consciousness and the unconscious, he was alone in an a-causal world. In the experience of his dreams and fantasies, he was in a very profound sense *Other to himself.*

This was the point at which the anima appeared – with the untrustworthiness, the seductiveness, the want of logic that were to remain among her characteristics, but also with the force of an inner reality which demanded relationship. Above all, she introduced Jung to the alchemical *opus* and everything it would have to teach him about the relation between masculine and feminine, soul and spirit, Sol and Luna, Eros and Logos. No wonder he called making out with the anima the masterwork! (1976: 481) And no wonder, either, perhaps, that we continue to be seized by the theories he spun round her, sometimes despite ourselves (e.g. Schwartz-Salant, 1992). People still experience that fearful disorientation when time is up for the once-comfortable collusions between ego and persona – and this is still the point at which the figures Jung called animus and anima will begin to demand attention. For as long as we humans sense that Otherness which is not only out there but also profoundly within, and long for and dread the experience of a unified self, or even a union with the Self, then we seem bound to be animated by images and intimations of figures whose function is precisely to bridge us to our own beyond.

And at the same time, we also seem bound to be driven crazy by the inadequacies of our formulations, limited as we must be whenever consciousness tries to speak of the unconscious. As Jung himself said (1976: 192), no philosopher in his senses would invent such irrational and clumsy ideas as animus and anima. And in our own inevitable clumsinesses as we engage with them, we may even be hampered in a way Jung simply was not. Our extraordinary contemporary reticence in speaking of 'difference' – for fear of falling into actual or implied judgement of the Other as inferior, or damaging individuals by generalization, or provoking attack – makes for difficulties of its own. We know the bitter histories that our current sensitivities seek to assuage. But at the same time too, perhaps, we can see in such huge contemporary oppositions as globalism and nationalism and the devastations of civil wars, that engagement with issues of difference and similarity, separateness and union, is a collective as well as an individual demand from which we cannot escape.

So Jung's writings on 'the feminine' and the contrasexual archetype are bound to evoke animation and animosity. They speak directly to issues which are of central importance to both individuals and societies. The insistence of the debate around them suggests that neither the energy he tapped into nor what he crafted of it is by any means exhausted. So we find our own versions of the old scholastic questions: not whether woman has a soul, but whether everybody has both animus and anima and whether each is bound to appear in contrasexual guise. Is it even answers we seek, or rather is it through a continual testing of the questions against experience that we work towards forging bridges between consciousness and the unconscious?

For debate as we will, it seems, women still dream of and conjure male figures of extraordinarily insistent energy, just as men dream of and conjure female ones of comparable intensity. And these figures continue to present themselves in a multitude of moods, guises and aptitudes –sometimes wondrous, often problematic, yet always somehow drawing us to the not-me but of-me that we call the unconscious. Then too, people also dream of and conjure same-sex figures of comparable energy and function, for whom the textbook definition as 'positive shadow' seems too feeble and as 'Self-figure' seems too grand. Consider, for an extraordinary collective example of this, the huge international response to the death of Diana, Princess of Wales (Haynes and Shearer, 1998). That event was archetypal. Through it, literally millions of people came to glimpse, however briefly, their own and the collective unconscious – and their guide was the image of a woman unknown, yet somehow deeply familiar, to them all. Who was the Princess then but the carrier of anima, of soul – and every bit as much for women as for men?

Of course women have soul – and 'anima' broodings and emotionalities as well! And of course men have spirit –as well as 'animus'-opinionatedness and unrelated intellectuality! We are all also our own 'second-rate' selves. So I am drawn by suggestions that both animus and anima are at work in us all (e.g. Hillman, 1986; Kast, 1986) – not, I hope, out of any politically correct even-handedness or fear of difference, but because this can seem to fit psychological experience. I am interested in the associated imaging of anima as a same-sex figure (e.g. Hopcke,

1990). I am attracted by the idea of polarity *within* both 'feminine' and 'masculine': of a 'yang' femininity that takes its thrusting, birthing power from the action of the exertive rather than the receptive womb (Pauli Haddon, 1987, 1991) and of a 'lunar' masculinity that is the receptive twin of the aggressive 'solar' one (Beebe, 1995).

There is room enough in Jung's framework, it seems to me, for any amount of such discussion – and even incentive for it. 'What is not-I, not masculine, is *most probably* feminine', says Jung, 'and because the not-I is felt as not belonging to me and therefore as outside me, the anima-image is *usually* projected upon women' (1954b: para. 58; my italics). And, as he emphasizes, it is only because we are not yet able to use animus and anima purposefully as *functions* that they remain personified complexes in the forms in which we meet them (1938: para. 339). (See Colman (1998) for further exploration of these themes.)

Yet I also wonder whether I am losing something here, some difference in the psychologies of women and men that might even be called essential. So I take note of those who insist on the distinction, and on the part played by the contrasexual archetype in that (e.g. Ulanov, 1992), or who emphasize that though spirit and soul are indeed present in both women and men, it is in distinctive ways (Tougas, 2000). I am interested in how qualities once labelled 'masculine' may become felt as inherent to a 'feminine self' (Stevens, 1992). And I find I want to look again at the rather central notion of 'consciousness'.

Not many people who read and write this sort of book, I suspect, will follow Jung's description of 'feminine consciousness', that 'lunatic logic', let alone attribute it to women as he does. The idea of 'consciousness' as a neutral sort of 'human potential', however gender-specific its content, might appear more comfortable (Kast, 1986). Yet Athene is not Apollo. The goddess whose very being is engagement in human affairs, from marketplace to citadel, whose hands-on interventions transform the stuff of the practical arts, is absolutely not the same as the god whose shining arrows shoot from afar, that solar brilliance of the discriminations of pure thought and form. Can we play, then, with the idea of a 'feminine consciousness' that is above all related to the reality of the world as it is, and contrast it with a 'masculine consciousness' that must soar above such limitations in search of the absolute? We come near to Jung's understanding of the ways of Eros and Logos here. We might go further to observe them at work in the findings of Carol Gilligan and her colleagues on the very different styles of moral decision-making among actual women and men. The first, it seems, tend to operate mostly from an 'ethic of care', the second from an 'ethic of justice' (Gilligan, 1982; Beebe, 1995). 'True nature'? Culture?

So I seem to return to the place from which I started and to know it not much better at all. Two final reflections, however. The first is how extraordinarily difficult I find it (as this piece shows) to consider 'the feminine' without also 'the masculine'. I am not at all sure, either, that I even want to. 'Shiva without Shakti is *shava*', as the sages have it: the god without the goddess is a corpse – and so, I would add, is the goddess without the god. The insistent images for me now are those of the syzygy: that is where the *animation* is. I am seized again by the wealth of playfulness, intensity, majesty and mystery in Eastern images of the divine pair, and the want of that essential union in Western images of the Godhead. Jung's engagement with the alchemical imagery of union becomes the more important, and the energy he found in the constant separations and unions of Eros and Logos becomes the more charged.

The empowerment of shaman and shamaness, we are told, their ability to travel through the upper and lower worlds, came through their marriage to their spirit wife or husband (Eliade, 1970). Contemporary women and men, it seems, still know something of that inner energy:

> 'I dreamed I was myself, and also a man with a penis, making love to a woman who was also myself'.

> 'I dreamed I was myself making love to a woman – and then realized I also had female genitalia'.

In the imagery and energy of such dreams – the first a woman's, the second a man's, both of them heterosexual – people can experience extraordinary transformative power. At the same time, of course, there is the knowledge that the fullness of the most fundamental and pre-existent union of all – that between the conscious and unconscious worlds – can never be more than intimated by consciousness. So it seems to me all the more important to stoke the imaginal fires of transformation, and to attend to psyche by animating the play of intimations.

'My aim', said Jung, 'is to bring about a psychic state in which my patient begins to experiment with his own nature – a state of fluidity, change and growth where nothing is eternally fixed and hopelessly petrified' (1931: para. 99). And hers, I would only add. And hers.

REFERENCES

Beebe, J. (1995) *Integrity in Depth*. New York: Fromm International.

Bennet, E. A. (1982) *Meetings with Jung*. London: Anchor Press.

Colman, W. (1998) 'Contrasexuality and the unknown soul', in I. Alister and C. Hauke (Eds), *Contemporary Jungian Analysis*. London: Routledge.

Eliade, M. (1970) *Shamanism*, trans. W. Trask. Princeton, NJ: Princeton University Press.

Gilligan, C. (1982) *In a Different Voice: Psychological Theory and Women's Development*. Cambridge, MA: Harvard University Press.

Goldberg, N. (1976) 'A feminist critique of Jung'. *Signs: Journal of Women in Culture and Society*, Vol. 2, no. 2, 433–449.

Haynes, J. and Shearer, A. (Eds) (1998) *When a Princess Dies: Reflections from Jungian Analysts*. London: Harvest Books.

Hillman, J. (1972) *The Myth of Analysis*. New York: Harper & Row.

Hillman, J. (1986) *Anima: An Anatomy of a Personified Notion*. Dallas, TX: Spring.

Hopcke, R. (1990) *Men's Dreams, Men's Healing*. Boston, MA: Shambhala.

Jung, C. G. (1929) 'Freud and Jung: Contrasts' in *Collected Works*, Vol. 4. London: Routledge & Kegan Paul.

Jung, C. G. (1931) 'The Aims of Psychotherapy' in *Collected Works*, Vol. 16, London: Routledge & Kegan Paul.

Jung, C. G. (1934) 'Anima and Animus', in *Collected Works*, Vol. 7. London: Routledge & Kegan Paul.

Jung, C. G. (1954a) 'Psychological Aspects of the Mother Archetype' in *Collected Works*, Vol. 9i. London: Routledge & Kegan Paul.

Jung, C. G. (1954b) 'Archetypes of the Collective Unconscious', in *Collected Works*, Vol. 9i. London: Routledge & Kegan Paul.

Jung, C. G. (1956) *Symbols of Transformation, Collected Works*, Vol. 5. London: Routledge & Kegan Paul.

Jung, C. G. (1963a) *Mysterium Coniunctionis, Collected Works*, Vol. 14. London: Routledge & Kegan Paul.

Jung, C. G. (1963b) *Memories, Dreams, Reflections*. London: Fontana.

Jung, C. G. (1976) *Letters*, Vol. 2, London: Routledge.

McGuire, W. and Hull, R. F. C. (Eds) (1980) *C. G. Jung Speaking: Interviews and Encounters*. London: Picador.

Kast, V. (1986) *The Nature of Loving: Patterns of Human Relationship*, trans. B. Matthews. Wilmette, IL: Chiron.

Paris, G. (1986) *Pagan Meditations*. Dallas, TX: Spring.

Pauli Haddon, G. (1987) 'Delivering yang femininity', *Spring*, pp. 133–141. Dallas: Spring Publications.

Pauli Haddon, G. (1991) 'The personal and cultural emergence of yang femininity', in Zweig (Ed.), *To Be a Woman: The Birth of Conscious Femininity*. London: Mandala.

Schwartz-Salant, N. (1992) 'Anima and animus in Jung's alchemical mirror', in N. Schwartz-Salant and M. Stein (Eds), *Gender and Soul in Psychotherapy*. Wilmette, IL: Chiron.

Shearer, A. (1998) *Athene: Image and Energy*. London: Penguin Arkana.

Showalter, E. (1987) *The Female Malady: Women, Madness and English Culture, 1830–1980*. London: Virago.

Stevens, C. (1992) 'What is the animus and why do we care?' in N. Schwartz-Salant and M. Stein (Eds), *Gender and Soul in Psychotherapy*. Wilmette, IL: Chiron.

Tougas, C. (2000) 'What is the difference between spirit and soul? Jungian reflections'. *Harvest: Journal for Jungian Studies*, Vol. 46, 1.

Ulanov, A. (1992) 'Disguises of the anima', in N. Schwartz-Salant and M. Stein (Eds), *Gender and Soul in Psychotherapy*. Wilmette, IL: Chiron.

Wehr, D. (1988) *Jung and Feminism: Liberating Archetypes*. London: Routledge.

Wilhelm, R. (1968) *The I Ching or Book of Changes*, trans. C. Baynes. London: Routledge & Kegan Paul.

Young-Eisendrath, P. (1992) 'Gender, animus and related topics', in N. Schwartz-Salant and M. Stein (Eds), *Gender and Soul in Psychotherapy*, Wilmette, IL: Chiron.

Zinkin, L. (1992) 'Anima and animus: an interpersonal view', in N. Schwartz-Salant and M. Stein (Eds), *Gender and Soul in Psychotherapy*, Wilmette, IL: Chiron.

Frequency of sessions and the analytic frame

Introduction

This chapter makes a valuable and highly original contribution to the field. In it Moira Duckworth and Martin Stone assess the results of a survey they have conducted among analysts concerning the frequency of analytic sessions. Although issues around frequency have been widely discussed, surprisingly little has actually been published on the subject before, and equally little is known about the effect of frequency on the outcome of therapy. The authors argue that the reasons for choice of frequency are not straightforward nor always based on perceived therapeutic need. Having established the frequency at which an international population of analysts actually works, they go on to discuss the psychological and political factors that may be influencing those choices.

The format of this chapter is somewhat different from the rest of this book. Although the case for both high- and low-frequency work are examined in separate sections, these occur within the main body of the chapter and are co-authored. Both authors are currently involved in further ongoing research on the subject of frequency.

Frequency of sessions and the analytic frame

Martin Stone and Moira Duckworth

Summary

The subject of frequency has been surprisingly little written about, considering its importance in analytic work in relation to patient needs, outcome, training requirements and preferred method of working. This chapter examines the case for working at different frequencies from theoretical and historical viewpoints, and looks at the results of a questionnaire sent to analysts and therapists to seek their attitudes and experiences. It starts with an historical overview of how the issue has become embedded in the theoretical framework of psychoanalysis and analytical psychology. The case for working at a high frequency is followed by the case for lower-frequency work, or a more flexible approach, and the advantages and disadvantages are considered. In discussion of the important theoretical, clinical and political questions, it is noted how concern about training standards has become focused on frequency of sessions.

This leads to consideration of why the subject has been surrounded by so much silence, and to how this is connected with the hierarchical and political structures of British psychotherapy.

INTRODUCTION

A prospective patient comes for an initial, exploratory or assessment session. One of the first things to be agreed on, if the therapist and patient are going to work together, is the frequency of the therapy. Usually the patient has come because something is troubling them. This may be an external factor in their lives, or inner conflicts which create unmanageable feelings. Presumably what the patient (the consumer) consciously wants is to feel better, for something to change. Their primary objective will be the *outcome* at the end of the therapy.

At this point it is the therapist rather than the patient who is interested in the process, and has to decide what may be needed in order for the person to feel more whole. What is going to be the frequency of the therapy? Unless the answer to this question is determined by training needs, or preferences held by the therapist, then a decision has to be made before regular sessions can commence.

Although some therapists change the frequency in the course of the work, the answer to this question may set the pattern for years of work, and may contribute to the nature, depth, and quality of the therapy, and to its outcome. The frequency is part of the analytic frame, the container, the temenos. It is possibly the most important decision to be taken at the outset.

The authors' interest in the subject has arisen in different ways. Moira Duckworth's has arisen from a fascination with 'process' in her own work as an analyst and as a supervisor, and from a thought that there might be shadow issues involved in how often and how long we work with people. Martin Stone's interest has emerged from a paper he wrote, 'Splits between Jungian groups: diversity and division', and from his work in the United Kingdom Council for Psychotherapy and in the London Jungian Umbrella group. In both these settings 'frequency' became a focus for disagreement.

WHY IS THE ISSUE IMPORTANT?

At first sight the decision about frequency appears to be an important practical one, related to process and to the therapist's preferred way of working, but it has become infused with theoretical importance, and complicated through its relationship with outcome and how we measure or define this. One of the most difficult aspects of any discussion about the subject is what is meant by 'outcome' and how it might be measured. There is a range of questions which need to be considered before we can make more realistic sense of the importance of the issue of frequency in therapy. What criteria do we apply? How objective is it possible to be? How valuable are subjective criteria? How generally applicable are outcome criteria, e.g. to work with adults, or children, or hospital inpatients? If a greater consensus can be found among therapists with regard to outcome (for example in finding ways of valuing it subjectively), can we then begin to be more objective about how we decide the appropriate frequency to work with an individual patient, so that their preference, the therapist's preference, and outside demands (e.g. for training) are all taken into account?

Some of the criteria quoted are that borderline patients benefit from being seen twice a week, not more frequently; that highly narcissistic patients need at least three times a week, preferably more; that borderline psychotic patients, or patients who have recently recovered from a psychotic episode, should be seen either once a week, or five times a week, but not anything between, as this would open them to being flooded by uncontainable unconscious material. Another view is that the frequency should be altered to take into account more or less psychotic elements, with sometimes quite complex formulations relating levels of neurotic, or psychotic, behaviour to different levels of frequency. But for every view expressed, there seems to be a contradictory view expressed elsewhere. This is anything but an exact science.

An internet search of 30,000 books, articles, and papers showed only eight with a reference to frequency. Of these eight only three were related to frequency of sessions. For a matter supposedly so central in the therapeutic process, the lack of written material or research on the subject is surprising. A little has been written in the last few years, often buried in issues to do with supervision, and there are references in literature on assessment. Virtually none of the papers refer specifically to the relationship of frequency to outcome, mainly, we believe, because research into the question is so difficult and beset with problems.

Given the importance of frequency in therapeutic work, the fact that there are more questions than answers and more assumptions than proven facts gives cause for concern. In an age when therapists are being challenged to substantiate the efficacy of their work, the subject of 'Frequency and the Analytic Frame' merits research. The authors have made a start with a research questionnaire to get some basic information from therapists: how they themselves actually work, what relationship, if any, they experience between frequency and outcome, and how they view the whole concept of outcome, subjectively and objectively. The results of the research so far are discussed in this chapter, and we look at how further exploration might address some of the questions raised by this controversial issue. Whether it is possible to separate outcome from process remains an open question, but if it is not, many of the assumptions which are made about working at different frequencies are themselves open to question.

The questionnaire was sent to 342 therapists in the UK, Germany, Italy and the USA, with a covering letter explaining the background to our request for information. Replies were received from 120 people, a response rate of just over 35 per cent. In addition to our request for information about the frequency at which therapists actually work compared to how they would like to work, we asked the following question: 'What are the main differences you personally experience working at different frequencies from the point of view of content, depth, duration, relationship between you and the patient, and outcome – as a quantifiable measurement, and as a qualitative experience'.

Their responses indicate that therapists themselves believe there is no discernible quantifiable relationship between frequency of sessions and outcome, although the qualitative experience may be different. Of the 120 replies, 30 people did not reply to this question. A further 41 indicated they did not experience any relationship between the frequency at which they worked with a patient and the outcome, either quantitatively or qualitatively; i.e. a total of 71 respondents (59 per cent) could not positively relate frequency to outcome. Forty-seven people, i.e. 39.2 per cent of respondents, indicated that they felt there was a qualitative difference in outcome. Although this is clearly a highly subjective response, we believe it is important to value it as the personal experience of almost 40 per cent of analysts/ therapists.

In contrast to this, only seven of those replying, 5.8 per cent, thought that outcome could be quantifiably measured against the frequency at which they worked. This is a highly significant result from this preliminary survey. Outcome as an objective measurement has not been shown to be affected by frequency in any of the literature we have seen on the subject, and this response shows that over 94 per cent of respondents themselves do not believe there is any quantifiable relationship between frequency and outcome.

The following two comments from replies to the questionnaire may help to put the issue in perspective:

'are there *any* quantifiable studies on analysis? I don't think so. It feels better seeing more of each other, for me and for the patient.'

'no generalizations make sense to me. E.g. I have had a rare experience of transformation in just two sessions.'

THE HISTORICAL CONTEXT

The issue of frequency has become embedded in the theoretical framework of psychoanalysis. It has been used as a differentiating tool within psychoanalysis and psychotherapy, and this distinction may indeed be helpful when used purely descriptively to distinguish Freud's preferred way of working from other practitioners'. The difficulty arose with Freud's famous statement at the Budapest congress in 1918:

It is very probable, too, that the large scale application of our therapy will compel us to alloy the pure gold of analysis freely with the copper of direct suggestion . . . but, whatever form this psychotherapy for the people may take, whatever the elements out of which it is compounded, its most effective and most important ingredients will assuredly remain those borrowed from strict and untendentious psycho-analysis. (1919: 167–168)

This important statement placed psychoanalysis in a strict hierarchical relationship with other forms of psychotherapy, and although the frequency of weekly sessions has never as such been used to define 'psychoanalysis', it has been used as a simple distinguishing yardstick. In a paper at a conference on Psychoanalysis and Psychoanalytic Psychotherapy, held in London in 1988, Heinz Wolff (1988) pointed to the difficulty of using frequency as a defining criterion:

When asked to define the main differences between psychoanalytic psychotherapy and psychoanalysis one may at first resort to definition in terms of frequency of sessions and, to some extent, also, the duration of treatment. In analysis the patient is seen five or perhaps four times a week, while in psychoanalytic psychotherapy he is usually seen only once or perhaps twice a week. It is obvious that what I am tempted to call this 'number game' is hardly a satisfactory definition. One is in fact left with the question of whether seeing a patient three times a week constitutes analysis or analytical psychotherapy?

and he continues:

> This difficulty in distinguishing . . . in terms of numbers only leads me to suggest that a more meaningful distinction can be made in terms of the shared *experience* the patient and the therapist have in their relationship during the therapy in one of these two forms of psychotherapy . . . There can be no doubt that the experience of both patient and therapist (of working at different frequencies) will be very different. The more frequent the sessions, the more intense the relationship is likely to be.

Wolff's view is endorsed by a majority of the respondents to the questionnaire.

Some psychoanalysts adopt a more rigorous position: anything less than five times, or four times a week is deemed to be psychotherapy not psychoanalysis, with the UK holding to the more rigorous end of the scale in terms of numbers. The current requirement of candidates in training at the British Psycho-Analytical Society is five daily sessions a week, each of 50 minutes, both for their own analysis and for their work with training patients. In the USA, the standard requirement is four times a week, but some of the 28 societies there affiliated to IPA – The International Psychoanalytical Association – train at five times, and some only require three times. The IPA minimum requirement is still four times a week, but standards in other countries vary in terms of frequency and length of session time: most of Europe and South America generally require four times minimum, while the prerequisite in France is only three times a week, because of the influence of Lacan. However, many candidates there choose to undergo five times a week analysis during training.

Joseph Sandler (1988) in a paper at the conference mentioned above, wrote:

> Many authors have spelled out for us the differences between the two, and have provided us with long lists of criteria for differentiating one from the other. Yet in spite of all these helpful lists, which overlap substantially, problems of differentiation remain. . . . The whole area is . . . complicated by the 'political' issues involved, linked with our different trainings . . . Clearly the yardsticks of frequency and time are not suitable measures on their own for differentiating psychoanalysis from psychotherapy . . . there are analysts who will say, convincingly, that they have carried out successful analyses on the basis of four or three times a week – and even on the basis of less frequent sessions.

More recently Otto Kernberg (1999) wrote in a paper considering the differentiation of psychoanalysis and psychotherapy:

> The only additional characteristics of psychoanalysis that contribute to its differences from psychoanalytic psychotherapy are the frequency of sessions

and the use of the couch. It may be argued that psychoanalysis cannot be carried out below a certain frequency of sessions without becoming 'anaemic', and most psychoanalysts would agree that three or four sessions constitute the minimum for psychoanalytic work to be effective. But in my view neither the frequency of sessions nor the use of the couch is a conceptually significant defining feature of psychoanalysis. . . .

Psychoanalytic psychotherapy usually requires two to four, but no fewer than two sessions per week, in order both to explore transference developments and to follow the changing reality of the patient's daily life. It is not possible to carry out these tasks with patients with severe psychopathology on a schedule of weekly sessions: on a once-weekly session, the time would either be utilised completely by updating the therapist of developments in the patient's life, thus precluding transference analysis, or else, systemic transference analysis under these circumstances may foster the splitting off of important developments (and acting out) in the patient's external life situation.

During the 1940s when the British Psycho-Analytical Society was tearing itself apart in the conflict between the supporters of Anna Freud and those of Melanie Klein, the acrimonious debate was related to serious theoretical issues, even though driven by the highly narcissistic nature of the personalities involved. Grosskurth (1986: 325) says Katherine Whitehorn once described them as the Valkyries of the psychoanalytical movement, and quotes John Bowlby's comment that: 'Anna Freud worshipped at the shrine of St Sigmund, and Klein at the shrine of St Melanie'.

At no time was there any mention of the work of psychoanalysis being conducted at less than five times a week – anything less would have been unthinkable in terms of preserving the 'pure gold of analysis', or of abandoning the fundamental foundations of psychoanalysis which were published in a posthumous article of Freud's. Klein herself had no doubts that what she did was pure gold, and justified it in terms of frequency, in an interview she made in 1958, quoted by Grosskurth (1986):

There was a long discussion about the standard five-times-a-week analysis. Despite the objections of some of her younger colleagues, she was adamant about classical procedure. It is important, she emphasized, to analyze why the patient cannot manage to come five times a week: it might simply be a subterfuge. If he cannot afford to come on a daily basis, then one should reduce one's fees. But suppose, she was asked, owing to other commitments, either the analyst or the patient cannot manage a regular routine. Would it not be heartless, under the circumstances, not to make another arrangement, if the aim was to relieve suffering? She replied that she would describe it as psychotherapy. Well, then, how do you do psychotherapy? Stanley Leigh asked her. 'I really couldn't tell you,' she answered. 'I couldn't do it.' Yet she had already admitted that during the war it had been possible to see some patients only on an irregular basis. (She had told Hanna Segal that during the last part of Paula Heimann's analysis she had seen her three times a week, and Sylvia Payne had seen her only once a week in 1934.)

THE CASE FOR HIGH-FREQUENCY THERAPY

Theoretical considerations, confirmed by the results of our survey, link frequency of sessions to intensity of transference. Balint's view developed in 'The Basic Fault' is that patients who have missed out on a good-enough early infantile experience with their mothers need to regress to this level to repair the damage. He distinguished between benign and malignant forms of regression, where the former leads to healing, and the latter to repetitive, unsatisfied, addiction-like states which cannot be gratified. Winnicott's concept of the holding-environment and the absolute importance of the mother–child relationship led to his use of the term 'regression to dependence', which has much in common with Balint's phrase 'regression for the sake of recognition, in particular, of the patient's internal problems'. Guntrip also developed his own ideas about the value of regression in the therapeutic process, and Kris contrasted 'regression in the service of the ego' with 'the ego overwhelmed by regression', which closely parallel Balint's two forms of regression, benign and malignant.

The purpose of this regression was summarized by Jung in his phrase 'reculer pour mieux sauter' – to return to an earlier, damaged state in childhood to connect, or reconnect, with a healthy internal object, to grow beyond a place of previous stuckness. There is an overwhelming argument that regression to positive dependence can only be attained with increased frequency, and thus that the deep analysis which enables patients to fight their inner destructive, bad objects requires working at a high frequency. The actual relationship to outcome is hard to quantify, and only a small number of therapists who responded to our questionnaire (5.8 per cent of the respondents) thought that outcome could be measured against the frequency at which they worked.

We give below some of the comments of this 5.8 per cent who experienced a quantifiable change in their patients:

'patients who come twice a week conclude the analysis, those who come once a week return'.

'increase in frequency leads to intensification of transference. This leads to elaboration of resistant complexes, and hence to conscious mastery of them. The process can only be effectively tracked with a frequency of 3–4 times a week'.

'increase in frequency of treatment leads to decrease in time of antidepressant medication'.

'greater frequency provides the opportunity to integrate far more unconscious material' (note: there is no indication how this may actually be measured).

'in primary care work, outcome is better at once a week therapy' (note: outcome is not in fact quantified in this response).

'psychic shift seems more long lasting after more intense therapy, but some once weekly patients say it has made a great difference'.

It is significant that outcome as an objective measurement has not been shown to be affected by frequency in any of the literature we have seen on the subject, and the responses to our survey show that over 94 per cent of respondents themselves do not believe there is any quantifiable relationship between frequency and outcome. When we examine the comments above in detail, the result is even more significant, for none of the replies shows there to have been some objectively measurable change. There are, however, some interesting ideas about what differences there might be, related to working at different frequencies, and these could possibly be the subject of further research.

This does not mean that change, related to the frequency at which the work has taken place, has not occurred, merely that we have not until now found a way to measure it. Of our respondents, about 60 per cent could not positively relate frequency to outcome in any form, and only 39.2 per cent indicated they felt there was a qualitative difference in outcome. Although this was a highly subjective response, we believe it is important to value it as a personal experience of almost 40 per cent of analysts/therapists, and we quote below examples of the qualitative changes they noted in their work:

'more frequency equals greater structural change'.

'higher frequency leads to more long-lasting personality change. I increase the frequency when the anxiety level increases'.

'*usually* the outcome is much better if therapy is more frequent'.

'at 4×w, risk of greater dislocation/'breakdown' during the analysis, but also this means the deep problems are reached, the psychic structure can be rebuilt more thoroughly, so the patient gains *enormously* – in practical, external affairs, job, money management, marriage etc. – and in internal comfortableness, strength and peace'.

'real analytical development, as opposed to psychotherapeutic progress, is more likely at 3×w'.

'the more you give, the more they receive'.

The comments should also be seen in relation to the results of our survey about how analysts and therapists actually work in their own practices, and how they would like to work. Actual practice covers a very broad range and the answers have provided us with a mass of information about different working practices in different countries, and in different organizations. We could summarize by saying that current US Jungian practice is conducted mostly at once a week, with a small proportion of twice-weekly work, and with only a few analysts seeing patients more frequently. In Germany and Italy, practice is spread more evenly between once- and twice-weekly work, with a larger amount of three and four times therapy in Germany than in Italy. In the UK, the working practice within different organizations reflects their perceived closeness to the 'psychoanalytic' end of the spectrum; the proportion of once- and twice-a-week work varied between just under 60 per cent and about 85 per cent. Correspondingly, the amount of therapy conducted at more than three times a week was between 15 per cent and 40 per cent.

What we found more significant was that in almost every case therapists prefer working at a higher frequency than they actually practise for most of their work. This discrepancy is wider in the USA, where the average working frequency is once a week, and there is a clear preference for twice a week or more. In the UK, only in the SAP did preferences match working practice, according to those who replied. Approximately 65 per cent of SAP analysts saw their patients twice a week or more frequently, and their preference was mostly for three to five times weekly work (with about a third of those replying preferring to work at varying frequencies), corresponding to actual practice. In the authors' own organization, AJA, over 80 per cent of the analysts who replied see patients once or twice a week, and only 13 per cent work at three times or more frequently. The frequency they prefer to work, on the other hand, is almost entirely two to three times, or more. The pattern in other UK organizations surveyed, including BAP, LCP, IGAP, AGIP and FPC, precisely matched the practice and preference found in AJA. This is an important, but not unexpected, finding from the survey.

Both the authors themselves have mixed practices, partly by preference, but more because of the constraints of time and money. About half of our work consists of once- or twice-a-week work, whereas we both prefer seeing people more frequently – twice, and if possible three times or more. We also devote part of our practices to supervision. In some of the once-weekly therapy, the frequency feels absolutely right and appropriate to the patients, their needs, and their problems; in others, it can feel as if too much time is spent each week in getting through outer events and back into the inner world, which can be frustrating for both therapist and patient.

Our own personal experiences and the responses of other analysts, make us wonder about job satisfaction, and the stress from working with too many psyches. We also wonder how the responses might be coloured by the difference between how therapists actually run their practices, and how they would like to.

The responses point to the majority of therapists valuing the role increased frequency plays not only in facilitating regression, but in dealing with high levels of anxiety, and traumatic early childhood experiences. Judith Hubback in 'People who do things to each other' (1988: 25) writes that if the patient's anxiety cannot be contained at the frequency they are coming, it should be increased until the level of anxiety is manageable:

> The advantage of frequent sessions is that the analyst does not have to be so cautious about the patient getting very anxious and perhaps acting out, because the working through which is not completed by the end of the fifty minutes can be taken up again very soon without the defences having had time to reestablish themselves.

The respondent quoted above who wrote 'higher frequency leads to more long-lasting personality change. I increase the frequency when the anxiety level increases', confirms this view.

The role trauma plays in the therapy has also been considered a factor in determining frequency. If a patient is coming to terms with a frightening trauma, or series of traumas, e.g. child sex abuse or violence, it may be important to see them frequently to offer containment for the feelings that come up as a result of interpreting flashbacks, or repressed memories. A patient Withers (Controversy Seven, p. 236 in the present volume) saw only became able to risk contacting such repressed memories when she moved from once to four times a week.

It is arguable that many of Freud's early cases seem to have been with patients suffering from trauma. We bear this in mind when in Freud's 1918 speech in Budapest he referred to the 'pure gold of analysis' in comparison with the 'alloy' of psychotherapy. The implication of this is that his method of psychoanalysis was the best for every kind of patient, as well as the purest, and the standard of excellence by which all other methods are to be measured was established. Out of this arose the rather simplistic assumption that 'more is better'. In his 1913 paper Freud had stated his own preferred method of working:

> I work with patients every day except on Sundays and public holidays. That is, as a rule, six days a week. For light cases or the continuation of a treatment which is already well advanced, three days a week will be enough.

With the introduction of the 'weekend', standard psychoanalysis reduced to five days a week, and this level of frequency became established historically as one of the external criteria which distinguished psychoanalysis from other forms of psychotherapy. The point at which this became the orthodox established practice appears to be after the International Congress in Budapest in 1918, and the reasons for it were based on Freud's preferred method of working:

> Even short interruptions have a slightly obscuring effect on the work. We used to speak jokingly of the 'Monday crust' when we began work again after the rest on Sunday. When the hours of work are less frequent, there is a risk of not being able to keep pace with the patient's real life and of the treatment losing contact with the present and being forced into by-paths. (Freud, 1913: 127–128)

However, Freud had not valued regression in analytic treatment, seeing it mostly in what he thought were its negative aspects: as a defence mechanism, as a factor in psychogenesis, and as a potent form of transference resistance, and only lastly as an essential factor in analytic therapy. Freud's views were affected by his attitude towards the difficulties Ferenczi got into when working with regressed patients, and he believed 'treatment must be carried out in the state of abstinence or of privation'. The fact that increased frequency led to regression was thus an obstacle to the work, as in his view it would inevitably lead to the patient's insatiable demands for gratification. The experience of object relations' practitioners in distinguishing between the type and degree of internal damage in their patients, and the needs of some patients for recognition as opposed to gratification, has in the authors' view been one of the most important factors in assessing the frequency of working.

As mentioned in the introduction, a review of the literature surprised us with its paucity. There are more articles on frequency of dreams than analytic sessions. The little there is concentrates on process rather than outcome, a reflection we believe of the difficulty of separating them, which makes it correspondingly difficult to examine the theoretical or practical reasons for working at different frequencies, let alone to justify them.

Some of the most interesting writing on the relevance of frequency can be found in papers on supervision. In thinking with a supervisee about the appropriate frequency of work for a particular patient, the supervisor is freer of some of the potential shadow aspects on this subject. Gerrard (1998), in a paper on supervision, uses her personal experience of working at different frequencies, both in her own analysis, and as a supervisor, to discuss the issue in relation to supervision.

In once weekly work she stresses the patient's need for something to hold on to until the next session, whereas in more frequent work there is time to wait and watch themes and patterns develop, and to offer a more sustaining situation during difficult times in the therapy (e.g. negative transference). She also points out that in once weekly therapy the patient will have to do more of the work:

> That suggests the establishment of a strong working alliance, the internalisation of the therapist as a therapist rather than as a transference object and makes regression less likely.

Paul Gedo and Bertram Cohler (1992: 245–250) put forward a probabilistic argument that 'the quantitative increase in sessions per week usually creates a qualitative change in the data obtained'. They also argue that more sessions per week will increase the patient's sense of the holding environment. Both these, they suggest, make a deeper regression more likely, which will then lead to more recurrent repetitions of archaic behaviour as enactments in the transference. They suggest that patients are more likely to acquire missing psychological skills in more intensive therapy.

Christoph Heinicke (1965) hypothesized about outcome of therapy with children seen once a week and those seen four times a week, at the end of treatment and on two subsequent follow-ups. Heinicke stressed that this was work in progress, but his conclusion was that the children seen four times a week were on the whole ahead of the children seen once a week in terms of various aspects of their psychological development after two years.

THE CASE FOR LOWER-FREQUENCY WORK / A MORE FLEXIBLE APPROACH

Jung's own way of working never stressed frequency as being of central importance as a fundamental aspect of technique, and the little he has written about frequency shows him to have varied it according to the needs of his patients. In 'General Problems of Psychotherapy' (Jung, 1935 para. 26) Jung states:

> All methods of influence, including the analytical, require that the patient be seen as often as possible. I content myself with a maximum of four consultations a week. With the beginning of synthetic treatment it is of advantage to spread out the consultations. I then generally reduce them to one or two hours a week, for the patient must learn to go his own way. This consists in his trying to understand his dreams himself . . . hence the interval between consultations does not go unused. In this way one saves oneself and the patient a good deal of time, which is so much money to him; and at the same time he learns to stand on his own feet instead of clinging to the doctor.

Later in the same paper (para. 43) Jung writes:

> The psychoanalyst thinks he must see his patient for an hour a day for months on end; I manage in difficult cases with three or four sittings a week. As a rule I content myself with two, and once the patient has got going, he is reduced to one.

Fordham (1974), who was influenced by psychoanalytic theory and technique, favours a frequency between psychoanalysis and traditional Jungian:

> A study of the distribution of manifest energy released by analysis in relation to the interview bears upon such questions as interview frequency, fantasy, and active imagination, all of which are particularly relevant to analytical psychologists, if only because they have no prescribed standard of interview frequency, but rather relate it to the varying needs of patients under different circumstances. My usual practice is to start with three interviews a week, increasing or reducing the number as occasion requires.

Fordham (1978) also relates the question of frequency to that of fees:

> The subject of fees interrelates with the question of interview frequency. There is . . . a wide range of patients for whom three times a week will be sufficient,

though it is liable to lengthen the treatment; others may do quite well on four times but would do better on five times a week. Less than three times makes analysis, as it has been defined, almost impossible and the considerable range of other less intensive psychotherapies available must be considered.

This contrasts with the more classical approach of Gerhard Adler (1948: 16) who writes in *Studies in Analytical Psychology*:

As regards the frequency of treatment, it is usual to start with two or three hours a week. In certain cases of exceptional gravity it is sometimes desirable and occasionally necessary to increase this number. If there are fewer than two weekly interviews, the intervals are too long and the effect of the analysis suffers. Besides, decreasing the number of weekly interviews does not save the patient anything in the long run, since it merely prolongs the analysis. On the other hand, it is usual not to see patients more than two or three times weekly, because experience has shown that the rhythmical change between the analytical interview and a period of assimilation is most valuable. . . . With the passage of time, that is with the patient's growing independence and towards the end of the analysis, these intervals are increased till the interviews take place only once a week or even less frequently.

Camilla Bosanquet (1988) writes about the confusion caused by the different usage of the term 'analysis' among Jungians. Fordham had pointed out that after 1914 Jung used the word 'analysis' to mean reductive analysis, but this restricted definition has not been kept to, and

the term analysis has now become a colloquial term notable for its high prestige value rather than its specific meaning. This causes confusion. In using the term 'psychoanalysis' or 'Jungian analysis' we need to know whether we are referring to the aims, the process generated in the analysand, or the practice – what we do. . . The aims, the process and the practice all get mixed up in these arguments.

In Jungian circles in general, arguments centre round the frequency of sessions, concentration on the transference, attitude to regression and other factors in efforts to distinguish analysis from psychotherapy.

For Jung the goal of analytical psychology was individuation, the healing of the psyche and the attainment of greater wholeness, and he matched his approach to the needs of his individual patients. Details of frequency, or the use of the couch or chair were external issues which could be varied to further the process of individuation. Psychotherapy was not an inferior form of of analysis, but encompassed both Freud's reductive method of psychoanalysis, and his own symbolic-synthetic approach of analytic psychology: there was therefore no hierarchical relationship between 'psychotherapy' and 'psychoanalysis'.

Other references in the literature are Bertram Karon's (1990) in which he quotes the only known (at that time)

> . . . systematic research on the effects of the number of sessions per week per se on the nature and content of the hour or on the course of the treatment. The nearest to a systematic study was the report of Alexander and French (1946) that reducing the number of sessions per week seemed more compatible with effective treatment than cutting down on calendar time.

In a paper at the 1980 IAAP conference, Crittenden Brookes (1983) writes that '. . . analysts have often been hard pressed to demonstrate a correlation between increased frequency and increased efficacy of therapy'. This paper was written over twenty years ago and little has been written about outcome since then. In his view, therapeutic change cannot take place without relationship and he states his criteria for the setting of frequency with that centrally in mind, but the change/outcome theme is not pursued.

In a paper 'The dose–effect relationship in psychotherapy' (Howard *et al.*, 1986) research showed that with weekly sessions, the greatest improvement in the patients was very early on the therapy, i.e. after only eight sessions. This concurs with other researches which report the major impact as being early on in the therapy, although the point was not specifically made by any of the respondents to our questionnaire, as indicated in the comments quoted below. This could, however, be due more to the way we framed our questions and is something we could take up in a future survey.

Gertrud Mander (1995) writing about once-weekly work, refers to the situation in the UK where frequency has become an issue in relation to registration, where it seems that status is attached to numbers (i.e. working at higher frequencies). She suggests there is a general assumption that more sessions equal deeper and better work, and questions a widely held assumption that deeper analytic work cannot be done consistently in once-weekly work. She wonders whether we know how to correlate disturbance levels and frequency, and whether we therefore rely on our intuition and prejudices. She suggests,

> that it may not be the *quantity* but the *quality* that counts, the quality of the relationship with the therapist and the quality of experience that happens within it and through it,

i.e. the difference in varying frequencies lies in the method not in the goals. If we take Freud's suggestion that the outcome is an elimination of neurotic misery, and a better ability to bear the ordinary unhappiness of life, then the patient and therapist have achieved what was implied in the original request for help. An underlying premise in her paper seems to be that the frequency of work needs to be related to each individual patient, not dictated by prejudices, inflexible theories and need for status either in the patient or the therapist.

Ruth Barnett (1992) explores whether there are any definable differences between two- and three-times-weekly therapy. She questions the assumption that more is better and wonders how this could be evaluated. She raises issues which link with our own thinking, wondering

> . . . whether there might be an optimum number of sessions per week which was best for the particular patient or whether it was more a matter of what the therapist had been brought up to think best and feel most comfortable with, and . . . whether training at more sessions a week also equips a therapist to work at fewer sessions.

She compares her experience in working with four patients who changed frequency in the course of their work with her. In her evaluation her comments are of a qualitative nature, and she suggests that some of the changes she noticed in the work, such as increase in clarity and intensity of how the patients were using the therapy, might also have happened over a period of time if twice-weekly work had continued.

John Beebe, in a private communication, looked at the situation from a slightly different perspective. His formulation is that the patient needs to be seen as frequently as necessary for him or her to sustain, or maintain, a *psychological* attitude towards the material. If patients are capable of maintaining a psychological attitude they can come less frequently. He noted that some patients, if not seen frequently enough, substitute other attitudes, e.g. acting out, or hedonistic, instead of psychological ones.

Amongst our respondents, the majority would like to see their patients more frequently than they do, as stated in the previous section. It is they, and the analysts who work at higher frequencies, who have valued the qualitative difference they experience they find in this kind of work, and whose comments we have previously noted. There are many others who indicate a preference for having a varied practice with patients coming for once-, twice- or more frequent weekly therapy. There are also a large number of people who have commented inversely on frequency/outcome, or who express clearly their preference for working less frequently. Others see a relationship to other extrinsic factors, such as duration of the therapy, not affected by the frequency of the work. There are also comments about the lack of any relationship at all between frequency and outcome, of any kind, and if we add this latter group to those who did not answer this question, they are in a large majority.

We quote below some of the views expressed by the therapists who have a clear preference for less frequent therapy for the different reasons mentioned above:

> 'I have seen the greatest depth at the greatest *in*frequency – patients need space to digest and metabolize sessions'.

> 'psychic shift seems more long lasting after more intense therapy, but some once weekly patients say it has made a great difference'.

'some of the less frequent patients have the most impressive outcomes' (note: these are not specified).

'higher frequencies risk collusion. Any frequency works – frequency is *not* a measure of these criteria of a patient's inner world'.

'greater frequency fosters delusional transference and dependency, less is inadequate, and the work unravels. Twice a week work is easier on me than once a week'.

'more often is easier for me. Some excellent depth work can be accomplished at 2×w, whilst some massive resistance exists at 5×w. It all depends on the patient–therapist fit and motivation'.

'I prefer the minimum frequency which enables the process to continue.'

'once a week working preferred, because I don't want the burden of the client's psyche. Clients can work on their own material in the rest of the week'.

'it's the length of work which counts, not the frequency'.

'in primary care work, outcome is better at once a week therapy' (note: outcome is not in fact quantified in this response).

A word often used by patients, when discussing the frequency which feels right for them to work most effectively, is rhythm. A young woman reported that until she went into therapy she had always assumed that people who came more often did so because they were more disturbed and therefore needed more support. She initially started once weekly, and found it took her almost until the end of the session to open up. She left feeling raw and, out of self-protection, had to close up until the following week to cope with work pressures. Soon she found it impossible to open up at all, and knew she needed to come more frequently. On her initiative she increased to twice a week, and found this rhythm suited her needs; it felt startlingly different, more than double the once-weekly session, and she could let herself sink into the therapy, and feel held and more confident in it.

A more traditional therapist might have proposed three times, or even more frequent treatment for this young woman, and undoubtedly greater depths of regression would have been reached, assuming she had not reacted against it. But she clearly felt that twice-weekly therapy was the right rhythm for her and she stuck to it, tailing off to once a week before ending what she experienced as successful therapy. In Jungian terms, we might say it was privileging individuation over regression.

There is also the rather different Jungian perspective, where regression is a move towards the deeper levels of the unconscious, and for this to be achieved a different kind of intensity may be needed. The ability to enter deeply into dialogue with one's own unconscious, through relationship with one's dreams, or engaging in active imagination, may be done in three-times-, two-times-, or once-a-week analysis. What happens between the sessions may be as important as what happens in them.

QUESTIONS ARISING – THEORETICAL, CLINICAL AND POLITICAL

When we came to look at the questions which arise from the issue of frequency, we found it helpful to think about some of the following areas in the light of the responses to our survey:

• What criteria do we commonly apply for working at a given number of sessions a week, or for changing this frequency?
• How might we examine the difference for both analysts and analysands, of the effect of working at different frequencies, with regard to outcome, content, duration and depth of analysis, as well as the relationship between analyst and analysand?
• What might be the unconscious factors affecting the decisions about frequency?

It is thus with the following theoretical questions in mind that we approach this section:

• Can perceived outcome differences be quantified?
• Can qualitative differences be measured?
• How do we value anecdotal evidence?
• How much do we impose our ideas and theories about frequency on our analysands?
• How much are we willing to listen to what analysands want and value?

The desire of many Jungians to get closer to their original roots has had a major impact on the development of the analytic landscape in the UK. Fordham's work with children led him to the belief that the split between Freud and Jung was a disastrous loss for both of their followers and he worked for good relations between the Society of Analytical Psychology in London, and the British Psycho-Analytical Society. The influence was felt not only in theoretical aspects of the training, but also in the training requirements. By the mid-1970s the SAP had formulated the rule that candidates for training must be in at least four times a week analysis, on consecutive days (this latter stipulation was subsequently dropped), whereas candidates at the C. G. Jung Institute in Zurich at this time were seeing one, or two, analysts concurrently, once or twice a week.

This situation allows the interesting possibility of conducting a blind comparison of Jungian analysts trained at the same time at different frequencies. It raises questions about the quality of analytic experience and the quality of the people trained: is there a discernible difference between candidates trained at different institutes at different frequencies? To what extent is the analytic experience a product of the personalities of the training analyst and the candidate, rather than of the frequency at which they worked?

Gedo and Cohler's argument (referred to above) that 'the quantitative increase in sessions per week usually creates a qualitative change in the data obtained' could provide a possibility for quantitative outcome research but again the focus in their paper is on the difference made to the process, not the outcome. We are led irrevocably to a modernist/postmodernist debate, focusing on the value of quantitative as opposed to qualitative outcome data.

We might expect that papers on assessment in psychotherapy would address the issue of frequency and outcome. Not so. Even in the most recent books and papers on assessment, such as those by Judy Cooper and Helen Alfille (1998) or by Chris Mace (1995), when there is consideration of frequency the thoughts immediately turn to process, rather than to the presenting problems of the patients, and what they might want as a result of the therapy. 'What the patient needs' is a favourite phrase, but the 'goals of treatment' seem to be more related to the therapists' ideas than to the patients'. There is a parallel here with medicine. The patient has an illness and wants to be cured. The doctor decides on how that can happen. The need to be cured is very much in the mind of both doctor and patient. In psychotherapy the patient wants to be healed and the therapist has to decide how that could happen, but somehow the end point often gets lost in the fascination with the process.

In a tripartite paper on outcome studies given to the 1997 IAAP Conference in Zurich, Georgia Lepper, Wolfram Keller and Seth Rubin (1997) made individual contributions on this topic. Lepper wrote about research methods and potential areas of enquiry but frequency is not mentioned. Keller noted that Jungians are not part of the tradition of empirical psychology, as they see the nature of research and claims of generalization in research results to be in conflict with the focus on the individuality of patients. He has been involved in a study in Berlin on the effectiveness of long-term Jungian analysis. Using several means of assessment the results show the effectiveness of this work. There is no reference to the place of frequency except that

> More than three-fourths of the patients examined here underwent analysis (rather than psychotherapy): thus there was empirical proof of effectivity for long-term analysis which is still demonstrable after a mean of six years.

By implication a distinction is being made between 'psychotherapy' and 'analysis', presumably on the basis of frequency, but in this paper there is no comparison of outcome results for these two modes of working.

Few analysts would, in theory, disagree with the notion that the frequency at which therapy is to be conducted must be guided by the needs of the patient. A decision about this may have to take place in an initial assessment interview, often when the analyst has very little information available about the patient's condition and inner needs. What the patient consciously wants from the therapy needs to be considered, as well as the unconscious situation. The frequency recommended for therapy ought also to be determined by the state of mind of the patient, and the degree of infantile regression appropriate to treating the patient's condition.

For the therapy to work successfully, there must not be too great a mismatch between the patient's needs and the analyst's preferred way of working. If we apply this formula to the profession as a whole, we should, in theory, find that patients who would most benefit from five-times-a-week work would all end up in psychoanalysis, and those more at ease working once a week would find an analyst who prefers this way of practising. To some extent this probably happens. If there is no *quantifiable* difference in outcome at different frequencies, then it could be argued that the right people end up working at the right frequency to suit their needs!

Because both analyst *and* patient are involved in the decision on how they are going to work together, and importantly, how frequently, the analyst's personal preferences and pathology can no more be left out of the process than the patient's. On a straightforward, psychological, level, it is likely that many analysts prefer working at higher frequencies, because they are interested in deep exploration of the psyche. Regression to infancy, through an intimate unfolding of their patients' lives, is a way of achieving this. It is the normal human condition to desire intimate relationships rather than superficial ones. This desire, when extended to the analytic situation, might be more connected to satisfying the analyst's narcissistic needs than to healing the patient. There appears to be no quantifiable difference in outcome when working at different frequencies, according to the responses to our questionnaire. We must therefore look for other reasons to determine why analysts favour different frequencies, and why higher status seems to be attached to higher frequency.

It seems possible that standards of excellence have become conflated with frequency of sessions, demands of training have become confused with clinical needs of patients, and assumptions have been made regarding outcome, none of which have been substantiated by research.

We have examined briefly the needs of the patient, in assessing how often they come, and how the natural desire for intimacy may be achieved. The criteria we use are highly subjective, for however objective we try to be, we cannot leave ourselves as analysts out of the equation. We also know that, however well we have been analysed ourselves, we carry our shadows with us, and aspects of our own pathology will be triggered by our patients, and we wonder to what extent our narcissistic wounds may influence the whole issue of frequency.

A letter from one of the respondents to the questionnaire raises similar questions. Her own training included work with patients at frequencies of from once to three times a week, and she commented that although depth can undoubtedly be reached and sustained at once a week, in her view it can also constitute an evasion on the part of both the therapist and the patient, permitting a level of disengagement. The demand for greater frequency can, however, constitute a hopeless quest for an idealized level of intimacy on both their parts. She continues:

I wonder whether the psychology of the practitioner will emerge as a factor in your survey. It seems to me that it is a factor too often overlooked. Are we all that well analyzed? I sometimes think that frequency, both less and more, is implicated in the narcissism of the practitioner. Personally I wonder whether the fact that I feel most comfortable with twice a week work is due to my training or to the space I maintain in most of my relationships!

Reading this reminded us of a question we have sometimes asked: are prospective therapists in some way unconsciously attracted to trainings which satisfy their own personal psychological needs? Finding the right balance between intimacy and distance is one of the problems that challenge all humans in their relationships with others. Too much space leads to fear of abandonment, too much intimacy to fear of envelopment, and there is a constant dynamic between these in all relationships, including analytic ones.

Deeper, more intimate relationships may be more easily forged when we see people more frequently. The respondent quoted above may be accurately perceiving her desire to work less frequently as a reflection of her preference for more space in her other, non-analytic relationships. There is, however, also the possibility that those of us who fear, or are uncomfortable with, intense, intimate relationships in our daily lives may be able to satisfy this need more safely in an analytic framework bounded by the certainty, and limitations of five-times-a-week analysis. In this situation we do not, after all, have to live with the other person for the remaining 163 hours each week. Sustaining a deep involvement with someone for a well-bounded four or five hours a week can be just as satisfying for the analyst as for the patient. Partners and children often complain that analysts have richer relationships with their patients than with their own families.

When we decide the frequency at which a patient should work, there are a number of external constraints, in addition to the internal assumptions we consciously or unconsciously make. Money, where the patient lives in relation to the analyst, work or job demands, and the times each of them have available all play a very real part in the initial decision about frequency. These may be external rationalizations on the part of either patient or analyst to justify coming less or more frequently, and however well we work with our patients' unconscious motives, we may not be free of our own. In the paper referred to earlier, Gerrard suggests that discussions about frequency between supervisor and supervisee, where the frequency is not dictated by issues of training, are a 'luxury'. Surely this should be a necessity rather than a luxury? The decision about what frequency to work at is one of the most important decisions to be made at the beginning of the therapy, and Gerrard refers to the many variables which need to be taken into account.

If demands of training dictate the frequency, the implication is that the variables, such as the ones Gerrard refers to, are not given the consideration they deserve during training. Candidates may lose the opportunity of learning through personal experience, about the needs of patients to work at a particular frequency, if they have to see them more often purely for training purposes. In addition, the candidate's own experience during training may have been restricted to one frequency, both with their patients and in their own analysis. This can only leave the newly qualified therapist lacking in the necessary knowledge and experience to make informed decisions about the frequency to work with patients.

In our questionnaire we analysed the replies of people from those training organizations which require training to be carried out at a frequency of three times a week or higher, to look at the numbers of their patients therapists see at this frequency, and to calculate how many of these patients (i.e. those seen at the minimum training frequency) are candidates in training, or have some connection with training. A summary of responses from all those organizations requiring training at three times a week or higher, shows that only 16 per cent of therapists actually work regularly at this level, and of the patients in three-times-weekly analysis, 58 per cent are in training or are connected with the training, and only 42 per cent have no connection. There is reason to believe that the proportion of patients in training would be even higher in those organizations with a four- or five-times-weekly training requirement, and this could be the subject of future study as the size of our sample did not provide us with any accurate information.

Some trainings do include work at different frequencies, and perhaps there is a case for more of this. There seems to be a general untested assumption that therapists should not work at a greater frequency than their training, but that it is all right to work at a lower one. To our knowledge, there is no objective evidence to support this view, although in the UK the ethical guidelines of some training organizations actually prohibit members from working at higher frequencies than they have been trained at, whereas they are free to work less frequently. Perhaps we should heed Mander's warning that:

> . . . once-weekly work is in some respects more rather less difficult than twice- or three-times-weekly work because of the need to make the hour memorable and meaningful for the clients to encourage them to persist, and because of the pressure of numbers on the therapist who has to hold in mind many people's stories and process more diverse clinical material.

We should like now to look at some of the more unconscious motivations which may surround the question of the frequency at which therapists work, to try to understand better the 'silence' on this subject.

WHY THE SILENCE?

We return to the point that surprisingly little has been written about frequency, despite the implicit assumption that 'more is better'. The issues related to it are often highly political, and have become the focus of divisions and splits within, and between, training societies. It is as if there is an unconscious silence on the subject which gives pause for thought.

Our thoughts on the subject, combined with the responses to the preliminary questionnaire, lead us to the postmodernist view that the issue of frequency is contextually bound to the whole analytic process. We suggest that decisions we make about frequency cannot be free from the interrelationship between the pathology of the patient and that of the analyst. Moreover we suggest that the issue is bound up with the analyst's own individual needs and preferences, with economic issues, with training and with the hierarchical structures of training institutes, and with issues of power, control and politics.

However much we wish to have our patients' best interests as our prime concern, there can be no denying the presence of our own self-interests. When these are conscious we can choose to grapple with any possible conflicts which arise, but when they are semi-conscious or unconscious, then it is possible that decisions we make may not always be in our patients' best interests. The fact that we need our patients in order to make our livelihood may not be a comfortable thought. We need the fees; we need patients; the more often they come, the fewer patients we need; and the longer they stay the fewer new patients we need to take on. Consciously or unconsciously there is the possibility of our personal shadows influencing decisions we make.

We wondered when we started researching this paper why the issue was apparently so much more important in UK than in USA, or the rest of Europe. We should like now to look at some of the possible unconscious reasons for this situation.

The psychotherapy profession in UK is a strong lay profession, and it is not a training requirement for psychoanalysis, or any other form of psychotherapy, for candidates to be members of the core professions of medicine or psychology. Although there are many medically qualified analysts, there is no separate medical register of psychoanalysts or psychoanalytic psychotherapists.

In the UK there is almost no therapy paid for by insurance companies, and the main source of salaried sessional work for psychotherapists has, for the last 50 years, been the National Health Service. High status is attached to consultancy posts in the NHS, and consultants traditionally have a say in the appointment of the staff working under them. In recent years the consultant psychotherapy posts in UK have been dominated by members of the British Psycho-Analytical Society (BP-AS), and membership of BP-AS, or association with it, has therefore been a useful qualification for regular work in the NHS. Psychotherapy posts are sometimes open to all analytically trained members, not just to the medical profession.

Some of the psychoanalytical psychotherapy organizations rely almost totally on the psychoanalysts for their trainings, as they require their training analysts to have themselves been trained at a level of five times a week, even though their own members' training is only, say, three times a week. This effectively locks the psychoanalysts, and the less frequently trained psychoanalytical psychotherapists, together into a position of dependency. Transference issues may continue to bind the two together, and may not always be easy to work through, when the training analyst may also be required to report on the candidate to the training committee regarding their assessment and qualification.

The envy of other therapists not involved in the system is evident, when they describe it as 'jobs for the boys', set up to protect positions and jobs within the NHS.

The results of the questionnaire confirm that the majority of therapists prefer to see their patients more, rather than less, frequently than they actually practise, and the often-quoted view is that it is harder working once a week than three to five times a week. Working with the psyches of seven or eight people, four or five times a week, getting to know them intimately, people generally regard as easier than working with the psyches of 25 or more people. The authors, and other colleagues to whom they have spoken, also note that it is much harder remembering all the biographical details of numerous people seen at weekly intervals, than of fewer people seen every two or three days when the details of the session are fresher in the mind.

When working privately it is not easy to find patients with the time and money at their disposal to attend analysis five times a week, and much of this work appears in practice to be restricted to candidates in training, or with training in mind. Arlene Kramer Richards (1997: 1241–1252) writes of the dilemma of an analyst needing to see a patient four times a week for requirements connected with a desire to become a training analyst. The patient can only afford a set amount a week. Does the analyst see the patient four times a week for the usual price of three sessions to satisfy the institute's requirements, and if so, how is that justified to the patient?

The status of a therapist is linked to frequency by the assumption, within psycho-analytical circles, that a therapist can work with someone at a lower frequency than they themselves have trained at, but not at a higher one. Inevitably this means that the therapist of someone in training must have undergone a training requiring equal or higher frequency than the candidate. A candidate in a psychoanalytical psychotherapy training in the UK, with a three-times-weekly therapy requirement, may want to increase the therapy to four or five times during the course of the training, for their own needs. Their own graduates would therefore not be eligible to become training analysts in their own organization, as their training would have only been carried out at a minimum level of three times.

A similar situation applies to supervisors, as to become one requires going over similar hurdles as to become a training analyst. The profession may then become locked into a rigid hierarchical structure, with three times-a-week (or less) trained therapists on the bottom rung, and five-times-a-week trained analysts, with the status of training analyst or supervisor, at the top. In this 'class' system there is no way a three-times-a-week trained therapist can acquire the status of a supervisor of psychoanalysts.

In addition to the status attached to analysis carried out at higher frequency, professional development continually demands that therapists should improve their skills with further training, therapy, supervision and courses. All too often 'develop-ment' becomes equated with higher-frequency work, and quality is confused with quantity. The whole question of why we work at the frequencies we do is understandably an uncomfortable subject for therapists, containing many shadow aspects of the pursuit of rigour and excellence.

In focusing now on the current UK scene, it will be noted how attitudes towards frequency have become used in a divisive way. The difficulties within the

United Kingdom Council for Psychotherapy, an umbrella organization for UK psychotherapists, which led to the formation of the British Confederation of Psychotherapists, reflected this.

POLITICAL ISSUES IN RECENT BRITISH HISTORY

The extent to which the BP-AS aspire to the pinnacle of analytical excellence is expressed in quite concrete terms in the frequencies at which they train, compared with other psychotherapy organizations, in the UK.

The question of frequency requirement in training is a political issue in the UK. One senior UK psychoanalyst questioned the five-times-a-week requirement for analysis during training, and said that in his view frequency should be chosen, not imposed clinically. For that reason he had decided not to take on any more students.

In the UK, however, there is strong resistance to reducing the IPA minimum to less than four times a week, although the actual application of the five-times-a-week requirement is more flexible than might be supposed. Candidates from Scotland and the North of England only have to have four times weekly analysis, and in Northern Ireland the current candidates have all completed their five-times-a-week analysis with one psychoanalyst prior to training, and do not have to continue it during training. 'Condensed analysis', with double sessions, or two sessions on the same day, is now acceptable in place of the five-times-weekly, equally spaced, 50-minute sessions, especially for candidates from Eastern Europe and in parts of Latin America where long distances have to be travelled to attend analysis.

A fear among British psychoanalysts, which is reflected within the IPA, is that if the general requirement is reduced to three times a week, twenty to thirty thousand people, many from South America, could apply for immediate membership of the IPA. If this were to happen, the important question would be how they could all be vetted so that standards would be maintained.

The view of a senior member of the BP-AS, from his experience outside the UK, was that the British society was the most respected in the world. It is interesting that it is also the most dedicated to five-times-a-week analysis. Standards of excellence have become equated with the rigour of five-times-a-week analysis. In the minds of many people, not only the psychoanalysts who practise this way, there is a strong connection between intellectual rigour, professional standards, psychological clarity and the pursuit of excellence, and the maintenance of five-times-weekly work. The pursuit of intellectual excellence and the exclusion of some members with unorthodox or heretical views may contribute to the view that there is a 'right' way to work if standards are to be maintained.

There is no doubting the commitment and dedication with which many analysts strive for the highest standards, but we wonder if the outer may have become confused with the inner. We are reminded of the British living abroad during colonial times, keeping up standards by dressing for dinner, served on the dot of seven o'clock. Standards were indeed maintained: British justice was imposed, men behaved correctly towards women or each other in the club or in public, and corruption was a serious offence. But there was a shadow side too.

UKCP/BCP (UNITED KINGDOM COUNCIL FOR PSYCHOTHERAPY/BRITISH CONFEDERATION OF PSYCHOTHERAPISTS)

The history of UKCP, and the split within it which led to the formation of BCP, shows how important theoretical differences can become focused on the issue of frequency. The UKCP is a broad-based professional association of about eighty member organizations, each of which is deemed to be a reputable psychotherapy organization in Britain. The Royal College of Psychiatrists, and the British Psychological Society are also members. It evolved out of an earlier association UKSCP, and, in its own words, 'exists to promote and maintain the profession of psychotherapy and high standards in the practice of psychotherapy for the benefit of the public, throughout the UK'. Within the UKCP are many organizations of very different backgrounds, and the early days were spent trying to find a structure which would accommodate them under one roof.

Disagreements among the disparate groups within UKSCP were based on fundamentally different approaches to the theory and practice of psychotherapy, and in particular to the importance of individual therapy for practitioners. The disagreements became focused on training, and the very real differences in standards became equated with the frequency requirements for seeing training patients. This inevitably led to stalemate as the differences were so great in concept as well as in numbers. The simple assumption that more was better made it difficult to examine the underlying differences.

In an attempt to resolve the impasse a federated structure was implemented, with separate sections for different types of therapy. This enabled most of the sections to proceed with the work of establishing standards, and vetting member organizations. It has undoubtedly resulted in higher standards within the profession in the UK.

The largest section was composed of psychodynamic therapists, psychoanalytic therapists, psychoanalysts and analytical psychologists all grouped together. Different ways of working, and in particular, different frequency requirements for training, were too great for them to coexist together. The BP-AS finally decided to leave, taking with them those psychotherapy organizations dependent on them for training, and to form the British Confederation of Psychotherapists. The BCP was formed to represent psychoanalytic and analytical psychotherapy only, and to uphold and strengthen the rigorous training standards prevailing in those organizations they represented. From the start, membership was restricted to associations trained at minimum of three times a week.

BCP felt that their view and approach to psychotherapy was sufficiently different from the general one in UKCP, that dual membership would not be viable. Member institutions could be represented as following one policy by BCP, and another by UKCP, as in their view the two organizations spoke with such different voices. BCP could therefore only adequately represent their members if they alone spoke for them.

Those member associations caught up in this conflict were thus asked to choose between membership of the BCP, with its roots in psychoanalysis and analytical psychology, where many of them felt at home, and the broad-based UKCP. Many of these same associations had been involved in the formation of UKCP and a dialogue was developing across sections of the federally structured UKCP between Freudians, Jungians, and non-psychoanalytic therapists in other sections. Standards of practice within the profession as a whole had been raised, and there had been benefits from the cross-fertilization of ideas and influences, but it has been traumatic for those institutions forced to choose between two organizations offering very different but important connections to the psychotherapy world.

CONCLUSION

If we are to bring greater understanding to why the frequency at which different therapists work has acquired an importance far beyond the apparently straight-forward clinical needs of the patient, then we need more information.

We have been encouraged during the writing of this chapter to think creatively about the symbolic meaning of frequency in our work, why it has acquired such importance yet has had so little written about it, and how this has led to a number of untested assumptions. This paper outlines some of the difficulties we have encountered in trying to untangle the complex, interwoven issues. We hope that further research will give us the information lacking in the literature: how analysts actually work, how they decide the frequency for individual patients, and what effect this has on the therapy.

The response to the questionnaire shows that therapists are willing to cooperate in thinking about why they prefer working at one frequency rather than another, about how they personally experience this in the transference and counter-transference, and what difference (if any) it makes to the 'outcome'. There was some acknowledgement of their own interests and of their patients' needs in their choices. Economic and training demands, questions of status, and politics were implicit in the replies. The difficult issue of outcome was engaged with, and the respondents were clearly concerned about the qualitative and quantifiable aspects: whether it is possible to measure outcome – of primary importance to the patient – objectively in individual analytic work, and if not, how do we best think about it.

There are two interlocking issues here. Analysts are almost certainly more interested in the process of analysis and what this means, than in an outside, 'objective' assessment of 'outcome'. The process of making the unconscious conscious, and of experiencing the inner change and transformation in their patients during the work, is an immediate emotional reward for therapists. Seeing how the process of analysis can lead to this change also brings the intellectual satisfaction of the validity of its theoretical basis. This 'qualitative' valuation of outcome, experienced by patients and analysts, was acknowledged by respondents to the questionnaire.

Our investigations to date have led us to recognize the following important points. Outcome cannot be measured quantitatively in a purely 'objective' way; it is unrealistic to try and separate qualitative from quantitative aspects of outcome; and process cannot be separated from outcome (however it is measured).

We are still left with the unresolved issue of how to approach the question of outcome, of how to know whether the work we are doing is generally seen by our patients to be worthwhile. A retrospective subjective assessment by patients, after the analysis has ended, would we believe be neither convincing nor informative. Problems related to memory of how they were at the start of the analysis, and unresolved transference issues, among others, would invalidate the study. A similar self-assessment before and after, would still have to deal with transference issues, and the question might only be compounded by the analyst's own assessments of the case.

What we need is a research tool which can be applied in a more detached way to each case, involving both analyst and patient before and after the analysis, which takes into account process and transference and gives them full subjective value in the assessments. It is beyond the scope of this paper to formulate what this tool might be, and how it could be applied. We believe, however, that any assessment should be done by both patient and analyst, and cover each of their experiences of the work. It would have to include: tests regularly used in clinical psychology and psychiatry; a description of the presenting problem(s) brought by the patient, and the underlying problems which emerged from these (as experienced by the patient); how these had changed by the end of analysis; the process by which change had occurred; how the patient, and the analyst felt at the beginning and at the end; changes in external life, both related to the original problems, and apparently unconnected to them; changes in the patient's inner world, as seen by each of them, including valuation of highly subjective aspects like meaning, purpose, the numinous, religious feelings, inner connection and the ineffable. It would be implicit that the relationship between analyst and patient would have to be central to such an assessment for there to be a meaningful understanding of 'outcome' in its fullest sense.

We hope the questions we have raised will stimulate further thought and debate on the whole subject.

NOTE

The authors acknowledge with gratitude support from the International Association for Analytical Psychology in a grant for funding the research questionnaire.

REFERENCES

Adler, G. (1948) *Studies in Analytical Psychology*. London: Routledge & Kegan Paul.

Barnett, R. (1992). 'Two or three sessions? A discussion of some ideas about the frequency of sessions in psychotherapy'. *British Journal of Psychotherapy*, Vol. 8, no. 4, 430–441.

Bosanquet, C. (1988) 'The confusion of tongues and the Rugby Conference'. *British Journal of Psychotherapy*, Vol. 5, no. 2, 228–240.

Brookes, C. (1983) 'The effect of frequency of sessions on the analytic process', in J. Beebe (Ed.), *Money, Food, Drink and Fashion and Analytic Training*. Fellbach: Bonz.

Cooper, J. and Alfille, H. (1998) 'Once-weekly or more intensive therapy', in J. Cooper and H. Alfille (Eds) *Assessment in Psychotherapy*. London: Karnac.

Fordham, M. (1974) *Technique in Jungian Analysis : Library of Analytical Psychology*, Vol 2. London: Heinemann.

Fordham, M. (1978) *Jungian Psychotherapy*. Chichester, UK: John Wiley.

Freud, S. (1913) 'On beginning the treatment: further recommendations on the technique of psycho-analysis 1'. *Standard Edition*, Vol. 18. London: Hogarth Press.

Freud, S. (1919) 'Lines of advance in psycho-analytic therapy'. *Standard Edition*, Vol. 17. London: Hogarth Press.

Gedo, P. and Cohler, B. (1992) 'Session frequency, regressive intensity and the psychoanalytic process'. *Psychoanalytic Psychology*, Vol. 9, 245–249.

Gerrard, J. (1998) 'Supervision, its vicissitudes and issues of frequency', in P. Clarkson (Ed.), *Supervision: Psychoanalytic and Jungian Perspectives*. London: Whurr.

Grosskurth, P. (1986) *Melanie Klein*. Cambridge, MA: Harvard University Press.

Grosskurth, P. (1991) *The Secret Ring*. Reading, MA: Addison-Wesley.

Heinicke, C. M. (1965) 'Frequency of psychotherapeutic session as a factor affecting the child's developmental status'. *Psychoanalytic Study of the Child*, Vol. 20, 42–98.

Howard, K., Kopta, S., Krause, M. and Orlinsky, D. (1986) 'The dose–effect relationship in psychotherapy'. *American Psychologist*, Vol. 41, 159–164.

Hubback, J. (1988) *People Who Do Things to Each Other*. Wilmette, IL: Chiron.

Imber *et al.* (1957) 'Improvement and amount of therapeutic contact'. *Journal of Cons Psychology*, Vol. 21.

Jung, C. G. (1935) 'General problems of psychotherapy'. *The Practice of Psychotherapy. Collected Works*, Vol. 6. London: Routledge & Kegan Paul.

Karon, B. (1990) 'Psychoanalysis, psychoanalytic therapy, and the process of supervision', in R. C. Lane (Ed.), *Psychoanalytic Approaches to Supervision*. Philadelphia, PA, Brunner Mazel.

Kernberg, O. F. (1999) 'Psychoanalysis, psychoanalytic psychotherapy and supportive therapy: contemporary controversies'. *International Journal of Psycho-analysis*, Vol. 80, no. 6, 1075–1092.

Lepper, G., Keller, W. and Rubin, S. (1997) 'Research and Jungian psychotherapy: outcome studies', in M. A. Mattoon (Ed.), *Open Questions in Analytical Psychology*. Einsiedeln: Daimon.

Lorr, M., McNair, D. M., Michaux, W. W. and Raskin, H. (1962) 'Frequency of treatment and change in psychotherapy'. *Journal of Abnormal Social Psychology*, Vol. 64, 281–292.

Mace, C. (Ed.) (1995) *The Art and Science of Assessment in Psychotherapy*. London: Routledge.

McNair, D. M., Lorr, M., Young, H., Roth, I. and Boyd, W. (1964) 'A three-year follow-up of psychotherapy patients'. *Journal of Clinical Psychology*, Vol. 20, 258–264.

Mander, G. (1995) 'In praise of once-weekly work: making a virtue of necessity or treatment of choice?' *British Journal of Psychotherapy*, Vol. 12, no. 1, 3–14.

Richards, A. K. (1997) 'The relevance of frequency sessions to the creation of an analytic experience'. *Journal of American Psychoanalytic Association*, Vol. 45, 1241–1251.

Sandler, J. (1988) 'Psychoanalysis and psychoanalytic psychotherapy: problems of differentiation'. *British Journal of Psychotherapy*, Vol. 5, no. 2, 172–177.

Wolff, H. (1988). 'The relationship between psychoanalytic psychotherapy and psychoanalysis: attitudes and aims'. *British Journal of Psychotherapy*, Vol. 5, no. 2, 178–185.

The role of interpreting and relating in analytic therapy

Introduction

In an excellent republished chapter the psychoanalyst Robert Caper explains why he believes that the analyst's task is to address the splits in the patient's psyche without giving in to the omnipotent fantasy he can somehow heal them. This healing is something outside the analyst's control that takes place within the patient and is largely determined by unconscious processes there. The proper analytic attitude is therefore to interpret split-off or repressed material and leave the rest to 'God'.

Analytical psychologist Warren Colman agrees that it is essential for the analyst to resist the temptation to become an omnipotent healer, but asserts that the analytic relationship has a much more important role to play in the therapeutic process than Caper acknowledges. He uses a clinical example to illustrate how unconscious factors *within the relationship* can be crucial in determining outcome. He also believes that the analyst's genuine care, concern, and even love can be crucial in maintaining that relationship in the face of the patient's fear of relating.

Caper replies that there is less difference between the two positions than first meets the eye. The analyst expresses his care, he says, specifically by remaining interested in the patient's material and interpreting it. This factor is crucial in maintaining the analytic relationship. Colman agrees and arguably this rapprochement illustrates a common shift in both analytical psychology and psychoanalysis away from a purely individualistic towards a more relational world-view in recent years. It also reveals the existence of enough common ground between analytical psychology and psychoanalysis to make genuine dialogue possible on these issues.

(a) Does psychoanalysis heal? A contribution to the theory of psychoanalytic technique

Robert Caper

INTRODUCTION

In his 'Recommendations to physicians practising psycho-analysis' (1912), Freud admonished psychoanalysts to 'model themselves during psycho-analytic treatment on . . . a surgeon of earlier times [who] took as his motto the words: 'Je le pansai, Dieu le guérit'' (p. 115).[1]

If he fails to adopt this attitude, Freud warned, the analyst 'will not only put [himself] in a state of mind which is unfavourable for his work, but will make him helpless against certain resistances of the patient, whose recovery, as we know, depends on the interplay of forces in him'. Freud was cautioning his colleagues against a belief that psychoanalysis can, or should, heal the patient. The fate of the analysis is determined ultimately not by the analyst's interventions per se, but by the dynamics of the patient's unconscious. The analyst can only probe the unconscious like a surgeon, while recognizing that the factors governing the patient's ultimate recovery are beyond his control (*Dieu le guérit*).

Far from being the call for indifference to the patient's pain that it has often been misunderstood to be, Freud's analogy between the psychoanalyst and the surgeon is a piece of technical advice based on a realistic modesty, aimed at putting the analyst into a state of mind that is very important, if not essential, for the practice of psychoanalysis. As I will try to show, this modest state of mind also seems to distinguish the practice of psychoanalysis from that of most psychological therapies other than psychoanalysis.[2] Since Freud made this recommendation, certain developments in the theory of psychoanalytic technique have allowed us to see

---

1 Ambroise Paré, the sixteenth-century French military surgeon, when praised for his skill in preventing soldiers' wounds from becoming gangrenous, is supposed to have replied: 'I dress the wound, God heals it'.
2 The distinction I am discussing of course does not depend on frequency or length of sessions, use of the couch, or particular arrangements for payment. These are merely practical arrangements whose purpose is only to facilitate what is essential to the practice of analysis, namely the analyst's adoption of a specific state of mind, one characteristic of which this paper describes.

more clearly its basis in the to and fro of the analytic session. I would like to review some of these, beginning with James Strachey's classic paper on 'The nature of the therapeutic action of psychoanalysis' (1934).

According to Strachey, the patient in analysis perceives the analyst as what he calls an 'external phantasy object' – a phrase that beautifully conveys the fact that what the patient unconsciously sees in the analyst is a mixture of external reality and projected pieces of the patient's internal reality, the two not being clearly distinguished in the patient's mind. One fairly common example of this occurs when the patient projects his own omnipotence into the analyst, so that the latter becomes a magical healer in the patient's eyes.

The patient's tendency to form external phantasy objects is not confined to the analytic setting, but occurs in all of his object relationships. The neurotic's world is full of such external phantasy objects, and, to the extent that the analyst becomes one in the patient's mind, his utility as an analyst – that is, someone on whom the patient can rely for an experience of external and internal reality in which the two are not confused – may be considerably diminished.

Despite this hazard, the analyst must become an external phantasy object for the analysis to proceed. An external phantasy object is simply a transference figure, and when the patient makes the analyst into one by projecting his omnipotence into him, the analyst has merely assumed a transference value. *What is crucial is that the analyst should not join in the patient's phantasies about his omnipotence.* Freud's recommendation seems to me to be directed precisely at this point, the necessity for the analyst to be realistic about his healing powers, if he is to maintain the proper analytic state of mind.

PROJECTIVE IDENTIFICATION IN THE ANALYTIC PROCESS

Since the publication of Strachey's paper, work by Klein (1946) and a number of her followers, including Bion (1959), Rosenfeld (1971) and Meltzer (1966) on the theory of projective identification has allowed us to understand Strachey's observations about the analyst as an external phantasy object in the transference. We now recognize that in forming the transference, the patient projects a part of himself (in fantasy) into the analyst and subsequently feels that the analyst has become identified with this part. That is, he believes that the projected part is no longer an attribute of himself, but of the analyst instead. When the patient elevates the analyst to the status of a healer, he does so by projecting his omnipotence into the analyst, leading himself to believe that the analyst possesses magical curative powers, and that the analytic process is somehow a longed-for realization of his belief in the particular external object called a personal god.

We also know that projective identification in the transference is more than a mere fantasy of the patient. The patient actually provokes (through verbal and non-verbal communication) a state of mind in the analyst that corresponds to what the patient is projecting into him in fantasy. This state of mind is a type of counter-transference that Grinberg (1962) has called projective counteridentification.[3]

Under the impact of the patient's projected omnipotence (and for reasons of his own as well), the analyst may unconsciously agree with the patient that analysis, interpretations or insight are magical, that is, *that they can act as a substitute for the patient's actually solving his problems himself.* If the analyst fails to gain insight into this countertransference, he is in danger of losing sight of his real function, which is only to bring the patient into fresh contact with himself, or, to follow Freud's analogy a bit further, to débride and approximate psychic tissue that has been unnaturally sundered by splitting.

I should make explicit at this point what my assumptions are about the real function of the psychoanalyst. It is to assist the patient to integrate repressed or split-off parts of his personality. This idea has a long lineage, going back to Freud's '*wo Es war, werde Ich sein*' and beyond, but while Freud was probably thinking about something like integrating split-off impulses or affects, I take the role of the psychoanalyst to be helping the patient integrate split-off parts of the personality. By this I mean that the interpretation must ultimately concern the patient's unconscious phantasies of himself in relation to some object, including who the object is, what he is doing to the object, and why he is doing it. This internal object relationship is 'doubled' in the transference, and may be approached by the analysis of what Klein (1952) and Joseph (1985) have called the 'total situation' in the transference.

To the extent that the analyst unconsciously agrees that interpretation or insight can act as a substitute for the patient's actually solving his problems himself, he will abandon his function of helping the patient to integrate split-off parts of his personality and become a magical healer instead. The point to be borne in mind here is that this 'healing' takes place by a process that is precisely the opposite of psychoanalysis: that is, by the analyst endorsing the fantasy, consciously or unconsciously, that analysis, interpretation, insight, catharsis or getting in touch with one's feelings can in itself resolve intrapsychic conflicts and thereby act as a substitute for the patient's actually struggling with these conflicts himself. This helps the patient to split off his problems, rather than helping him to come into fresh contact with them within himself.[4]

---

3   This is perhaps an oversimplified statement of a complex issue. The fact that the patient's fantasy – for example, that the analyst is a magical healer – may find a corresponding fantasy in the analyst's mind does not mean that the patient's fantasy has become more than a fantasy. It remains a fantasy, but has now been joined by another one – the analyst's. A *folie à deux* is no less a *folie* than a *folie à un*, and even mass delusions, for all their impact on reality, are still delusions. How it is that the patient's projective identification can have a real impact on the analyst is an important and complex matter, but to pursue it further here would take us too far afield.

4   The analyst and the patient who are thus in collusion each have their own reasons for believing that the analyst can be ultimately responsible for the patient's mind: the analyst because it supports the fantasy that he can heal the patient, and the patient because it

I would like to illustrate this tendency of analysts to become healers through splitting, and its sequelae, with a case history published by Kohut in 1979 ('The two analyses of Mr Z'). In Mr Z's first analysis, Kohut, as he later recognized, was dominated by a 'health and maturity morality' that led him into 'taking a stand against' the patient's demands on him. This countertransference activity was an attempt to cure the patient of his demandingness. It appeared at the time to work, probably because it forced Kohut to become demanding himself, and this provided the patient with a receptacle into which he could split off and project his own demandingness.

By the time Kohut undertook Mr Z's second analysis, his approach had changed significantly. He was able to demur from the coercive tactics that had formed such an important part of the first analysis. This was clearly a substantial technical improvement, and one that brought obvious and justified relief to both patient and analyst. But now Kohut, having abandoned a technique that unintentionally encouraged the patient to split off something bad into his analyst, began to encourage the patient to do the same thing with his mother. He took at face value the patient's assertions that his psychopathology must have stemmed entirely from his mother's destructive frustration of his healthy attempts to develop. This technical stance was another way of encouraging splitting in the patient. It prevented both analyst and patient from exploring the patient's own contributions to his difficulties, either with his mother or in his first analysis. Kohut's approach interfered with the patient's being able to integrate the destructive aspects of his own personality.

Both Kohut's therapeutic morality and his 'empathic' approach were attempts at healing. Neither addressed or respected the hard reality of the conflict between the patient's constructive and destructive impulses; both attempted to deal with this conflict by splitting off or suppressing the patient's destructiveness. In these analyses, Kohut seems to have crossed over the line of wound-dresser, and to have become something like the god that heals. On one hand, this reinforced the patient's resistance-fantasy of an omnipotent object that will, by 'healing' him, relieve him of the responsibility of finally coming to terms with himself. And on the other, it reinforced his fear that his destructiveness is too powerful even to contemplate, and deprived him of the freedom to communicate about it that he would have had if it had been interpreted.[5]

supports the fantasy that he need never himself assume responsibility or feel the need for reparation and preservation of a good internal object.

5   Kohut indicated that Mr Z's object relationships remained on a rather 'narcissistic' level at the conclusion of his second analysis. This is what one would expect if his destructive impulses were still being projected into his objects, rendering them too dangerous to depend on.

ORIGINS OF THE ANALYST'S NEED TO CURE

The transference, expressed in the patient's projective identification into the analyst, exerts a pressure on the analyst to be an omnipotent healer. But what makes the analyst go along with this process, to act in the fantasy with the patient? Freud considered the analyst's need to cure, which forces him to abandon his realistic analytic modesty, to be a defence against his own sadistic impulses: '. . . I have never been a doctor in the proper sense', he wrote in his Postscript to 'The question of lay analysis' (1927), 'I have no knowledge of having had any craving in my early childhood to help suffering humanity. My innate sadistic disposition was not a very strong one, so that I had no need to develop this one of its derivatives . . . in my youth I felt an overpowering need to understand something of the riddles of the world . . . and perhaps even to contribute something to their solution' (p. 253).

The state of mind that Freud had recommended in his paper on technique can be achieved only if the analyst has come to terms with his own sadism and destructive impulses. The reason for this is that the analyst who refrains from suppressing or splitting off the patient's destructiveness, but instead restricts himself merely to bringing the two sides of the conflict between constructive and destructive impulses closer together in the patient's mind, leaves the outcome of the analysis hostage to the patient's ability to resolve this conflict, a resolution that is, of course, by no means guaranteed. If the analyst has himself not succeeded in coming to terms with his own omnipotently destructive impulses, he will have little belief in the adequacy with which such conflicts may be addressed and encompassed. He will then be loath to risk letting the outcome of all his work rest on someone else's ability to do so.

But if the analyst can recognize the sources of his need to relieve the patient's suffering in his own unconscious conflict between loving and destructive impulses, and in his doubts about the adequacy of the former in the face of the latter, he will (at least temporarily) be free of his need to heal the patient. This will allow him to make an interpretation that simply brings together the disparate parts of the patient – that only describes the immediate emotional situation in the analysis as it is, including the patient's unconscious role in it, without needing to prod the patient into health. This is one of the meanings of psychoanalytic containment: the analyst must contain his need to cure the patient.

If the function of the analyst is to help the patient integrate split-off parts of his personality, a psychoanalytic interpretation would not be an attempt to cure the patient of anything (except perhaps self-deception), but only a communication about the patient's state of mind. In this view, the analyst would make an interpretation because he believes he sees something of the patient's unconscious clearly enough to communicate about, not because he can judge or direct the interpretation's curative impact on the patient. No one can really predict beforehand what it will mean to the patient if one succeeds in one's interpretive attempts to help him integrate split-off parts of his personality. This makes a true analytic interpretation unsuitable as a therapeutic tool in the conventional sense – as a means of bringing about psychic change in any specific 'therapeutic' direction.

THE EMOTIONAL DIFFICULTIES OF PSYCHOANALYSIS FOR THE ANALYST

This constraint on the analyst's therapeutic potency (in the conventional sense of the term) brings to mind Melanie Klein's observation (1937) about a painful reality that parents must accept about their relationship to their children:

> the child's development depends on, and to a large extent is formed by, his capacity to find the way to bear inevitable and necessary frustrations [of life] and conflicts of love and hate which are in part caused by them: that is, to find a way between his hate, which is increased by frustrations, and his love and wish for reparation, which bring in their train the sufferings of remorse. The way the child adapts himself to these problems in his mind forms the foundation for all his later social relationships, his adult capacity for love and cultural development. He can be immensely helped in childhood by the love and understanding of those around him, but these deep problems can neither be solved for him nor abolished. (p. 316)

In the same way, we can say that integration of split-off parts of the patient's personality helps the patient to deal with his difficulties by letting him know what they are, but it doesn't solve or abolish them for him.

This brings us to the difference between working through in analysis and being cured. If the aim of psychoanalysis is to help the patient integrate split-off parts of his personality, then working through would have to mean something like the patient's accepting his unconscious as a part of himself, mourning the attendant loss of self-idealization, and facing the depressive anxieties that follow from this. This contrasts with 'curing' oneself of the newly discovered piece of the unconscious by getting rid of it. Working something through means first facing the fact that one cannot get rid of it.

A dream will illustrate this point. The patient, a woman who had developed an eroticized transference primarily as a defence against awareness of her dependency on her analyst, and who had done a considerable amount of painful and productive work to understand it, had a dream in which

> she approached the analyst 'like a little girl', sat on his lap, put her head on his shoulder, and began to kiss him tenderly on the neck. He then kissed her on the mouth, which left her feeling confused.

In her associations, she made no mention of the erotic element in the dream, focusing instead only on the tender one, and on her confusion about the analyst's reaction, which persisted even after she awoke.

When the analyst asked her if she would be confused in waking reality by a man reacting in that way if she sat on his lap and began to kiss his neck, she realized immediately that her confusion stemmed from a denial of her continued erotization of the analysis. This insight made her quite sad, because, as she said, she thought she had 'gotten rid of that' in the previous work.

This turned out to be precisely the problem. By assuming that this powerful aspect of her personality could be 'gotten rid of' by being interpreted and discussed, she had failed to realize that it was an important reality, not to be dissolved merely by being named. Having now realized this, she was better able to take her unconscious seriously as a real part of her personality, to come to terms with its reality instead of imagining she could get rid of it, which turned out to be an important development in her analysis. This limitation of psychoanalysis as a tool for ridding oneself of unwanted parts of the personality is humbling for both the patient and for the analyst, and this disappointment of one's therapeutic ambitions is one of the emotional difficulties of psychoanalysis.

A second emotional difficulty with recognizing that an interpretation of the unconscious does not rid the patient of it is that it offers no safeguard against the eruption of destructive impulses, guilt and feelings of persecution into the analysis.[6] There is then the constant risk that painful and frightening transferences and countertransferences may arise, without any certainty that they can be contained. This is terribly anxiety-provoking. It is difficult to realize that one has such limited powers in the face of such frightening things.

These difficulties, the sense of therapeutic limitation, and the danger of destructive impulses erupting into the analysis at any moment, are consequences of the analyst's decision to analyse rather than heal and, in psychotherapies other than analysis, tend to be circumvented rather than confronted. In my experience, these painful emotions are reliable clinical indicators that the work of analysis is progressing. If these indicators are consistently absent from what is supposed to be an analysis, the analyst should consider the possibility that a pseudo-analysis has taken over.

A third emotional difficulty for the analyst stems from the fact that psychoanalysis is a very peculiar activity and even, in a certain way, an unnatural one: one is unable to do the natural thing, which is to offer immediate solace, support or reassurance in the presence of obvious suffering. One can offer only support for the patient's attempts to integrate his mind, and the solace that comes from that. And, while this solace is quite profound, it is often quite slow in arriving, and to refrain from offering the more immediate (if less profound) forms of relief is one of the most difficult injunctions of the rule of abstinence. However, if the analyst is to do his job, he must accept the fact that, by withholding immediate solace, he is in a way 'causing' real suffering in the short run for the sake of the greater long-term relief that comes from psychological integration.

---

6 More cure-oriented approaches to the patient prevent the emergence of primitive, psychotic transferences. But in this case they are merely split off into the patient's parents, children, spouse, friends and colleagues, who are left to cope with them.

Viewed in this light, the analytic rule of abstinence – that the relationship between patient and analyst cannot really be that of friends (or even family, despite our frequent use of the parent–child analogy to describe the transference) – is not simply a procedural rule and in fact not a procedural rule at all, but a consequence of the fact that analysis as an activity must necessarily exclude too many of the elements that are vital to any ordinary, natural human relationship. Its power stems from its intense, exclusive and dispassionate focus on the passions of the unconscious. This exclusive intensity produces what Bion called the 'sense of isolation within an intimate relationship' that prevails when each party is aware of his own responsibilities and limits in the analysis.

THE PSYCHOANALYST AS A REAL OBJECT

While it may seem that the analyst's lack of responsibility for whether or not his interpretations heal the patient is a rather cold and inhuman attitude, and perhaps even an irresponsible one, I would argue that precisely the opposite is true – that only by resisting the urge to achieve a cure with an interpretation can the analyst discharge his primary responsibility to the patient, which is not to heal him, but to help him recover himself.

In the long term, this approach brings great relief to patients, even, or rather especially, to more disturbed ones. I believe that this sense of relief arises from the patient's gradual recognition of the analyst's single-minded, even-handed focus on the business at hand, which is to see what is active in the patient's unconscious at the moment, and why. The effect of this is to relieve the patient of a profound anxiety that his inner world cannot be explored realistically, in a balanced way, without evasion, splitting, or the need to fix it immediately.

However, while the healthy part of even disturbed patients feels relief and gratitude at the analyst's ability to bear the patient's projections (as manifested by his ability to do no more than calmly interpret all aspects of the patient's unconscious), a disturbed part of even healthy patients feels that the analyst's exclusive commitment to even-handed interpretation is nothing more than a pointless, artificial device. This part of the patient seems to regard transference figures that act out their roles as external phantasy objects as absolutely real, and the real figure of the analyst as artificial. Such patients will often refer to their relationship with external phantasy objects as 'real relationships', in contrast to the supposed 'artificiality' of the relationship with a real analyst.

What leads the patient to feel that the analytic relationship is artificial is, paradoxically, the analyst's very insistence on being real – his careful avoidance of the manifold collusions with the patient's unconscious fantasies that the patient expects of him in his role as an external phantasy object. The patient may perversely idealize these collusions as ordinary sociability or friendliness, common human decency, or warmth and empathy. This leads him to feel that when the analyst is actually analysing (rather than colluding with) this state of mind, he is not a real person, not friendly, warm or empathic. It is therefore quite important to keep in mind, when the patient feels that one is being 'real' and empathic, that one may be unwittingly colluding with the patient's perverse attack on the analyst's, and his own, reality sense.

While the analyst's real function is to help the patient to integrate split-off parts of his personality, we must also of course recognize that both the patient and the analyst may have unconscious fantasies of a relationship different from this – for example, that when the analyst is doing analysis, he is a lover, child, adversary, spouse, parent or persecutor. But these are still just fantasies. Of course, these fantasies are real fantasies, and they have real effects on the quality of the relationship between analyst and patient (which is saying no more than that transference and countertransference have a real and undoubted impact), but the real job of the real analyst is to identify and understand the meaning of both the transference and countertransference fantasies in terms of split-off parts of the patient's personality, and to communicate this understanding to the patient. In this view, providing the patient with anything else, such as love, advice, guidance, or support for his self-esteem is the analyst's acting in his countertransference, and represents his resistance to analysis.

This is not, of course, to suggest that the analyst should be free of counter-transference, which would be like saying that the patient should be free of resistance. Even if this were possible, it would be antithetical to the interests of the analysis. Resistance is a valuable indicator that we are nearing an important unconscious fantasy, and we would be lost without it. The same is true of countertransference, as manifested by the analyst's urge to do something other than give a non-partisan interpretation.[7]

Partly in response to our patients' transferences, and partly for reasons of our own, we always unconsciously wish to influence our patients rather than analyse them, and quite regularly we put this wish into effect. But one of the things that distinguishes psychoanalysts from psychotherapists is that when we do use suggestion or influence it is unintentional, whereas such deliberate attempts to alter the patient's state of mind is the major therapeutic currency of psychotherapy. And, although we constantly fall short of our goal of simply analysing our patients, we treat these shortcomings not as something we must simply resign ourselves to as inevitable manifestations of our human fallibility (though they certainly are that), but as opportunities – fuel for further analysis. In this view, the analyst is not someone who maintains a 'neutral' stance above the fray, but someone who is always being drawn

---

7 Another, rather striking, connexion between resistance and countertransference is the fact that, when we become aware of a countertransference reaction while doing analysis, our initial reaction is often to feel guilty (or rather persecuted), just as we feel when we become aware of our resistance when having analysis. The forces behind these feelings of persecution, which arise in response to our awareness of what is after all only human in ourselves, are an important obstacle to psychological integration, and need to be understood in detail in each analysis.

into the fray, could not do analysis if he were not in the fray, and who does analysis largely by figuring out what kind of fray he is in.

Klein (1952) and Joseph (1985) have referred to this as the analysis of 'total situations' in the transference, which Joseph described in the following terms:

> Much of our understanding of the transference comes through our under-standing of how our patients act on us to feel things for many varied reasons; how they try to draw us into their defensive systems; how they unconsciously act out with us in the transference, trying to get us to act out with them; how they convey aspects of their inner world built up from infancy – elaborated in childhood and adulthood, experiences often beyond the use of words, which we can often only capture through feelings aroused in us, through our countertransference, used in the broad sense of the word. (p. 447)

Heimann (1950), Money-Kyrle (1956), Segal (1977) and Pick (1985) have also helped to form this view of the interplay of transference and countertransference as a vital element in the psychoanalytic process.

TECHNICAL CONSIDERATIONS

One implication of the view I am proposing, namely that the purpose of psycho-analysis is only to help the patient integrate split-off parts of his personality, is that it is not the business of analysis to deliberately bring about the predominance of one or another part of the patient that the analyst regards as healthy. Success in analysis is measured by the degree of integration, not by the degree to which the patient approximates a standard of normality.

To extend Freud's surgical analogy even further, the task of the psychoanalyst might be thought of as freshening the patient's experience of the unconscious by removing the defensive structures that prevent integration of the unconscious, just as the surgeon would freshen the margins of a traumatic wound by removing the dead tissue that prevents healing. This delicate débridement is obviously to be done with a delicate hand; the dead, defensive tissue must be carefully dissected from the patient's living unconscious experiences, both 'good' ones and 'bad' ones, which are themselves to remain as untouched as possible.

The analyst can only help the patient to think about and experience himself impartially. We may hope that when this integration occurs, good internal objects will in the end predominate over bad ones. We may reassure ourselves by recalling past experiences in which this has indeed happened. But we have no way of guaranteeing it. An analyst, as Meltzer has observed, is like a gardener, weeding and watering the garden so each plant might develop to its full potential. But he does not convert a plane tree into a fir tree or vice versa.

This sobering view of analysis highlights its limits as a therapeutic modality. I believe that these limits are real, and that we should keep them constantly in the backs of our minds. Analysis, like all real objects, is less than we would like it to be.

In a way, this view greatly simplifies the technical demands that the analyst places on himself. He need not worry about the likely therapeutic impact of an interpretation, but only concern himself with giving an accurate, intelligible description of what the patient is doing in the transference and in his internal world, to whom he is doing it, and why. Although I have called this a technique, it would be better to call it an absence of tactics.

In 'Envy and gratitude' (1957), Melanie Klein returned to the technical issue that Freud had addressed in 1912. She wrote:

> It makes great demands on the analyst and on the patient to analyse splitting processes and the underlying hate and envy in both the positive and negative transference. One consequence of this difficulty is the tendency of some analysts to reinforce the positive and avoid the negative transference, and to attempt to strengthen feelings of love by taking the role of the good object which the patient has not been able to establish securely in the past. This procedure differs essentially from the technique which, by helping the patient to achieve a better integration of his self, aims at a mitigation of hatred by love. (p. 225)

This observation touches on the heart of the matter. Omnipotently healing a patient means reinforcing his attempts to split off his destructive impulses, to reassure him that he is after all a good person, and that the therapist, as the source of this reassurance, is also a good person, without ever seriously exploring that possibility that either one may not be. This is a common feature of many psychotherapies. Analysis contrasts strongly with these therapies in that it takes all sides of the patient seriously, so that he may own them rather than merely be reassured about them.

Klein continues,

> There is indeed an ingrained need for reassurance in everybody, which goes back to the earliest relation to the mother. The infant expects her to attend not only to all his needs, but also craves for signs of her love whenever he experiences anxiety. This longing for reassurance is a vital factor in the analytic situation and we must not underrate its importance in our patients, adults and children alike. We find that though their conscious, and often unconscious, purpose is to be analysed, the patient's strong desire to receive evidence of love and appreciation from the analyst, and thus to be reassured, is never completely given up . . . the analyst who is aware of this will analyse the infantile roots of such wishes; otherwise, in identification with the patient, the early need for reassurance may strongly influence his counter-transference and therefore his technique. This identification may also easily tempt the analyst to take the mother's place and give in to the urge immediately to alleviate the child's (the patient's) anxieties. (pp. 255–6)

CONCLUSION

In keeping with the title of this chapter I have concluded with some remarks on the analyst's technical stance. But the line of thought I have been following leads to the conclusion that the stance I am recommending is not a stance at all, in the sense of being a technique that one can simply adopt. It is a consequence of the analyst having attained a state of mind that results from having worked through certain emotional difficulties of being an analyst.

If, as I have assumed, the analyst's role is simply to help the patient experience neglected aspects of himself and his objects as fully and accurately as possible, then the analyst must face the fact that this does not *in itself* provide the patient with a corrective emotional experience, mitigate the severity of his superego, or guide him along the correct developmental path. The analyst's acknowledgement of this limitation – which is equivalent to acknowledging that he can help the patient to grow, but he cannot 'grow' him – places a psychological burden on the analyst that is painful and frightening, but that he must take up over and over again at each step in the analysis, since it is part of a state of mind that the analyst must have to do analysis. It requires him to recognize that his ever-resurgent belief in his healing powers is a countertransference reaction that defends him against his fear that destructiveness – either his own or the patient's – will predominate over loving impulses if the two are brought together and simply left to their own devices. The analyst's belief in these healing powers, in conjunction with the patient's transference fantasies of an object that will cure him omnipotently, forms a *folie à deux* between patient and analyst, a joint delusion that is a vehicle of 'cure' in many types of psychotherapy, but is antithetical to the integrative goal of psychoanalysis.

Finally, to return to Freud's warning that the analyst's failure to adopt the attitude towards the patient that he recommended will put him 'in a state of mind which is unfavourable for his work' and will 'make him helpless against certain resistances of the patient, whose recovery, as we know, depends on the interplay of forces in him'; we can see that the analyst who needs (rather than hopes) to cure the patient is searching for reassurance that his own creativity has not fallen victim to his own destructiveness. The 'resistances of the patient' that this makes him helpless against is the patient's corresponding need for reassurance about his destructiveness. But the patient's recovery, Freud reminds us, depends on the interplay of forces in the patient's unconscious, which are, ultimately and in the final analysis, beyond the reach of the analyst.

The limits that 'dressing the wound' rather than healing it places on the analyst gives an additional meaning to the term psychoanalytic containment: to contain the patient analytically, the analyst must first contain his anxieties about *his* own destructive impulses, and his omnipotent beliefs about analysis that serve as a defence against them. Only then can he be free of the particular derivative of his omnipotence that makes its appearance as an urge to heal, and only then can he be free to do psychoanalysis.

SUMMARY

Beginning with Freud's controversial admonition to psychoanalysts to model themselves on the surgeon who 'dresses the wound, but does not heal it', the author attempts to explore the limits of the therapeutic effect of psychoanalysis. After briefly reviewing the role of projective identification in the transference, and the origin of the analyst's need to be a healer in his anxieties about the strength of his own destructive impulses, he describes certain emotional difficulties that arise in the analyst when he accepts the fact that he can only do analysis. He goes on to suggest that, while psychoanalysis is able to reduce the psychic distance between parts of the patient's mind that have been separated by splitting, this in itself does not provide the patient with a corrective emotional experience, mitigate the severity of his superego, or guide him along the correct developmental path. He further suggests that the analyst's acknowledgement of this limitation – which is equivalent to acknowledging that he can help the patient to grow, but he cannot 'grow' him – is part of a state of mind that the analyst must have to do analysis, and that this state of mind helps to distinguish the practice of psychoanalysis from that of other psychotherapies.

NOTE

This is a revised and expanded version of a paper read at the 37th Congress of the International Psychoanalytical Association, Buenos Aires, July 1991. which was first published in *The International Journal of Psycho-analysis*, Vol. 73, p. 283 (1992). Copyright © Institute of Psycho-Analysis, London, 1992.

REFERENCES

Bion, W. R. (1959) 'Attacks on linking'. *International Journal of Psycho-analysis*, Vol. 40, 308–315.

Freud, S. (1912) *Recommendations to Physicians Practising Psycho-Analysis.* Standard Edition, Vol. 12. London: Hogarth Press.

Freud, S. (1927) Postscript to 'The question of lay analysis'. Standard Edition, Vol. 20. London: Hogarth Press.

Grinberg, L. (1962) 'On a specific aspect of countertransference due to the patient's projective identification'. *International Journal of Psycho-analysis*, Vol. 43, 436–440.

Heimann, P. (1950) 'On countertransference'. *International Journal of Psycho-analysis*, Vol. 31, 81–84.

Joseph, B. (1985) 'Transference: the total situation'. *International Journal of Psycho-analysis*, Vol. 66, 447–454. Also in E. Spillius and M. Feldman (Eds), *Psychic Equilibrium and Psychic Change, Selected Papers of Betty Joseph*. London: Routledge.

Klein, M. (1937) 'Love, guilt and reparation', in *Love, Guilt and Reparation and Other Works, 1921–1945*. New York: Macmillan, 1984, pp. 306–343.

Klein, M. (1946) 'Notes on some schizoid mechanisms', in *Envy and Gratitude and Other Works, 1946–1960*. London: Hogarth Press, 1975, pp. 1–24.

Klein, M. (1952) 'The origins of transference', in *Envy and Gratitude and Other Works, 1946–1960*. London: Hogarth Press, 1975, pp. 48–56.

Klein, M. (1957) 'Envy and gratitude', in *Envy and Gratitude and Other Works, 1946–1960*. London: Hogarth Press, pp. 176–235.

Kohut, H. (1979) 'The two analyses of Mr Z'. *International Journal of Psycho-analysis*, Vol. 60, 3–27.

Meltzer, D. (1966) 'The relation of anal masturbation to projective identification'. *International Journal of Psycho-analysis*, Vol. 47, 335–342.

Money-Kyrle, R. (1956) 'Normal countertransference and some of its deviations'. *International Journal of Psycho-analysis*, Vol. 37, 360–366. Also in E. Spillius (Ed.), *Melanie Klein Today, Developments in Theory and Practice*, Vol. 2, pp. 22–33.

Pick, I. (1985) 'Working through in the countertransference'. *International Journal of Psycho-analysis*, Vol. 66, 157–166. Also in E. Spillius (Ed.), *Melanie Klein Today, Developments in Theory and Practice*, Vol. 2, (1998) pp. 34–47.

Rosenfeld, H. R. (1971) 'Contribution to the psychopathology of psychotic states: the importance of projective identification to the ego structure and object relations of the psychotic patient', in E. Spillius (Ed.), *Melanie Klein Today, Developments in Theory and Practice*, (1988) Vol. 1, pp. 117–137.

Segal, H. (1977) 'Countertransference', in *The Work of Hanna Segal*. New York: Jason Aronson, 1981, pp. 81–87.

Strachey, J. (1934) 'The nature of the therapeutic action of psychoanalysis'. *International Journal of Psycho-analysis*, Vol. 50, 275–292 (1969).

(b) Interpretation and relationship: ends or means?

Warren Colman

INTRODUCTION

Robert Caper's chapter contains a specific argument about analytic practice and technique embedded in a more general outline of the nature of psychoanalysis per se. The specific argument warns against the dangers of therapeutic omnipotence which he associates with a need to cure in the analyst, derived from the analyst's own unresolved conflicts about his or her destructiveness. As a result, the analyst may be drawn into unhelpful collusions with the patient and/or be unable to tackle the more destructive aspects within the therapeutic relationship. The argument is put with great lucidity and is persuasive and enlightening. The difficulty to which he refers is a common one and the paper is to be strongly recommended (especially to trainees) on these grounds.

My disagreement with Caper concerns the more general argument about 'healing' which gives the paper its title. Here I believe that Caper overstates the case by arguing that the specific critique of therapeutic omnipotence must necessarily be embedded in a view of analytic practice which entirely eschews the positive value of the relationship between therapist and patient. Where Caper sees the argument as being concerned with differing aims, I see it as being concerned with differing means. That is, I wish to argue that it is possible to maintain a broader view of therapeutic practice while still being committed to essentially the same aims.

In particular, Caper privileges interpretation as the only proper activity of the analyst and therefore the only means by which psychic change may be brought about. In my view, this restrictive definition fails to offer an adequate conceptualization of the therapeutic process. I shall argue that the therapeutic action of psychoanalysis occurs directly through the relationship between analyst and patient, rather than through the interpretation of its transference elements. Analysis of the transference then becomes the means by which the relationship is furthered as opposed to the Kleinian view espoused by Caper in which the relationship is seen only in terms of its transference elements and therefore as grist to the mill of interpretation. This then leads to an alternative view of the *site* of therapeutic action/change: where Caper places this *within* the patient in terms of what use (or not) is made of interpretations, I would argue that the purpose of interpretation is to foster the conditions in which something takes place *between* patient and analyst that may be called healing. This does not imply that such healing constitutes 'cure', let alone that it is within the omnipotent control of the analyst. While this in no way reduces the emotional difficulties of being an analyst outlined by Caper, it does suggest that the analyst's role is considerably more than that of an interpreter. This carries with it anxieties of its own which, arguably, may be greater than those of Caper's 'interpretation only' model.

THE AIMS OF ANALYSIS: NON-OMNIPOTENT HEALING

It is not the case, as is sometimes asserted, that psychoanalysis has no aims other than 'simply analysing' (Dreher, 2000). Rather, as Caper points out, true psycho-analysis does not have *methodological* goals, i.e. the use of specific techniques to bring about specific results. Although Caper argues that psychoanalysis does not heal, he does propose that the aim of psychoanalysis is to assist the patient to 'recover himself' by the integration of split-off and neglected parts of his person-ality. These aims seem to me to be fully congruent with those proposed by other analysts, including Jung, who do regard analysis as a healing procedure. For example, 'integration' is essentially similar to Jung's concept of individuation, defined as 'becoming the person you already are', 'becoming an individual' and 'becoming whole'. A similar emphasis on self-discovery can be found in the British Object Relations School where, for example, Guntrip, perhaps following Winnicott refers to the patient 'finding his own true self' (Guntrip, 1974: 839) and Balint describes a process whereby the patient is 'able to find himself' (Balint, 1968: 179).

Balint is particularly significant here since he explicitly refers to 'the healing power of relationship'. He goes on to state: 'we are compelled to recognise that the two most important factors in psychoanalytic therapy are interpretations and object relationship' (Balint, 1968: 159). Yet Balint is also assiduous in his warnings against the dangers of omnipotence, amongst which he includes the dangers of omnipotent interpretation, as well as the idea of 'corrective emotional experience'. Caper rather throws the baby out with the bathwater here: it is not *healing* that is the problem, it is *omnipotent* healing (or, rather, the fantasy of it). Since Caper does not distinguish between healing and a magical fantasy of omnipotent healing, he is led to conclude that healing depends entirely on the forces at work within the patient's unconscious, rather than in the quality of relationship that includes not only the patient's but also the analyst's unconscious. It may indeed be God that heals, but the fact that the analyst is not God does not mean he has no part in healing. For healing to take place, both patient *and* analyst must be open to the 'Holy Spirit' that is constellated between them. This process is strikingly represented in metaphorical form in Jung's commentary on *The Rosarium*, especially figure 9 'The return of the soul'. In this picture the soul is pictured as a naked child, the *aqua divina* descending through the clouds to breathe life into the fused dead body of the 'King and Queen' (Jung, 1946: 283–287).

DESTRUCTIVENESS AND DEPENDENCE ON A GOOD OBJECT

It is clear that Caper regards his main interpretative thrust as being directed towards the way the patient defends himself against knowing about his own destructiveness. Resistance to analysis therefore is primarily the patient's resistance to *knowing the truth about himself*. While this is undoubtedly important, and is indeed the central issue for some analysands, I consider that the defensive structures which are restricting the patient, both in their internal life and in their relation to other people ('external objects') may also concern their fear of dependence on a good object. As it happens, Caper does himself give an example of a patient who defended against her dependency on the analyst by means of an eroticized transference but it is significant that he describes this as 'a defence against *awareness* of her dependency' – i.e. that the issue is not the avoidance of dependency itself but the avoidance of *knowing* about it. In my view, such defences are not merely defences against *awareness* but against *relationship* – the patient does not actually allow herself to be dependent in the first place This is because the patient suffers from a paralysing doubt about the existence of a good object with whom she can have a loving relationship – that is, a relationship in which she is able both to love and to be loved.

The demand that the analyst 'take the role of the good object' as Klein puts it, may be seen as an aspect of this anxiety and the defence against it. What such patients require is not a good object at all but an *ideal* one – a distinction that Caper, following Klein, fails to make. Thus Klein says 'this identification may also easily tempt the analyst to take the mother's place and give in to the urge immediately to alleviate the child's (the patient's) anxieties' (Klein, 1957: 226; quoted in Caper). This is hardly a recipe for good mothering, any more than good analysis. The fantasy of all-providing 'ideal' mother, whether in the infant or in the patient is actually a defence against the fear of the bad mother: it reflects an inner doubt whether a truly good object exists at all. While anxieties about their own destructiveness or 'badness' often play a part in this, the central issue is whether a good object exists that can be relied upon to contain and sustain the patient or whether they are condemned to the loneliness of their narcissistic isolation. The primary anxiety is the fear of annihilation, a state of non-being, and it is to avoid this potential catastrophe that the patient maintains his/her defensive state. This means that the patient is fundamentally and primarily defended, not against knowledge of their own destructiveness but against a relationship which is seen as threatening their existence.

This obviously has an impact on the kind of interpretations the analyst makes. It is not enough to interpret the patient's resistance to relating to the analyst as 'destructive attacks' for example (Symington, 1985): the most important thing is to analyse the anxieties which underlie the attacks, thereby facilitating the patient's capacity to let go of his defensive limitations and allow himself to engage in depth with another person. In my view it is this engagement at depth which is the therapeutic factor, enabling change to take place within the patient through the influential impact of another person, the analyst.

PROJECTIVE IDENTIFICATION AND TWO-PERSON RELATIONSHIPS

Although the Kleinian school do take the relationship between analyst and patient very seriously, they do so purely in terms of the way it enacts the phantasies of the patient's internal world. The analyst's emotional involvement is then seen only in terms of the way he is in 'drawn in' to participating in the patient's phantasies (Joseph, 1985). In other words, the analytic relationship is construed entirely in terms of its phantasy elements. Beyond this, there is, as Strachey (1934) originally defined it, a 'real analyst' and the more the patient emerges from his or her transference, the more s/he will be able to recognize the reality of the analyst's activity. But does the real analyst *actually* care about the patient – is the real analyst *actually* warm and empathic, for example? Apparently, this is of no importance since, even if he does care, Caper regards anything which demonstrates it as 'resistance':

> In this view, providing the patient with anything else [other than interpretation], such as love, advice, guidance, or support for his self-esteem is the analyst's acting in his countertransference, and represents his resistance to analysis.

In which case, it hardly makes any difference whether the analyst cares or not and it is perhaps better if he does not. Actually, this is hogwash. In reality, I believe that all successful analysts *do* care about their patients a great deal and are personally involved with them at a deep level. The point I am making concerns how this is theorized. In my view, far from 'resistance', the analyst's care and, frequently, love for his patient makes an enormous difference to the outcome of the treatment (Gerrard, 1996). While this view, which emphasizes the importance of the actual relationship can accommodate the success of a 'transference is all' approach insofar as the latter does include a deep emotional relationship, the reverse is not the case. The 'transference is all' model which disregards the analyst's actual behaviour as a caring figure ('good object') for the patient cannot account for the success of any approach which does not lay the same stress on interpretation of the transference. Proponents of this model, including Caper, are then reduced to denigrating alternative approaches as merely 'psychotherapy' and disparaging their results. As I have already shown, there are many analysts who take a quite different view of the analytic process yet in all essential respects are wholly psychoanalytic in their thinking, attitude and practice.

What is missing in Caper's conceptualization of the analyst's function is that element which *requires* a two-person relationship – the interrelationship of two subjective persons which is not reducible to the phantasies that one person has about the other. The patient seeks not only knowledge of himself but also the recognition, understanding and intimacy within which that knowledge may be realized and through which it may develop and grow. In theory, a patient might come to knowledge of himself through some such heroic self-analysis as that which Freud famously undertook, if only he were sufficiently able to see through his own defences. But no-one can have the *experience* of recognition, understanding and intimacy except through a relationship with another person. This dimension of intersubjectivity plays no part in Kleinian theory due to the hegemony of the theory of projective identification as the explanatory model for two-person interactions. There is simply no other means of conceptualizing the influence and impact that one person can genuinely have on another. Furthermore, this kind of influence is then eschewed as being inherently tied to pathological, narcissistic states in which, due to a failure of differentiation between self and object, the reality of the other is abrogated. This is one of the reasons why Caper eschews any influence that the analyst may have on the patient other than via his interpretations.

EMPATHY, COLLUSION AND MUTUAL INFLUENCE

In his zeal to prevent the analyst acting as the patient's external phantasy object, Caper explicitly argues against any kind of real empathy on the part of the analyst as a collusion:

> The patient may perversely idealize these collusions as ordinary sociability or friendliness, common human decency or warmth and empathy. . . . It is therefore quite important to keep in mind, when the patient feels that one is being 'real' and 'empathic', that one may be unwittingly colluding with the patient's perverse attack on the analyst's and his own, reality sense.

This is rather confusing and I believe, potentially dangerous, since it may lead some analysts/therapists to stifle any expression of empathy in the misguided belief that this makes them more 'analytic'. They avoid colluding with the positive transference only at the price of colluding with the negative one – and with the demands of their own analytic superego for adherence to the 'correct' position. Caper's statement is, at best, ambiguous, if not misleading. On the one hand, he implies that the analyst *is* a real person, friendly warm and empathic, and it is only that the patient feels he is not. But he then warns that if the analyst actually displays that warmth and empathy he may be colluding with the patient. Surely it is bound to have an inhibiting effect on the analyst's relation to the patient if he is all the time worrying whether any warm and positive feeling between them is 'unwittingly colluding with the patient's attack'? How is the analyst to know? In fact, there is a way to know but Caper does not say what it is – the way to know is for the analyst to trust his countertransference.

In my experience there is a real and obvious difference between perverse collusion and real empathy, warmth, kindness and love for the patient. In the former, the analyst always feels anxious, guilty and resentful and feels himself to be under a compulsion to act in certain ways. This is strikingly different from situations in which loving feelings occur in the context of a freedom from compulsion and a sense of space to think with the patient. Then the analyst feels that his activity stems from his own internal free choice and this creates a benign circle of mutual affection and gratitude between him and his patient which may go beyond 'positive trans-ference' into an acknowledgement of the *reality* of the good experience that is taking place. For this to happen, though, the analyst does need to be free of his own superego demands and this does very much include the kind of 'need to cure' that Caper defines so well. It is unfortunate then that Caper's argument takes such a prescriptive and proscriptive form. In my view, this obscures his efforts to release analysts from the internal demand to be 'positive' by seeming to offer an alternative injunction that they should not be.

I think Caper's remarks could more usefully be put the other way around, viz.: 'it is important to keep in mind that when the patient accuses the analyst of *not* being warm and empathic, that the patient may be trying to press the analyst into colluding with the patient's perverse idealizations etc.' This I think *is* helpful since it relieves the analyst of guilt and enables him to keep his bearings under this kind of pressure. But it is also important to bear in mind that when the patient feels one is being real and empathic it may be because one *is* being warm and empathic and the patient is able to recognize it and be grateful for it. In these circum-stances I believe that the transference is transcended and it becomes more appropriate to speak, as Jung does, of transformation produced by a process of mutual influence.

> By no device can the treatment be anything but the product of mutual influence, in which the whole being of the doctor as well as that of his patient plays its part. . . . Hence the personalities of doctor and patient are often infinitely more important for the outcome of the treatment than what the doctor says and thinks. For two personalities to meet is like mixing two different chemical substances: if there is any combination at all, both are transformed. (Jung, 1929: para. 163)

Jung emphasizes that the influence proceeds from the actual personality of the analyst ('doctor'), that is it arises from the *self*, from who the analyst *is*, and is not under the control of the ego. I believe that the patient, often unconsciously, attends closely to the whole manner of the analyst's being-with-the-patient and that the way the analyst is makes a deep impression on the patient beyond anything that the analyst says or overtly does. This is something quite different from 'suggestion' in which the patient is more or less unconsciously bamboozled into getting better by the analyst's conscious or unconscious persuasion. Effectively, 'suggestion' is a kind of collusion involving the patient unconsciously identifying with the analyst's projections.

Real influence is also far more extensive than any process that might occur directly through the analyst's interpretations (presumably even Caper could not object to 'influence' of this nature). To paraphrase an aphorism originally about education, 'Analysis is what is left after the interpretations have been forgotten'. This may constitute a further emotional demand of analytic work in that the analyst cannot control or even know what kind of influence he is having. Apart from not knowing what the fate of his interpretations may be, he does not even know whether it is his intentions that are likely to be the most effective factor in the treatment. He does not have the security offered by Caper's model that as long as he is 'simply analysing' he is bound to be on the right track. Other factors, he knows not what, why or wherefore, may be called forth from him and for long periods or even permanently, he may not know or understand why he is doing what he is doing or what impact it is likely to have. In a very real sense, the analyst must put his trust in the 'god that heals', in the Self that is constellated between him and his patient. This is also what I take Bion to mean by 'being in O'.

For this reason, I am wary of a stance which continually warns of the dangers of enactment and the need to analyse projections. The danger is that the analyst will become over-zealous in his endeavours to convert enactments and projections into interpretations and will not allow sufficient time for the spontaneous development of the unconscious process between analyst and patient. In Bion's terms, K must defer to O; in Jung's terms, the ego must give way before the greater (and unknown) wisdom of the Self.

CLINICAL EXAMPLE

Ms A was in analysis with me for many years. During that time she consistently treated me as a feared and dangerous object that she felt she needed to control since, by the mirror image of projective identification, she felt that I was trying to control her. By a projective reversal, I also felt myself to be under attack from a very powerful but invisible destructive part of her and my response was dominated by a sort of 'heroic' endurance and a determination not to give up hope but to go on believing in her and the analysis despite her repeated insistence that it was damaging her. There was no doubt in my mind that she had got inside me in a big way and I would certainly see this in terms of projective identification. However, I was perplexed by the fact that her conviction was exactly the opposite: she was convinced that she could have no impact on me whatever and this was precisely what made me so threatening and made her feel so hopeless.

Eventually, without any of this being resolved, we agreed to end the analysis, leaving me with a sense of disappointment and relative failure, since Ms A seemed almost as depressed and hopeless at the end as she was at the beginning. It seemed that she had been unable to allow herself to come together with me into any fruitful intercourse, that we had not been able to achieve a *conjunctio* – the process that Jung describes as 'mutual influence'.

A few years later, she came to see me again following a further bout of depression and therapy was resumed on a once-weekly basis. Gradually it became apparent that the main purpose of this was to review and, hopefully, to resolve the difficulties that had been left unresolved when the analysis ended. In the interval, various experiences had helped her to feel that she could risk allowing herself to be influenced and 'still be me' – i.e. her existential dread of non-being had lessened. She was now able to acknowledge the positive feelings she had for me, especially that I had 'hung on in there' and showed that I could stand her hatred and despair in a way she had felt her parents had been unable to do. The fact that she had come back to see me – and that I had been prepared to take her on again – showed both of us that this was a relationship of mutual value and enabled her to feel, as I put it, that 'it's alright with me for you to be not alright'. In saying this, I understood for the first time the meaning of my 'heroic' endurance. This was what Ms A had called forth from me, from the core of my own inner being, in order for her to discover that the good object could survive the worst of her destructive attacks. And now she was able to return in order to make reparation to me and express her gratitude for what I had done. This in turn, of course, transformed her internal state since, instead of a feared and dangerous object who had to be resisted, I had now become a good object who could love her and whom she could love.

It is important to stress that this was not a process occurring only in phantasy or in the patient's internal world. My actual psychic survival was vital in the process and depended on the mobilization of my own capacities for determination and endurance. Behind the negative transference in which I was hated and feared, Ms A had needed me to be the good object for her. Interpreting this was by no means enough – I had actually to *be* the good object and the fact that I did really care about my patient, that she could actually make me suffer terribly when I saw her destroying herself and that I did not give up on her – all this was vital in the eventual rapprochement that enabled her to feel that she had the capacity to go on being herself. Since this was an unconscious process it could not be interpreted since, by the time it had become available for conscious understanding, the necessary work had already been done.

'THE FRAY'

I have had several experiences of this kind where it is only much later in the work that I have come to understand why I have felt or behaved the way I have, and on each occasion it has been apparent that my way of being with the patient has been what the patient needed. In my view, it would be a travesty of the truth to describe this in the terms used by Betty Joseph and quoted by Caper to describe 'how patients try to draw us into their defensive systems, how they unconsciously act out with us in the transference, trying to get us to act out with them' (Joseph, 1985: 447). My endurance and so forth was certainly a countertransference response but how can something so obviously therapeutic, so deeply valued by the patient as to be the source of her gratitude and love and the occasion for the restoration of her good object, how can this be described as 'acting out with the patient'? And yet what choice does the Kleinian model leave us? Let us attend very closely to what Caper does say about the emotional involvement which characterizes every analysis.

> . . . although *we constantly fall short of our goal of simply analysing our patients*, we treat these *shortcomings* not as something we must simply resign ourselves to as inevitable manifestations of our human fallibility (though they certainly are that), but as opportunities – fuel for further analysis. In this view, the analyst is not someone who maintains a 'neutral' stance above the fray, but someone who is always being drawn into the fray, could not do analysis if he were not in the fray, and who does analysis largely by figuring out what kind of fray he is in. (italics added)

While Caper makes a full acknowledgement of the analyst's emotional involvement in 'the fray' this involvement is nevertheless seen as a 'shortcoming' as 'falling short of our goal'. The ideal situation to which the analyst is constantly referring in his mind is one in which he does *not* get drawn into the fray and it is this hypothetical point to which he is continually trying to return as a means of orienting himself to what is happening in the fray and guiding his interpretative behaviour. The fray the analyst is in is not regarded as the therapeutic process itself but simply a means to the true end of analysis, as the 'fuel' for 'simply analysing'. This point is brought out even more strongly by Betty Joseph:

> Throughout the history of psychoanalysis, the need for *an uncontaminated transference* has been stressed. If we allow ourselves to be manipulated in this way, the transference situation becomes blurred and then we are cut off from parts of the ego with which we need to make contact. (Joseph, 1975, italics added)

It is quite clear from these remarks that Joseph is recommending an implicit injunction to analysts *not* to get drawn into the fray, even while acknowledging that they do.

I believe that the ideal of 'an uncontaminated transference' is not merely impossible – it is also undesirable. In fact, the situation is the reverse of the one advocated by Joseph: in cases such as the one I have described, it is only by their analysts allowing themselves to become 'contaminated' that our patients are able to make contact with lost or undeveloped parts of themselves.

This turns Caper's view of the fray on its head. The fray is not merely 'fuel for further analysis' – it *is* the analysis, not a means to an end but the end itself. I suggest that the experience of mutual interaction and involvement that goes on between analyst and patient *is* the goal of analysis and that interpretation is merely the means by which this goal is promoted. The aim of interpretation is to make possible an experience of the *conjunctio*, the coming together of patient and analyst in an intersubjective whole of mutual relatedness.

This shifts the model of the analytic container from the analyst's mind, as Bion thinks of it, to the analytic relationship itself, the analytic *vas*, as Jung calls it, in which containment occurs via the relationship, the emotional struggle and toing and froing that takes place between patient and analyst – in other words, via the fray. The fray is the container, as well as that which is contained. The analyst's task is to manage the boundaries of the container so that is both sufficiently firm and sufficiently flexible for the patient's needs while applying 'heat' in the form of interpretations. The resulting ferment does not merely take place within the patient's mind but in the intersubjective field between the two participants. Out of this ferment, if all goes well, the patient finds what he or she needs.

ACKNOWLEDGEMENT

With gratitude to Elizabeth Gee who taught me more than either of us knew at the time.

REFERENCES

Balint, M. (1968) *The Basic Fault: Therapeutic Aspects of Regression*. London: Routledge.

Dreher, A. U. (2000) 'Changing aims in psychoanalysis'. *British Journal of Psychotherapy*, Vol. 16, no. 4, 434–446.

Gerrard, J. (1996) 'Love in the time of psychotherapy'. *British Journal of Psychotherapy*, Vol. 13, no.2, 163–173.

Guntrip (1974) 'Psychoanalytic object relations theory: The Fairbairn–Guntrip approach', in *American Handbook of Psychiatry*, Vol. 1: *The Foundations of Psychiatry*. pp. 828–842. New York: Basic Books.

Joseph, B. (1985) 'Transference: the total situation'. *International Journal of Psycho-analysis*, Vol. 66, 447–454.

Jung, C. G. (1929) 'Problems of modern psychotherapy'. *Collected Works*, Vol. 16. London: Routledge & Kegan Paul.

Jung, C. G. (1946) 'The psychology of the transference'. *Collected Works*, Vol. 16. London: Routledge & Kegan Paul.

Joseph, B. (1975) 'The patient who is difficult to reach', in M. Feldman and E. B. Spillius (Eds), *Psychic Equilibrium and Psychic Change: Selected Papers of Betty Joseph*. London: Routledge, 1989.

Klein, M. (1957) 'Envy and gratitude', in *Envy and Gratitude and Other Works, 1946–1960*. London: Hogarth Press, 1975, pp. 176–235.

Strachey, J. (1934) 'The nature of the therapeutic action of psychoanalysis', *International Journal of Psycho-analysis*, Vol. 15, 127–159. Reprinted: Vol. 50, 275–292 (1969).

Symington, J. (1985) 'The survival function of primitive omnipotence'. *International Journal of Psycho-analysis*. Vol. 66, 481–486.

(c) Response to Coleman

Robert Caper

Warren Colman's discussion is partly a consideration of what I wrote in my paper and partly a dispute with what he calls the Kleinian view. Since I am unsure of what the 'Kleinian view' encompasses, I will respond only to what he said about my views, leaving the Kleinian view to fend for itself except insofar as it seems to correspond to my views. The first thing that strikes me about Colman's discussion is that, between my position and his, there is much less disagreement than meets his eye. I agree with him that the problem I am addressing in this chapter is not healing per se, but omnipotent healing. I indicate this at the beginning of the chapter when I write that, when the patient wishes for the analyst to be a magical healer, what is crucial is that the analyst not join in the patient's phantasies about his omnipotence. I make this same point in various ways throughout the chapter. I also agree that, as he says, there is a real and obvious difference between perverse collusion and real empathy, warmth, kindness and love for the patient and that one of the ways this difference shows itself is in the analyst's feeling about what he is involved in with the patient. I agreed that the ideal of an uncontaminated transference is not merely impossible, but also undesirable when I wrote in my paper that 'it would be a mistake to think that the analyst should be free of countertransference, which would be like saying that the patient should be free of resistance. Even if this were possible, it would be antithetical to the interests of the analysis'.

I also agree with Colman (and Symington) that it is incorrect to interpret the patient's resistance to relating to the analyst as destructive attacks rather than focusing on the anxieties which underlie the resistance (I am not sure I know anyone who would disagree with this). I would go even further and say that, if a patient is resisting a relationship with the analyst, he may have good reason for doing so. Recall Freud's account of watching Bernheim attempt to hypnotize a non-compliant subject: when Bernheim said to the patient 'What are you doing? *Vous vous contre-suggestionnez*!', Freud remarked that the patient had every right to give himself counter-suggestions when someone was trying to subdue him with suggestions.

The main point of Colman's disagreement with me is the importance of interpretation as against the relationship between analyst and patient as an agent of therapeutic change. But even this disagreement seems to me to be more apparent than real, since the dichotomy that Colman sets up between interpretation and the analyst–patient relationship is a false one. I think I can explain what I mean by this by referring to the clinical illustration Colman presents in his discussion. He describes a patient who 'consistently treated [him] as a feared and dangerous object that she felt she needed to control, since . . . she felt [he] was trying to control her'. he felt himself to be 'under attack by a very powerful but invisible destructive part of her', and his 'response was dominated by a sort of "heroic" endurance and a determination not to give up hope but to go on believing in her and the analysis despite her repeated insistence that it was damaging her'. Despite the fact of her enormous impact on him, she insisted that she made no impact on him at all, and this was precisely what made him so threatening to her and made her feel so hopeless.

The patient broke off the treatment (with the analyst's agreement). What makes this example so interesting and useful is that she came back to him a few years later in a different frame of mind, which allowed her to acknowledge for the first time the positive feeling she had for his having 'hung in there' and shown her that he could stand her hatred and despair in a way that her parents had been unable to. One of the things that seemed most positive for her was that, as Colman said to the patient, it was alright with him for her not to be alright. Colman then says that when he said that, he understood for the first time the meaning of his 'heroic' endurance. It was what the patient had called forth from him, in order for him to discover a good object that could survive the worst of her destructive attacks.

This example illustrates some important points. One is that Colman's 'heroic' endurance, which I gather he feels was a curative factor in the treatment, consisted of his ability to accept that the patient was not alright, and could continue not being alright, despite his desire to help her. I agree with him that this factor contributes in an important way to the patient's analytic development, and I would say further that Colman's ability to accept that the patient was not alright meant that he had succeeded in overcoming his need to heal the patient (that is, in a magical way). But this example illustrates beautifully the major point of my paper.

Why then does Colman disagree with it? I think the point of disagreement is located in our respective views of the role of interpretation in establishing and maintaining the therapeutic relationship. The question is, given Colman's 'heroic' maintenance of an analytic stance despite the patient's destructive attacks, how does the patient *know* he is doing this? That is, how does Colman *convey* to the patient that he is 'a good object who could love her and whom she could love'? I suggest that this is conveyed precisely by the analyst maintaining an interested, concerned and curious attitude in the face of the patient's destructive attacks, that is, by the analyst really only interpreting what the patient is saying and doing. In this way, he shows that he can survive the patient's attacks as an object who can still remain interested and still think in the face of them. But this he can do only by interpreting. Only in this way does he convey that he really is able to be interested and thoughtful (that is, to demonstrate it, rather than just claim it).

There are many kinds of good, loving relationships, but an analytic relationship is good in a very specific way. One of the things that makes it not just a good relationship, but good in a special way is that it is an interpreted relationship, that is, a relationship with someone who can be in contact with one, even the most feared and hated parts of one's personality, and still think and be concerned. But to make this kind of contact, the analyst must, among other things, accept that the patient has a right not to get better, that she is not there to satisfy the analyst's need to heal. This is what Colman did, much to his patient's benefit.

(d) Reply to Caper

Warren Colman

I am not entirely surprised to find that the gap between myself and Robert Caper is not so wide as I might have suggested. I very much welcome his clarification of his views which read (at least to me) as substantially different in tone from his original argument. It is particularly illuminating to see the way he addresses the clinical material in my chapter, although this example was deliberately chosen as one which would meet his criteria for psychoanalysis while demonstrating that something *additional* to these was also in operation.

I accept what Caper says about interpretation being the means by which the nature of the relationship is conveyed. This may not be a shift from what he *meant* in his original chapter but I think it is certainly a shift from what he *conveyed*. The debate between us will have amply fulfilled its purpose if it enables others to think further about these difficult but vital clinical issues.

Index